Targeting the Microbiome for Disease Diagnosis and Therapy: New Frontiers for Personalized Medicine

Targeting the Microbiome for Disease Diagnosis and Therapy: New Frontiers for Personalized Medicine

Editor

Lucrezia Laterza

MDPI • Basel • Beijing • Wuhan • Barcelona • Belgrade • Manchester • Tokyo • Cluj • Tianjin

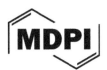

Editor
Lucrezia Laterza
CEMAD Digestive Diseases Center
Fondazione Policlinico
Universitario "A. Gemelli" IRCCS
Università Cattolica del Sacro Cuore
Rome
Italy

Editorial Office
MDPI
St. Alban-Anlage 66
4052 Basel, Switzerland

This is a reprint of articles from the Special Issue published online in the open access journal *Journal of Personalized Medicine* (ISSN 2075-4426) (available at: www.mdpi.com/journal/jpm/special_issues/targeting_microbiome).

For citation purposes, cite each article independently as indicated on the article page online and as indicated below:

LastName, A.A.; LastName, B.B.; LastName, C.C. Article Title. *Journal Name* **Year**, *Volume Number*, Page Range.

ISBN 978-3-0365-5612-3 (Hbk)
ISBN 978-3-0365-5611-6 (PDF)

© 2022 by the authors. Articles in this book are Open Access and distributed under the Creative Commons Attribution (CC BY) license, which allows users to download, copy and build upon published articles, as long as the author and publisher are properly credited, which ensures maximum dissemination and a wider impact of our publications.

The book as a whole is distributed by MDPI under the terms and conditions of the Creative Commons license CC BY-NC-ND.

Contents

About the Editor . . . . **vii**

Lucrezia Laterza and Irene Mignini
The Microbiome Revolution: New Insights for Personalized Medicine
Reprinted from: *J. Pers. Med.* **2022**, *12*, 1520, doi:10.3390/jpm12091520 . . . . **1**

Cristina Graziani, Lucrezia Laterza, Claudia Talocco, Marco Pizzoferrato, Nicoletta Di Simone and Silvia D'Ippolito et al.
Intestinal Permeability and Dysbiosis in Female Patients with Recurrent Cystitis: A Pilot Study
Reprinted from: *J. Pers. Med.* **2022**, *12*, 1005, doi:10.3390/jpm12061005 . . . . **5**

Ekaterina Chernevskaya, Evgenii Zuev, Vera Odintsova, Anastasiia Meglei and Natalia Beloborodova
Gut Microbiota as Early Predictor of Infectious Complications before Cardiac Surgery: A Prospective Pilot Study
Reprinted from: *J. Pers. Med.* **2021**, *11*, 1113, doi:10.3390/jpm11111113 . . . . **23**

Rumi Higuchi, Taichiro Goto, Yosuke Hirotsu, Sotaro Otake, Toshio Oyama and Kenji Amemiya et al.
Sphingomonas and *Phenylobacterium* as Major Microbiota in Thymic Epithelial Tumors
Reprinted from: *J. Pers. Med.* **2021**, *11*, 1092, doi:10.3390/jpm11111092 . . . . **41**

Ryodai Yamamura, Ryo Okubo, Noriko Katsumata, Toshitaka Odamaki, Naoki Hashimoto and Ichiro Kusumi et al.
Lipid and Energy Metabolism of the Gut Microbiota Is Associated with the Response to Probiotic *Bifidobacterium breve* Strain for Anxiety and Depressive Symptoms in Schizophrenia
Reprinted from: *J. Pers. Med.* **2021**, *11*, 987, doi:10.3390/jpm11100987 . . . . **55**

Soukaina Boutriq, Alicia González-González, Isaac Plaza-Andrades, Aurora Laborda-Illanes, Lidia Sánchez-Alcoholado and Jesús Peralta-Linero et al.
Gut and Endometrial Microbiome Dysbiosis: A New Emergent Risk Factor for Endometrial Cancer
Reprinted from: *J. Pers. Med.* **2021**, *11*, 659, doi:10.3390/jpm11070659 . . . . **63**

Silvia Bellando-Randone, Edda Russo, Vincenzo Venerito, Marco Matucci-Cerinic, Florenzo Iannone and Sabina Tangaro et al.
Exploring the Oral Microbiome in Rheumatic Diseases, State of Art and Future Prospective in Personalized Medicine with an AI Approach
Reprinted from: *J. Pers. Med.* **2021**, *11*, 625, doi:10.3390/jpm11070625 . . . . **91**

Hai-Hua Chuang, Jen-Fu Hsu, Li-Pang Chuang, Cheng-Hsun Chiu, Yen-Lin Huang and Hsueh-Yu Li et al.
Different Associations between Tonsil Microbiome, Chronic Tonsillitis, and Intermittent Hypoxemia among Obstructive Sleep Apnea Children of Different Weight Status: A Pilot Case-Control Study
Reprinted from: *J. Pers. Med.* **2021**, *11*, 486, doi:10.3390/jpm11060486 . . . . **107**

Vincenzo Di Leo, Patrick J. Gleeson, Fabio Sallustio, Carine Bounaix, Jennifer Da Silva and Gesualdo Loreto et al.
Rifaximin as a Potential Treatment for IgA Nephropathy in a Humanized Mice Model
Reprinted from: *J. Pers. Med.* **2021**, *11*, 309, doi:10.3390/jpm11040309 . . . . **123**

Andrea Piccioni, Laura Franza, Mattia Brigida, Christian Zanza, Enrico Torelli and Martina Petrucci et al.
Gut Microbiota and Acute Diverticulitis: Role of Probiotics in Management of This Delicate Pathophysiological Balance
Reprinted from: *J. Pers. Med.* **2021**, *11*, 298, doi:10.3390/jpm11040298 . . . . **131**

Rumi Higuchi, Taichiro Goto, Yosuke Hirotsu, Sotaro Otake, Toshio Oyama and Kenji Amemiya et al.
Streptococcus australis and *Ralstonia pickettii* as Major Microbiota in Mesotheliomas
Reprinted from: *J. Pers. Med.* **2021**, *11*, 297, doi:10.3390/jpm11040297 . . . . **141**

Irina Grigor'eva, Tatiana Romanova, Natalia Naumova, Tatiana Alikina, Alexey Kuznetsov and Marsel Kabilov
Gut Microbiome in a Russian Cohort of Pre- and Post-Cholecystectomy Female Patients
Reprinted from: *J. Pers. Med.* **2021**, *11*, 294, doi:10.3390/jpm11040294 . . . . **151**

Abigail R. Basson, Fabio Cominelli and Alexander Rodriguez-Palacios
'Statistical Irreproducibility' Does Not Improve with Larger Sample Size: How to Quantify and Address Disease Data Multimodality in Human and Animal Research
Reprinted from: *J. Pers. Med.* **2021**, *11*, 234, doi:10.3390/jpm11030234 . . . . **169**

Yi-Ting Lin, Ting-Yun Lin, Szu-Chun Hung, Po-Yu Liu, Wei-Chun Hung and Wei-Chung Tsai et al.
Differences in the Microbial Composition of Hemodialysis Patients Treated with and without β-Blockers
Reprinted from: *J. Pers. Med.* **2021**, *11*, 198, doi:10.3390/jpm11030198 . . . . **193**

Xiubin Liang, Mohamad Bouhamdan, Xia Hou, Kezhong Zhang, Jun Song and Ke Hao et al.
Intestinal Dysbiosis in Young Cystic Fibrosis Rabbits
Reprinted from: *J. Pers. Med.* **2021**, *11*, 132, doi:10.3390/jpm11020132 . . . . **209**

Andrea Pession, Daniele Zama, Edoardo Muratore, Davide Leardini, Davide Gori and Federica Guaraldi et al.
Fecal Microbiota Transplantation in Allogeneic Hematopoietic Stem Cell Transplantation Recipients: A Systematic Review
Reprinted from: *J. Pers. Med.* **2021**, *11*, 100, doi:10.3390/jpm11020100 . . . . **223**

Zahra A. Barandouzi, Joochul Lee, Kendra Maas, Angela R. Starkweather and Xiaomei S. Cong
Altered Gut Microbiota in Irritable Bowel Syndrome and Its Association with Food Components
Reprinted from: *J. Pers. Med.* **2021**, *11*, 35, doi:10.3390/jpm11010035 . . . . **237**

Isabel Cornejo-Pareja, Patricia Ruiz-Limón, Ana M. Gómez-Pérez, María Molina-Vega, Isabel Moreno-Indias and Francisco J. Tinahones
Differential Microbial Pattern Description in Subjects with Autoimmune-Based Thyroid Diseases: A Pilot Study
Reprinted from: *J. Pers. Med.* **2020**, *10*, 192, doi:10.3390/jpm10040192 . . . . **257**

About the Editor

Lucrezia Laterza

Dr. Lucrezia Laterza's degree in Medicine and Surgery at the Catholic University of the Sacred Heart (Rome) in 2011 with 110/110 cum laude. Specialization in Gastroenterology and Digestive Endoscopy at the Catholic University of the Sacred Heart (Rome) in 2017 with 50/50 cum laude. Experience as a clinical observer at New York University (NYC, USA). PhD student in Nutrition Sciences. Her areas of research and interest including Chronic Inflammatory Bowel Diseases (IBD), irritable bowel syndrome, gastrointestinal and gynecological microbiota and dysbiosis, nutrition, digestive endoscopy, and ultrasound of the intestinal loops. Author of numerous abstracts presented at national and international conferences, as well as numerous publications in international journals (H-index: 14; citations: 593).

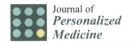

Editorial

The Microbiome Revolution: New Insights for Personalized Medicine

Lucrezia Laterza * and Irene Mignini

CEMAD Digestive Diseases Center, Fondazione Policlinico Universitario "A. Gemelli" IRCCS, Università Cattolica del Sacro Cuore, 00168 Rome, Italy
* Correspondence: laterza.lucrezia@gmail.com

Citation: Laterza, L.; Mignini, I. The Microbiome Revolution: New Insights for Personalized Medicine. *J. Pers. Med.* **2022**, *12*, 1520. https://doi.org/10.3390/jpm12091520

Received: 14 September 2022
Accepted: 14 September 2022
Published: 16 September 2022

Publisher's Note: MDPI stays neutral with regard to jurisdictional claims in published maps and institutional affiliations.

Copyright: © 2022 by the authors. Licensee MDPI, Basel, Switzerland. This article is an open access article distributed under the terms and conditions of the Creative Commons Attribution (CC BY) license (https://creativecommons.org/licenses/by/4.0/).

The availability of new culture-independent techniques to study microbes led to the explosion of the gut microbiota revolution in recent decades. Thanks to the information deriving from 16-RNA and metagenomics, we have begun to gain insight into a previously unexplored organ: the microbiome. Thus, we changed our ontological perspective of the human body, considering it as the result of the interaction between eukaryotic cells—the body as traditionally intended—and prokaryotic cells, consisting in the multiple microorganisms living in different body niches, which constitute the "mammalian holobiont" [1]. In fact, even if the gut microbiome is the first and most studied one, multiple microbiomes have been evaluated. Previously considered sterile districts have been questioned and new possible unexpected niches have been postulated. Beyond the biological interest, the knowledge on the microbiome offers a unique opportunity for personalized medicine as it constitutes the variable part of our genome, contributing to more than 90% of the variability among the individuals, whereas our traditionally intended genome shows a more than 90% identity among individuals [2]. Furthermore, beyond the mere characterization of microorganisms constituting the microbiome, thanks to proteomics and metabolomics, we can characterize the possible function that they have in physiologic and pathologic processes [3].

Considering these characteristics, the study of the microbiome will provide new opportunities to understand the pathogenesis of many non-communicable diseases, and it may be used for diagnosis, staging and tailoring different therapies on individual specific characteristics. Aiming at exploring the potential applications of microbiome in the personalization of medicine, we propose this Special Issue to collect new original data on the study of the microbiome and to offer the reader the main novelties in the landscape of the microbiome in the perspective of personalized medicine.

In such a context, the gut microbiome plays an undoubtedly pivotal role, not only in gastrointestinal but also extra-gastrointestinal disorders.

In gastrointestinal diseases, the contribution of the gut microbiota in the pathophysiology of both organic and functional disorders is now largely recognized. The review by Piccioni et al. underlined how dysbiosis, causing imbalance between pro-inflammatory and anti-inflammatory bacterial species, can trigger mucosal and peri-visceral inflammation leading to acute diverticulitis, and hypothesized a possible therapeutic role of probiotics in this setting, which is still to be confirmed by further evidence [4]. Grigor'eva et al. analysed fecal microbiota in patients affected by gallbladder stones and described how cholecystectomy can modify bacterial abundance [5]. Moreover, Barandouzi et al. showed that the microbiome composition was different in patients with irritable bowel syndrome and healthy controls and revealed the association between bacterial diversity and the consumption of specific foods such as caffeine, thus highlighting the interaction between microbiota and the environment [6]. This relationship has also been confirmed by data concerning non-gastrointestinal settings, as it is described in the study by Lin et al., which focused on a population of patients undergoing hemodialysis and analysed the impact of beta-blockers on the gut microbiome [7].

The potential link between the gut microbiome and apparently disconnected diseases has been investigated in multiple different contexts. Some districts, notably the urinary tract, can be more easily colonized by gut bacteria due to their intestinal contiguity. On this basis, our group examined how gut microbiome and intestinal barrier disruption can impact on the pathogenesis of urinary tract infections, particularly recurrent cystitis [8]. Nonetheless, the role of the gut microbiome is not limited to contiguous segments. As Cornejo-Pareja et al. showed in their pilot study about autoimmune-based thyroid diseases, gut microbiome alterations may contribute to the impairment of the immune system and subsequent onset of autoimmune disorders [9]. Furthermore, the pilot study by Chernevskaya et al. underlined the possible role of gut microbiota in identifying patients with a high risk of postoperative complications after cardiac surgery [10]. Similarly, Yamamura et al. demonstrated that the characteristics of lipid and energy metabolism of gut microbiota were able to predict a response to probiotic therapy in patients with schizophrenia [11].

However, the gut microbiome is not the unique target for diagnosis and therapy, and growing interest is rising around other microbiomes. In this context, it is worth noting that recent findings have also revealed the presence of bacterial species in some niches which were traditionally considered sterile, questioning an old paradigm and providing new potential therapeutic targets.

Indeed, Bellando-Randone et al. summarized current evidence about the contribution of oral microbiomes in the pathogenesis of different rheumatic diseases and propose to apply artificial intelligence, especially machine learning, to understand the link between oral microbiota and rheumatic diseases [12]. Chuang et al. observed that the tonsil microbiota composition was associated with chronic tonsillitis and oxygen desaturation in children affected by obstructive sleep apnea syndrome [13]. Moreover, in two different studies, Higuchi et al. evaluated the microbiome of two previously unexplored districts. They analysed in particular mesothelioma-specific [14] and thymoma-specific [15] microbiota, using resected or biopsied mesothelioma samples and resected thymoma samples, respectively, suggesting a possible microbial role in cancerogenesis. Similarly, based on emerging evidence that the uterus is not sterile, Boutriq et al. presented in their review the most recent data concerning the potential role of the endometrial microbiome in endometrial cancer and its possible interplay with the gut microbiome [16].

From diagnosis, research is now moving towards therapeutic objectives. Microbiome modulation through pre-biotics, pro-biotics and non-absorbable oral antibiotics (e.g., rifaximin) is an already a diffuse practice, especially but not only in gastrointestinal disorders, but further investigation is needed to identify more personalized treatments [17,18]. Di Leo et al. administered rifaximin to mice models for IgA nephropathy and observed symptom improvement, suggesting an unexplored therapeutic direction [19]. Fecal microbiota transplantion (FMT) usefulness in re-establishing intestinal eubiosis is widely recognized and recommended for specific indications, notably recurrent *Clostridioides difficile* colitis, but its role seems not to be limited to this setting, and it has been explored in multiple diseases, as Pession et al. showed in their review addressing the role of FMT in allogenic hematopoietic stem-cell recipients [20]. Not only *Clostridioides* infections, but also the treatment of gut graft-versus-host disease and prevention of gut dysbiosis or decolonization from antibiotic-resistant bacteria could be the main applications. Furthermore, in order to promote research and novel therapeutic strategies, Liang et al. developed a rabbit model of cystic fibrosis that, as well as cystic fibrosis human patients, was characterized by a dysbiotic microbiota compared to wild-type rabbits [21].

Giant steps have been made so far on microbiome investigation from the perspective of personalized medicine. However, certain aspects remain unclear. For example, as Basson et al. highlighted, poor study reproducibility is one of the current concerns [22]. They speculated on the possible causes of study irreproducibility and proposed some solutions, thus indicating lights and shadows on our current knowledge on this complex and challenging topic that the microbiome represents. As this Special Issue pointed out, actual data are very promising, but research should keep on exploring the various unsolved issues to perfect the use of microbiome data for the personalization of medicine.

Author Contributions: Conceptualization, L.L.; writing—original draft preparation, L.L. and I.M.; writing—review and editing, L.L. and I.M.; supervision, L.L. All authors have read and agreed to the published version of the manuscript.

Funding: This research received no external funding.

Institutional Review Board Statement: Not applicable.

Informed Consent Statement: Not applicable.

Data Availability Statement: Not applicable.

Conflicts of Interest: L.L. is a consultant for Actial Farmaceutica. I.M. has no conflict to declare.

References

1. Zwart, H. "Love Is a Microbe Too": Microbiome Dialectics. *Endeavour* **2022**, *46*, 100816. [CrossRef] [PubMed]
2. Adams, C.; Gutierrez, B. The Microbiome Has Multiple Influences on Human Health. *J. Microbiol. Biotechnol.* **2018**, *7*, 1–8.
3. Walker, M.E.; Simpson, J.B.; Redinbo, M.R. A Structural Metagenomics Pipeline for Examining the Gut Microbiome. *Curr. Opin. Struct. Biol.* **2022**, *75*, 102416. [CrossRef] [PubMed]
4. Piccioni, A.; Franza, L.; Brigida, M.; Zanza, C.; Torelli, E.; Petrucci, M.; Nicolò, R.; Covino, M.; Candelli, M.; Saviano, A.; et al. Gut Microbiota and Acute Diverticulitis: Role of Probiotics in Management of This Delicate Pathophysiological Balance. *J. Pers. Med.* **2021**, *11*, 298. [CrossRef]
5. Grigor'eva, I.; Romanova, T.; Naumova, N.; Alikina, T.; Kuznetsov, A.; Kabilov, M. Gut Microbiome in a Russian Cohort of Pre- and Post-Cholecystectomy Female Patients. *J. Pers. Med.* **2021**, *11*, 294. [CrossRef]
6. Barandouzi, Z.A.; Lee, J.; Maas, K.; Starkweather, A.R.; Cong, X.S. Altered Gut Microbiota in Irritable Bowel Syndrome and Its Association with Food Components. *J. Pers. Med.* **2021**, *11*, 35. [CrossRef]
7. Lin, Y.-T.; Lin, T.-Y.; Hung, S.-C.; Liu, P.-Y.; Hung, W.-C.; Tsai, W.-C.; Tsai, Y.-C.; Delicano, R.A.; Chuang, Y.-S.; Kuo, M.-C.; et al. Differences in the Microbial Composition of Hemodialysis Patients Treated with and without β-Blockers. *J. Pers. Med.* **2021**, *11*, 198. [CrossRef]
8. Graziani, C.; Laterza, L.; Talocco, C.; Pizzoferrato, M.; Di Simone, N.; D'Ippolito, S.; Ricci, C.; Gervasoni, J.; Persichilli, S.; Del Chierico, F.; et al. Intestinal Permeability and Dysbiosis in Female Patients with Recurrent Cystitis: A Pilot Study. *J. Pers. Med.* **2022**, *12*, 1005. [CrossRef]
9. Cornejo-Pareja, I.; Ruiz-Limón, P.; Gómez-Pérez, A.M.; Molina-Vega, M.; Moreno-Indias, I.; Tinahones, F.J. Differential Microbial Pattern Description in Subjects with Autoimmune-Based Thyroid Diseases: A Pilot Study. *J. Pers. Med.* **2020**, *10*, 192. [CrossRef]
10. Chernevskaya, E.; Zuev, E.; Odintsova, V.; Meglei, A.; Beloborodova, N. Gut Microbiota as Early Predictor of Infectious Complications before Cardiac Surgery: A Prospective Pilot Study. *J. Pers. Med.* **2021**, *11*, 1113. [CrossRef]
11. Yamamura, R.; Okubo, R.; Katsumata, N.; Odamaki, T.; Hashimoto, N.; Kusumi, I.; Xiao, J.; Matsuoka, Y.J. Lipid and Energy Metabolism of the Gut Microbiota Is Associated with the Response to Probiotic Bifidobacterium Breve Strain for Anxiety and Depressive Symptoms in Schizophrenia. *J. Pers. Med.* **2021**, *11*, 987. [CrossRef] [PubMed]
12. Bellando-Randone, S.; Russo, E.; Venerito, V.; Matucci-Cerinic, M.; Iannone, F.; Tangaro, S.; Amedei, A. Exploring the Oral Microbiome in Rheumatic Diseases, State of Art and Future Prospective in Personalized Medicine with an AI Approach. *J. Pers. Med.* **2021**, *11*, 625. [CrossRef] [PubMed]
13. Chuang, H.-H.; Hsu, J.-F.; Chuang, L.-P.; Chiu, C.-H.; Huang, Y.-L.; Li, H.-Y.; Chen, N.-H.; Huang, Y.-S.; Chuang, C.-W.; Huang, C.-G.; et al. Different Associations between Tonsil Microbiome, Chronic Tonsillitis, and Intermittent Hypoxemia among Obstructive Sleep Apnea Children of Different Weight Status: A Pilot Case-Control Study. *J. Pers. Med.* **2021**, *11*, 486. [CrossRef]
14. Higuchi, R.; Goto, T.; Hirotsu, Y.; Otake, S.; Oyama, T.; Amemiya, K.; Mochizuki, H.; Omata, M. Streptococcus Australis and Ralstonia Pickettii as Major Microbiota in Mesotheliomas. *J. Pers. Med.* **2021**, *11*, 297. [CrossRef] [PubMed]
15. Higuchi, R.; Goto, T.; Hirotsu, Y.; Otake, S.; Oyama, T.; Amemiya, K.; Ohyama, H.; Mochizuki, H.; Omata, M. Sphingomonas and Phenylobacterium as Major Microbiota in Thymic Epithelial Tumors. *J. Pers. Med.* **2021**, *11*, 1092. [CrossRef]
16. Boutriq, S.; González-González, A.; Plaza-Andrades, I.; Laborda-Illanes, A.; Sánchez-Alcoholado, L.; Peralta-Linero, J.; Domínguez-Recio, M.E.; Bermejo-Pérez, M.J.; Lavado-Valenzuela, R.; Alba, E.; et al. Gut and Endometrial Microbiome Dysbiosis: A New Emergent Risk Factor for Endometrial Cancer. *J. Pers. Med.* **2021**, *11*, 659. [CrossRef]
17. Ford, A.C.; Harris, L.A.; Lacy, B.E.; Quigley, E.M.M.; Moayyedi, P. Systematic Review with Meta-Analysis: The Efficacy of Prebiotics, Probiotics, Synbiotics and Antibiotics in Irritable Bowel Syndrome. *Aliment. Pharm.* **2018**, *48*, 1044–1060. [CrossRef]
18. Bloom, P.P.; Tapper, E.B.; Young, V.B.; Lok, A.S. Microbiome Therapeutics for Hepatic Encephalopathy. *J. Hepatol.* **2021**, *75*, 1452–1464. [CrossRef]

19. Di Leo, V.; Gleeson, P.J.; Sallustio, F.; Bounaix, C.; Da Silva, J.; Loreto, G.; Ben Mkaddem, S.; Monteiro, R.C. Rifaximin as a Potential Treatment for IgA Nephropathy in a Humanized Mice Model. *J. Pers. Med.* **2021**, *11*, 309. [CrossRef]
20. Pession, A.; Zama, D.; Muratore, E.; Leardini, D.; Gori, D.; Guaraldi, F.; Prete, A.; Turroni, S.; Brigidi, P.; Masetti, R. Fecal Microbiota Transplantation in Allogeneic Hematopoietic Stem Cell Transplantation Recipients: A Systematic Review. *J. Pers. Med.* **2021**, *11*, 100. [CrossRef]
21. Liang, X.; Bouhamdan, M.; Hou, X.; Zhang, K.; Song, J.; Hao, K.; Jin, J.-P.; Zhang, Z.; Xu, J. Intestinal Dysbiosis in Young Cystic Fibrosis Rabbits. *J. Pers. Med.* **2021**, *11*, 132. [CrossRef] [PubMed]
22. Basson, A.R.; Cominelli, F.; Rodriguez-Palacios, A. 'Statistical Irreproducibility' Does Not Improve with Larger Sample Size: How to Quantify and Address Disease Data Multimodality in Human and Animal Research. *J. Pers. Med.* **2021**, *11*, 234. [CrossRef] [PubMed]

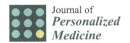

Article

Intestinal Permeability and Dysbiosis in Female Patients with Recurrent Cystitis: A Pilot Study

Cristina Graziani [1], Lucrezia Laterza [1,*], Claudia Talocco [2], Marco Pizzoferrato [1], Nicoletta Di Simone [3,4], Silvia D'Ippolito [5], Caterina Ricci [5], Jacopo Gervasoni [6], Silvia Persichilli [6], Federica Del Chierico [7], Valeria Marzano [7], Stefano Levi Mortera [7], Aniello Primiano [6], Andrea Poscia [8], Francesca Romana Ponziani [1], Lorenza Putignani [9], Andrea Urbani [6], Valentina Petito [1], Federica Di Vincenzo [1], Letizia Masi [1], Loris Riccardo Lopetuso [1], Giovanni Cammarota [1,2], Daniela Romualdi [5], Antonio Lanzone [5], Antonio Gasbarrini [1,2] and Franco Scaldaferri [1,2]

[1] CEMAD Digestive Diseases Center, Fondazione Policlinico Universitario "A. Gemelli" IRCCS, Università Cattolica del Sacro Cuore, 00168 Rome, Italy; cristina.graziani@guest.policlinicogemelli.it (C.G.); marco.pizzoferrato@policlinicogemelli.it (M.P.); francescaromana.ponziani@policlinicogemelli.it (F.R.P.); valentina.petito@policlinicogemelli.it (V.P.); federica.divincenzo30@gmail.com (F.D.V.); letizia.masi94@gmail.com (L.M.); lorisriccardo.lopetuso@policlinicogemelli.it (L.R.L.); giovanni.cammarota@policlinicogemelli.it (G.C.); antonio.gasbarrini@unicatt.it (A.G.); franco.scaldaferri@unicatt.it (F.S.)
[2] Dipartimento di Medicina e Chirurgia Traslazionale, Università Cattolica del Sacro Cuore, 00168 Rome, Italy; claudia.talocco@yahoo.it
[3] Department of Biomedical Sciences, Humanitas University, Via Rita Levi Montalcini 4, 20072 Pieve Emanuele, Italy; nicoletta.disimone@hunimed.eu
[4] IRCCS Humanitas Research Hospital, Via Manzoni 56, 20089 Rozzano, Italy
[5] Ginecologia ed Ostetricia, Dipartimento di Scienze Della Vita e Sanità Pubblica, Fondazione Policlinico Universitario "A. Gemelli" IRCCS, 00168 Rome, Italy; silvia.dippolito@policlinicogemelli.it (S.D.); caterina.ricci@policlinicogemelli.it (C.R.); daniela.romualdi@policlinicogemelli.it (D.R.); antonio.lanzone@policlinicogemelli.it (A.L.)
[6] UOC Chimica, Biochimica e Biologia Molecolare Clinica, Dipartimento di Scienze Biotecnologiche di Base, Cliniche Intensivologiche e Perioperatorie, Fondazione Policlinico Universitario "A. Gemelli" IRCCS, 00168 Rome, Italy; jacopo.gervasoni@policlinicogemelli.it (J.G.); silvia.persichilli@policlinicogemelli.it (S.P.); aniello.primiano@policlinicogemelli.it (A.P.); andrea.urbani@policlinicogemelli.it (A.U.)
[7] Multimodal Laboratory Medicine Research Area, Unit of Human Microbiome, Bambino Gesù Children's Hospital, IRCCS, 00165 Rome, Italy; federica.delchierico@opbg.net (F.D.C.); valeria.marzano@opbg.net (V.M.); stefano.levimortera@opbg.net (S.L.M.)
[8] UOC ISP Prevention and Surveillance of Infectious and Chronic Diseases, Department of Prevention-Local Health Authority (AUSR-AV2), 60035 Jesi, Italy; andrea.poscia@sanita.marche.it or andrea.poscia@unicatt.it
[9] Department of Diagnostic and Laboratory Medicine, Unit of Microbiology and Diagnostic Immunology, Unit of Microbiomics and Multimodal Laboratory Medicine Research Area, Unit of Human Microbiome, Bambino Gesù Children's Hospital, IRCCS, 00146 Rome, Italy; lorenza.putignani@opbg.net
* Correspondence: laterza.lucrezia@gmail.com; Tel.: +39-0630156265

Citation: Graziani, C.; Laterza, L.; Talocco, C.; Pizzoferrato, M.; Di Simone, N.; D'Ippolito, S.; Ricci, C.; Gervasoni, J.; Persichilli, S.; Del Chierico, F.; et al. Intestinal Permeability and Dysbiosis in Female Patients with Recurrent Cystitis: A Pilot Study. *J. Pers. Med.* **2022**, *12*, 1005. https://doi.org/10.3390/jpm12061005

Academic Editor: Jorge Luis Espinoza

Received: 30 April 2022
Accepted: 16 June 2022
Published: 20 June 2022

Publisher's Note: MDPI stays neutral with regard to jurisdictional claims in published maps and institutional affiliations.

Copyright: © 2022 by the authors. Licensee MDPI, Basel, Switzerland. This article is an open access article distributed under the terms and conditions of the Creative Commons Attribution (CC BY) license (https://creativecommons.org/licenses/by/4.0/).

Abstract: Recurrent cystitis (RC) is a common disease, especially in females. Anatomical, behavioral and genetic predisposing factors are associated with the ascending retrograde route, which often causes bladder infections. RC seems to be mainly caused by agents derived from the intestinal microbiota, and most frequently by *Escherichia coli*. Intestinal contiguity contributes to the etiopathogenesis of RC and an alteration in intestinal permeability could have a major role in RC. The aim of this pilot study is to assess gut microbiome dysbiosis and intestinal permeability in female patients with RC. Patients with RC (*n* = 16) were enrolled and compared with healthy female subjects (*n* = 15) and patients with chronic gastrointestinal (GI) disorders (*n* = 238). We calculated the Acute Cystitis Symptom Score/Urinary Tract Infection Symptom Assessment (ACSS/UTISA) and Gastrointestinal Symptom Rating Scale (GSRS) scores and evaluated intestinal permeability and the fecal microbiome in the first two cohorts. Patients with RC showed an increased prevalence of gastrointestinal symptoms compared with healthy controls. Of the patients with RC, 88% showed an increased intestinal permeability with reduced biodiversity of gut microbiota compared to healthy controls, and 68% of the RC patients had a final diagnosis of gastrointestinal disease. Similarly, GI patients reported a higher incidence of urinary symptoms with a diagnosis of RC in 20%. Gut barrier impairment seems to play a major role in the pathogenesis of RC. Further studies are necessary to elucidate the role of microbiota and intestinal permeability in urinary tract infections.

Keywords: intestinal permeability; gut microbiome; recurrent cystitis; dysbiosis

---

1. Introduction

Recurrent cystitis (RC) is defined as more than two episodes of bladder infection in a 6-month period or more than three episodes in a year. Generally, urinary tract infections (UTIs) are much more common in women than in men, involving over 50% of the female population, of which at least 20–30% develop a recurrence [1]. This increased incidence in women can be partially explained by the presence of anatomical, behavioral and genetic predisposing factors [2–4]. Most urinary tract pathogens consist of facultative Gram-negative anaerobic bacilli, common microorganisms of the intestinal microbiota, mainly *Escherichia coli*, but they also belong to other Enterobacteriaceae (such as *Klebsiella* spp. and *Proteus* spp.). However, even Gram-positive microorganisms, such as *Staphylococcus saprophyticus* and *Enterococcus faecalis*, can act as pathogens [5].

The main route of infection is the fecal–perineal–urethral route, also known as the ascending retrograde route, which consists of the colonization of the vaginal introitus and/or the urethral meatus by fecal microbiota-derived bacteria, and the consequent colonization of the bladder through the urethra [6]. Thus, the intestine could act as a reservoir of uropathogens and the cross-talk between the intestinal and urogenital microbiome, the "gut–bladder axis", could play a major role in UTIs' pathogenesis [7].

Changes in epithelial permeability may represent a novel mechanism for visceral organ crosstalk and it may explain the overlapping symptomology of painful bladder syndrome and irritable bowel syndrome (IBS) [8].

The pathophysiology of painful bladder syndrome (PBS) is poorly understood. However, there is evidence of female predominance and a high incidence of IBS in these patients: up to 30–50% of patients diagnosed with IBS show symptoms of PBS, while up to 40% of patients diagnosed with PBS show symptoms that meet the criteria for IBS. The hypothesis is that the cross-sensitization between the bladder and colon is due to altered permeability in one organ, which affects the other organ, but we do not know which one is the first. [9,10]. However, there is limited knowledge of the mechanisms that link these conditions. According to this hypothesis of cross-organ visceral communication between the colon and bladder, previous experiments in rodent models have shown that colonic irritation is capable of producing irregular urination patterns, such as early onset of urination and increased urethral sphincter activity in rats [11]. Furthermore, there is evidence that active colonic inflammation induces abnormalities in the detrusor-muscular contractility of the bladder [12], and can increase vascular permeability in the bladder of female rats [13]. Conversely, bladder irritation results in increased visceral sensitivity to colonic stimulation. The induction of permeability in the bladder induces increased permeability in the colon, and, on the other side, inflammation of the colon likewise induces permeability in the urinary bladder. These findings suggest that altered permeability has a key role in the visceral organ cross-talk [8].

Based on this rationale, it is possible to hypothesize a further route of colonization of the bladder by an anterograde route in RC, possibly by the transmigration of bacteria or bacterial fragments from the intestine, particularly in the presence of impaired permeability, as demonstrated in murine models [14]. However, little is known about the contribution of intestinal permeability in the pathogenesis of recurrent cystitis.

Intestinal homeostasis depends on the good health of the gut barrier, a complex defensive system capable of separating the intestinal contents from the host tissues, which regulates nutrient absorption and allows interactions between the resident microbiota and the local immune system [15]. The gut barrier is constituted and regulated by many factors, including, first of all, the intestinal microbiota itself, which could also influence the microbiota of nearby organs, the mucus layer, the integrity of epithelial cells and intercellular junctions, and the innate and adaptive immune system associated with the mucosa [16]. In this context, an important measure of barrier integrity is intestinal permeability, the property that allows the exchange of solutes and fluids between the lumen and the intestinal mucosa. The increase in intestinal permeability as a marker of gut barrier dysfunction has been implicated in the pathogenesis of many gastrointestinal and extra-gastrointestinal diseases [17]. However, little or nothing is known about the relationship between RC, dysbiosis and increased intestinal permeability.

Therefore, the aim of this pilot study is to evaluate the possible relationship between impaired gut barrier function and RC, through the investigation of the prevalence of increased intestinal permeability and dysbiosis in a cohort of female patients with RC (primary endpoint) compared to healthy women. To explore the possible crosstalk between the gut and the urinary tract and to support the rationale of a bi-directional gut–bladder dysfunction, we also evaluated the prevalence of RC in a cohort of patients with chronic gastrointestinal disorders.

2. Materials and Methods

2.1. Study Design and Patients

We recruited three cohorts of patients: the first cohort (cohort I) consisted of female patients, aged 18 and over, who reported at least two episodes of acute uncomplicated cystitis in the last 6 months or three episodes in the last year, and came to our attention at the Gynecology Unit of the Fondazione Policlinico Universitario "A. Gemelli" IRCCS Hospital. The exclusion criteria for this cohort were the presence of morpho-functional alterations of the genitourinary tract, the diagnosis of complicated acute or chronic cystitis, pregnancy and lactation. The second cohort (control group, cohort II) was composed of healthy female subjects from the age of 18, followed up by the Gynecology Unit of the Fondazione Policlinico Universitario "A. Gemelli" IRCCS Hospital for routine controls, without a history of recurrent cystitis or any gastroenterological symptoms/disorders, and in the same age range. The third cohort (cohort III) was composed of female patients who attended the General Gastroenterology and Breath Test Clinics of the Fondazione Policlinico Universitario "A. Gemelli" IRCCS Hospital for GI disorders. Enrolled patients did not undergo any therapy at the time of enrollment and execution of examinations and tests. In addition, patients were required not to change their eating habits.

The subjects in cohort I and II performed the Intestinal Permeability Test, based on the lactulose/mannitol ratio and, at the same time, on the measurement of exhaled H_2 (the Lactulose Breath Test) for the assessment of oro-cecal transit time and Small Intestinal Bacterial Overgrowth (SIBO). On the same day, they provided a fecal sample for metagenomic 16S ribosomal RNA (rRNA) analysis of the intestinal microbiome.

Subjects belonging to all three study cohorts were administered validated questionnaires for self-evaluation of urological symptoms—the Acute Cystitis Symptom Score (ACSS) questionnaire [18] and the UTI Symptom Assessment (UTISA) questionnaire [19]—and for gastrointestinal symptoms, the structured Gastrointestinal Symptom Rating Scale (GSRS) questionnaire was administered [20].

Enrolled patients and controls had no history of alcohol or drug abuse and they were not current smokers. Subjects participating in the study did not refer to any particular restricted dietary regimen (i.e., vegetarian or a low FODMAP diet) and they were asked not to change their dietary habits and to avoid the use of antibiotics 15 days before their enrollment in the study and microbiota analysis. Patients with RC were also required to provide the results of the last urine culture, in order to collect data about the causative agent of the urinary infection.

The study was approved by the Ethical Committee of Fondazione Policlinico Universitario "A. Gemelli" IRCCS Hospital and all the subjects participating in the study provided written informed consent to the study (Protocol Number 0011046/21 of 03/24/2021).

2.2. Intestinal Permeability Test

We developed a new method to evaluate the intestinal permeability index, according to our preliminary results (unpublished data). It showed the comparability of data on exhaled gas obtained from a standard H_2 Lactulose Breath Test compared to data obtained after the concomitant administration of lactulose and mannitol to perform a Lactulose/Mannitol urinary test. Thus, we developed a contemporary breath and urinary test that was able to provide combined information: the H_2 Lactulose/Mannitol Breath Test (L/M BT), thanks to the administration of two sugars, instead of lactulose alone. This method also allows the simultaneous determination of both H_2 and CH_4 measurements, providing information on oro-cecal transit time and SIBO, and at the same time, the determination of urinary lactulose/mannitol urinary ratio, for the estimation of intestinal permeability. This test has already been demonstrated to provide reliable information on the alteration of intestinal permeability [16,21–25] and it is currently part of the clinical practice in our center. In this way, by performing a single, simple, non-invasive, sensitive, reliable and repeatable test, it is possible to not only obtain information relating to the functionality of the intestinal epithelium, but also relating to any alterations in intestinal transit time or to the presence of SIBO. The L/M BT is performed through serial sampling of gases exhaled by the patient, such as hydrogen, carbon dioxide and methane, and the subsequent analysis of their concentrations, measured in parts per million (ppm) by means of a dedicated gas chromatograph. After the appropriate preparation the day before the test and an overnight fast, 17 samples of exhaled gas were obtained at time 0 (T0) and after taking 5 gr of mannitol (powder) dissolved in 200 mL of water and 10 gr of pure lactulose (15 mL of syrup), at intervals of 15 min in the following 4 h. An increase of ≥20 ppm in hydrogen within 90 min was considered the cut-off value for the determination of SIBO, according to the North American consensus criteria [26]. Patients also provided a urine sample at baseline (T0), before taking lactulose and mannitol. Then, they collected urine samples in the following 6 h to allow the measurement of the two sugars. The lactulose/mannitol ratio was considered increased and therefore indicative of increased intestinal permeability, for values ≥0.030 [27].

2.2.1. Chemicals and Reagents

Water and acetonitrile (LC-MS grade) was purchased from Merck (Merck KGaA, Darmstadt, Germany). Formic acid (98%, LC-MS grade) was purchased from Baker (Mallinckrodt Baker Italia, Milano, Italia) and D-Mannitol-1 ^{13}C, 1-1-d$_2$, Lactulose ^{13}C$_{12}$ and ammonium formate was purchased from Sigma-Aldrich (Merck KGaA, Darmstadt, Germany). Lactulose, mannitol and chlorhexidine were purchased from BioChemica (AppliChem GmbH, Darmstadt, Germany). Stock solutions of mannitol (4 g/L) and lactulose (4 g/L) were prepared in water and stored at −80 °C. Internal standards (IS) stock solutions containing 500 µg/mL D-mannitol-1 ^{13}C.1, 1-d$_2$ and lactulose ^{13}C$_{12}$ were prepared in water and stored at −80 °C. Working solutions were prepared in water/acetonitrile (20/80, v/v) at concentrations of 1600 µg/mL for mannitol and 640 µg/mL for lactulose. Serial dilutions from working solutions were used to prepare seven-point calibration curves for both mannitol and lactulose (10, 40, 80, 160, 320, 640 µg/mL; 2.5, 10, 20, 40, 80.,160 µg/mL, respectively) and kept at −20 °C until use. The calibration curve included a zero (only solvent) and a blank (solvent plus IS), which were not used for the construction of calibration curves. D-Mannitol-1 ^{13}C, 1-1-d$_2$ and lactulose ^{13}C$_{12}$ stock solutions were diluted with acetonitrile to achieve a final concentration of 5 µg/mL and 2.5 µg/mL for D-Mannitol-1 ^{13}C, 1-1-d$_2$ and lactulose ^{13}C$_{12}$, respectively.

2.2.2. Sample Collection and Treatment

Urine samples were collected at two time points: T0 (at the start of the Lactulose/Mannitol Breath Test when the patient had fasted from solids and liquids for at least 8 h, before the assumption of the two sugars) and at T6 (for 6 hours after the consumption of the two sugar solutions: 10 gr of lactulose and 5 gr of mannitol). An aliquot of the urine sample collected at 6 h was taken for analysis. Then, 150 μL of chlorhexidine (1.9 gr/100 mL) was added to the urine samples as a preservative. Samples were stored at −80 °C until analysis.

Before the analysis for the L/M ratio, urine samples were left to thaw at room temperature, then stirred for 1 min using a vortex mixer and centrifuged at $5000 \times g$ for 4 min to remove the sediment according to the laboratory procedure. IS solution (240 μL) was added to 10 μL of the urine samples, controls and standards, and after mixing, 200 μL was transferred into a glass vial for injection into the UPLC-MS/MS (Ultra Performance Liquid Chromatography Mass Spectrometry).

2.2.3. Instrumentation

The LC-MS/MS (Liquid Chromatography Mass Spectrometry) system consisted of an Acquity UPLC system interfaced with a triple quadrupole mass spectrometer (Xevo TQS-Micro, Waters, Milford, MA, USA) equipped with an electrospray ion source.

2.2.4. Chromatographic Conditions

The UPLC separation was performed using an ACQUITY UPLC BEH Amide 1.7 μm, 2.1×50 mm column (Waters Corporation, Milford, MA, USA) operating at a flow rate of 200 μL/min, and eluted with a 4 min linear gradient from 90 to 40% acetonitrile in water (2 mM ammonium formate). The oven temperature was set at 40 °C. The injection volume was 5 μL, and the total analysis time, including 1 min for equilibration of column, was 5 min.

2.2.5. Mass Spectrometer Conditions

The ESI (Electrospray Ionization) source operates in negative mode, with a capillary voltage of 2.0 kV and a desolvation temperature of 300 °C. The source of the gas was set as follows: desolvation at 200 L/h and cone at 0 L/h. The collision cell pressure was 3.50×10^{-3} mbar. The cone voltage and collision energy settings were established individually for each compound for Selected Reaction Monitoring (SRM) detection. The conditions for the detection of lactulose, mannitol and their internal standards obtained by direct infusion of a standard solution (1 μg/mL) were in line with the UPLC at initial mobile phase conditions [27].

2.3. Fecal Microbiome Analysis

For cohort I and II, stool samples were collected at a single timepoint, immediately before the L/M BT, and were stored at −80° until DNA extraction. Frozen stool samples were thawed at room temperature, and the DNA was manually extracted using the QIAmp Fast DNA Stool mini kit (Qiagen, Germany) according to the manufacturer's instructions. DNA was quantified using the NanoDrop ND-1000.

Targeted-Metagenomics

For each sample, the amplification of the V3-V4 region of the 16S rRNA gene was performed by polymerase chain reaction (PCR) to obtain bacterial amplicon libraries (630 bp), using primers reported in the MiSeq rRNA Amplicon Sequencing protocol (Illumina, San Diego, CA, USA) [28]. Internal PCR contaminations were excluded by using negative controls (no template). Moreover, a defined mixture of microbial standard DNA was used as a positive control for sequencing. The sequencing was performed on an Illumina MiSeqTM platform (Illumina, San Diego, CA, USA), where paired-end reads of 300 base-length were generated.

Trimmomatic v. 0.36 software was used to filter raw sequences for their quality and read length [29], and the ChimeraSlayer tool in QIIME 1.9.1 software was employed to filter chimera sequences [30]. Reads were clustered into Operational Taxonomic Units (OTUs) at 97% identity by UCLUST [31] against the Greengenes 13.8 database [32]. QIIME was used to calculate α- and β-diversity and statistical tests (Mann–Whitney U, Kruskal–Wallis, Benjamini–Hochberg tests) were applied on the OTUs' relative abundances.

2.4. Self-Evaluation of Urological Symptoms (ACSS/UTISA) Questionnaire

Generally, the diagnosis of acute uncomplicated cystitis is made based on a history of lower urinary tract symptoms in the absence of vaginal discharge; urine dipstick testing and urine cultures can be used only in particular situations [33]. Considering that the diagnosis of acute uncomplicated cystitis is mainly clinical, several dedicated questionnaires, in particular the Acute Cystitis Symptom Score (ACSS) and the UTI Symptom Assessment (UTISA), have been created and validated as diagnostic methods in many clinical settings [34–36]. Given the absence in the literature of a dedicated questionnaire for patients suffering from uncomplicated RC, we used a combined ACSS/UTISA questionnaire for this study. The combined ACSS/UTISA questionnaire (questionnaire N° 2 and 3 in the Supplementary Materials) consists of 13 questions. These questionnaires analyze three aspects of the urological manifestations. First, the "typical symptoms", which consist of urgency and increased voiding frequency, dysuria, incomplete emptying of the bladder, pelvic pain/discomfort, and lumbar pain. Second, the "atypical symptoms", and third, the subjective perception of how these symptoms have affected the patient's quality of life in the last year. For each response, a sub-sheet from 0 to 3 was assigned, according to increasing severity. The patients were considered to have a previous acute uncomplicated cystitis if they exceeded the cutoff value of ≥ 6 in the "typical symptoms" section. In the cohort of patients with GI symptoms, we tried to evaluate the prevalence of lower urinary tract symptoms. Therefore, we administered a combined ACSS/UTISA questionnaire to all patients in the three cohorts, to ascertain the presence or absence of recurrent urinary pathology.

2.5. Self-Evaluation of GI Symptoms (GSRS) Questionnaire

The GSRS questionnaire contains 15 questions related to five areas of interest in regard to gastroenterological symptoms such as diarrhea, constipation, abdominal pain, reflux, dyspepsia. In this case, each answer was scored from 0 to 3, representing increased severity [20]. All patients from the three cohorts were given this questionnaire. Furthermore, they were asked to qualify their most frequent stool consistency based on the Bristol stool scale.

2.6. Statistical Analyses

The demographic and clinical characteristics of the sample were described through descriptive statistical techniques. The qualitative variables were presented through tables containing absolute values and percentage frequencies. Quantitative variables were summarized through the following measures: minimum, maximum, range, mean and standard deviation. The normality of continuous variables was verified with the Kolmogorov–Smirnov test. The primary objective was evaluated by comparing the values of the lactulose/mannitol urinary excretion ratio in two groups of subjects (cohort I and II). The comparison was calculated with the Student's T-test if the variables were normally distributed and with the Mann–Whitney test in case of the absence of normality. The prevalence of RC in the gastrointestinal cohort (cohort III) was calculated as the percentage of patients who were reported to suffer from recurrent cystitis.

3. Results

We enrolled 16 patients in the RC cohort (cohort I) and 15 healthy controls (cohort II), whose characteristics are summarized in Table 1. Furthermore, we enrolled 238 female patients with gastrointestinal symptoms (III cohort) attending the General Gastroenterology and Breath Test Outpatient Clinic.

Table 1. The demographic characteristics and medical history of patients in the RC and gastrointestinal cohort and of healthy controls are summarized.

	Patient Affected by Recurrent Cystitis (RC, Cohort I)	Healthy Controls (Cohort II)	Patients Attending GI Outpatient Clinic (Cohort III)
Subjects number (f)	16	15	238
Mean age	44 (+/− 8 years)	42 (+/− 6 years)	42 (+/− 15 years)
Recurrent cystitis prevalence	100%	0%	20.2%
Gastrointestinal diseases prevalence	68% (11/16)	0%	48.7% (116/238)
IBD	18.75% (3/16)	0%	5.04% (122/238)
IBS and chronic functional bowel disorders	37.5% (6/16)	0%	16.4% (39/238)
Dyspepsia/GERD	43.75% (7/16)	0%	8% (19/238)
Lactose intolerance	37.5% (6/16)	0%	19.3% (49/238)
Diverticular disease	0%	0%	2.1% (5/238)

The prevalence of recurrent cystitis was 100% in cohort I, 0% in cohort II and 20% in cohort III (Table 1). Among the 16 patients in cohort I, 11 patients (68%) had a final diagnosis of GI disease, in particular IBS, inflammatory bowel disease (IBD), gastroesophageal reflux disease (GERD) and lactose intolerance. No GI disease was observed in healthy controls.

Finally, among 238 patients enrolled in cohort III, including patients seeking gastroenterological advice for GI symptoms, 116 patients (48.7%) had an established GI diagnosis, in particular IBD, diverticular disease, IBS and lactose intolerance.

No significant differences were found between patients affected by RC in cohort I compared to patients affected by RC in cohort III.

3.1. Self-Evaluation of Urological Symptoms (ACSS/UTISA) Questionnaire

All patients from cohort I with RC showed a significantly increased median score for the urological symptomatology questionnaire compared to controls (cohort II), for both typical and atypical symptoms ($p < 0.005$). Furthermore, significant differences were also found in 3 items of the ACSS/UTISA questionnaire, which dealt with daily discomfort, daily activity impairment and impairment of social activities ($p < 0.05$) (Figure 1A,B, respectively).

3.2. Self-Evaluation of GI Symptoms (GSRS) Questionnaire

Overall, 68% of patients from cohort I reported GI symptoms, as shown by an increase in the median values of all the items of the GSRS questionnaire (Figure 2A–C). On average, patients with RC showed more intense symptoms, such as diarrhea, constipation and abdominal pain, than controls. Patients with RC also showed great variability in their stool consistency compared to controls, who reported a more homogeneous consistency of type 3 or 4 on the Bristol Stool Scale (data not shown).

3.3. Intestinal Permeability Test

Eighty-eight percent of patients with RC from cohort I showed an increased intestinal permeability, with an average value of 0.05 ($p < 0.05$) compared to controls, who did not exceed the established cut-off of 0.03 (Figure 3A,B).

3.4. Alteration at Breath Testing

No statistically significant alterations among RC (cohort I) and controls (group II) were found at breath test analysis. In fact, the AUC of hydrogen and methane did not show any statistical significance. However, a clear trend towards an increased prevalence of SIBO and alterations in oro-cecal transit time were found in patients with recurrent cystitis compared to controls (p = ns, Figure 4A,B).

3.5. Gut Microbiota Profiling

Microbiota typing showed a trend toward a reduction in biodiversity, which was greater in patients than in controls, as seen from the graphs of α-diversity (i.e., observed species, CHAO 1 and Shannon indexes) (Figure 5A). The patients tended to cluster in a different way compared to controls (Figure 5B) (p = 0.02).

Furthermore, the phyla that was most represented in this distribution was Firmicutes, followed by Verrucomicrobia (Figure 5C, left side). At the genera level, potential markers of dysbiosis in RC seem to belong mainly to the phylum of Firmicutes, such as *Ruminococcus*, *Blautia*, *Veillonella* and *Streptococcus* spp. (Figure 5C, right side), while in terms of species, *Acinetobacter* showed particular abundance.

3.6. UTIs Etiology

Urinary tract infections appear to be mainly caused by agents derived from the intestinal microflora. The main representative was *E. coli*, but other widely present species include *Streptococcus agalactiae*, *Enterococcus faecalis*, and to a lesser extent, *Shigella* and *Proteus mirabilis* (Figure 6).

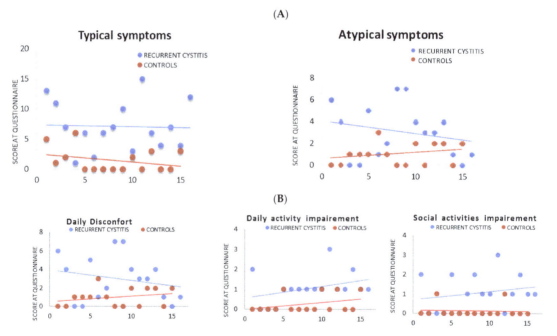

Figure 1. Symptoms and quality of life impairment in patients affected by RC (cohort I): ACSS/UTISA scores. (**A**) ACUTE CYSTITIS SYMPTOM SCORE (ACSS) AND UTI SYMPTOM ASSESSMENT (UTISA); (**B**) SELECTED ITEMS FROM ACSS/UTISA QUESTIONNAIRE. Patients with recurrent cystitis showed higher scores for the questionnaires compared to controls, both in the area of typical and atypical symptoms (**A**) Similarly, they scored significantly higher in items evaluating the perceived impact on quality of life. Selected items are reported in (**B**). All the differences were statistically significant (p < 0.05).

(A)

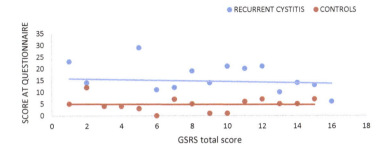

(B) GASTROENTEROLOGICAL COMPLAINTS: SELECTED AREA

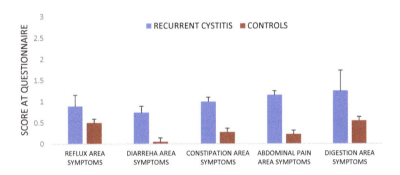

(C) GASTROENTEROLOGICAL COMPLAINTS: INTENSITY OF GI SYMPTOMS WITHIN SELECTED AREAS

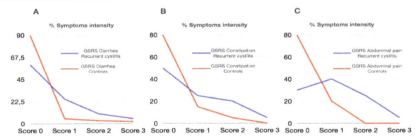

Figure 2. Gastroenterological complaints in RC patients (cohort I): Gastrointestinal Symptoms Rating Scale (GSRS) score. This questionnaire contains 15 questions related to five areas of interest in the gastroenterological clinic, concerning symptoms such as diarrhea, constipation, abdominal pain, reflux, dyspepsia. Among the enrolled patients, most showed an increased prevalence of all the items in the GSRS questionnaire. (**A**) Full GSRS score. (**B**) GSRS SCORE divided per gastrointestinal symptoms area score: reflux, diarrhea, constipation, abdominal pain, indigestion. (**C**) Intensity of symptoms according at GSRS for each single area: percentage of patients indicating a score of 3 (higher) or 2 or 1 or 0 (lower), respectively. Higher scores are consistent with increased severity of symptoms.

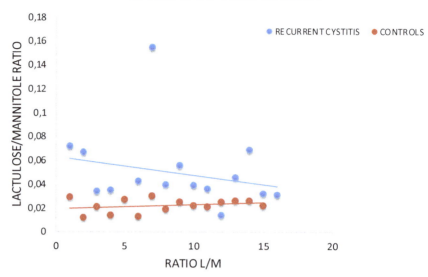

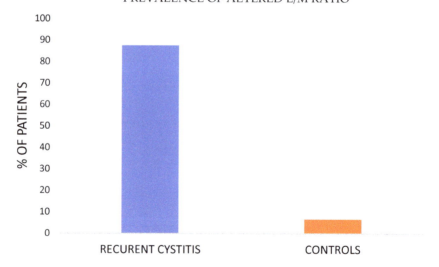

Figure 3. Intestinal permeability modification in patients with RC (cohort I). (**A**) Intestinal permeability. Patients affected by recurrent cystitis showed a statistically significant increase in intestinal permeability, measured as L/M ratio (lactulose/mannitol) with an average urinary ratio of lactulose/mannitol equal to 0.050 compared to 0.02 of controls. ($p < 0.05$). (**B**) Prevalence of altered L/M ratio. Of patients affected by recurrent cystitis, 88% displayed an altered L/M ratio compared to controls.

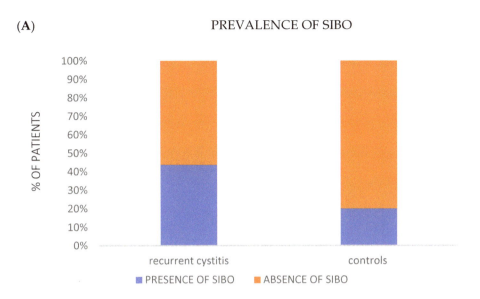

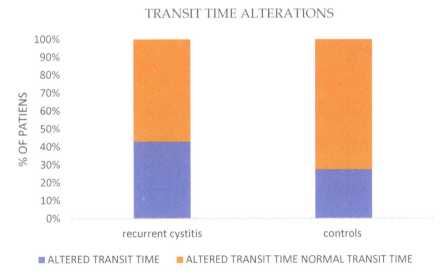

Figure 4. Increased prevalence of alteration at breath testing in RC (cohort I). Prevalence of SIBO (**A**) and prevalence of oro-cecal transit time alterations (**B**). The Breath Test showed that patients with recurrent cystitis showed a trend towards an increased prevalence of SIBO and alterations of the oro-cecal transit time, compared to the control population (differences were not statistically significant, $p > 0.05$).

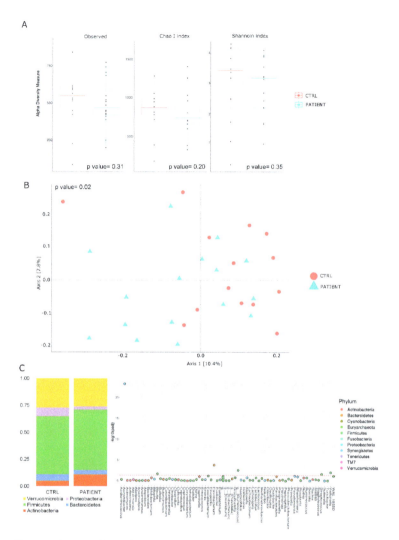

Figure 5. Gut microbiota alteration in RC patient (cohort I). (**A**) Boxplots representing α-diversity indices. The interquartile range is represented by the box and the line in the box is the median. The whiskers indicate the largest and the lowest data points, respectively, while the dots symbolize samples. The analysis of the gut microbiota showed a certain degree of reduction in the observed species and of the CHAO 1 and of Shannon indexes between the two groups. Furthermore, a greater degree of reduction in biodiversity seems more evident in the group of patients (cohort I) versus controls (cohort II). (**B**) β diversity analysis performed by Bray Curtis distance matrix and plotted by PCoA plot. Patients affected by RC (green, PTS, cohort I) tend to cluster differently than controls (red, ctr, cohort I). PERMANOVA *p* value = 0.02. (**C**) Phylum distribution (left side) and species distribution between RC patients (cohort I) and controls (cohort II) (right side). Firmicutes and Verrucomicrobia were the most represented phylum of gut microbiota (left side). In terms of prevalent microbial species, some species seem more abundant than others species. In the controls, particular abundance was found for *Acinetobacter*, while the most candidate species as potential markers of dysbiosis in the course of recurrent cystitis seem to belong above all to the phylum of *Firmicutes*, such as *Ruminococcus*, *Blautia*, *Veillonella*, *Streptococcus spp.* Mann–Whitney U test *p* values ≤ 0.05 (right side).

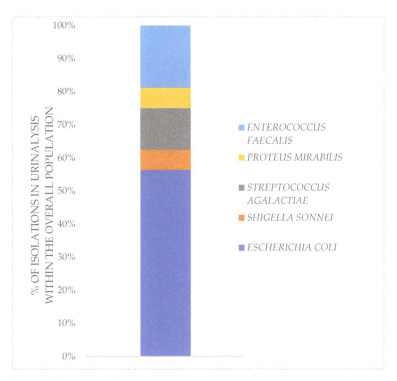

Figure 6. UTIs etiology. Urinary tract infections appear to be mainly caused by agents derived from the intestinal microflora. The main representative was *E. coli*, but other widely present species included *Streptococcus agalactiae*, *Enterococcus faecalis*, and to a lesser extent, *Shigella* and *Proteus mirabilis*.

4. Discussion

In this pilot study, patients with recurrent UTIs described a wide range of negative emotions related to the burden of experienced symptoms and to their impact on the quality of daily life, as well-described in the ACSS/UTISA questionnaire. We found some correlation with previous research on the experiences of patients with UTIs. A recent qualitative, interview-based study by Grigoryan et al. of German and US participants who experienced uncomplicated UTIs, showed a range of negative effects of UTI symptoms on the daily lives, sleep and relationships of the women involved, along with a feeling of helplessness and dread in the context of recurring infections and treatment failure [37]. Similar to this study and to a previous qualitative interview study by Eriksson et al. [38], our patients described a significant impact of urinary symptoms, such as pollakiuria, urgency, suprapubic pain/discomfort, small involuntary urine leakage or sensation of incomplete emptying of the bladder on their daily-life activities. In particular, they complained about daily discomfort and the consequent compromise and impairment of daily activities and social relationships.

As this pilot study has shown, patients with a previous diagnosis of RC not only experienced a significant increase in the incidence of urinary symptoms, but also, they frequently reported GI symptoms, such as dyspepsia, abdominal pain, bloating, flatulence, diarrhea or constipation (or mixed bowel habits), much more than controls, as evidenced by the scores of the GSRS questionnaire. For example, up to 20% of enrolled patients reported significant diarrheal symptoms. However, in most cases, patients with RC showed only mild to moderate symptom intensity.

The pathogenesis of urinary infections typically starts with contamination of the periurethral region by pathogen microorganisms of the gut, followed by colonization of the urethra and ascending migration to the bladder [39]. Dysbiosis and increased intestinal permeability could contribute to the onset of extra-intestinal disorders, such as RC. In order to better explore the potential role of gut barrier dysfunction in the pathogenesis of RC, we performed an evaluation of intestinal permeability with the H_2 Breath Test Lactulose/Mannitol, and subsequently, the metagenomic analysis of gut microbiota in the patient and control groups. These evaluations showed a higher incidence of impaired intestinal permeability. At the same time, breath test results showed a trend towards an increased prevalence of SIBO and alterations in the intestinal transit time in patients compared to controls, suggesting the presence of a certain degree of dysbiosis, even considering that urinary infections are mainly caused by components of the intestinal microbial flora, as emerged from our study.

In regard to a possible underlying pathogenetic explanation to our data, it can be assumed that the impaired intestinal permeability observed in the RC cohort, as well as the presence of a pro-inflammatory gut microbiota, could contribute to the dysregulation of enterocytes, with a reduction in the expression of tight junctions, increase in mucosal permeability and dysregulation of immune cells finally leading to an abnormal inflammatory state, which causes mucosal damage and subsequent translocation of microbial fragments in the inner layers of intestinal barrier. Then, the extraintestinal spaces and the areas next to the intestinal tract, such as the urogenital system, may be colonized by gut-derived bacteria, which finally cause the recurrence of cystitis once they reach the bladder [40,41]. Further studies will be required to test the validity of this hypothesis. Unfortunately, probably due to the relatively low number of enrolled patients, we were not able to identify specific bacteria associated with gut barrier dysfunction in this cohort of patients (data not shown).

Conversely, a significant number of patients with GI symptoms reported lower urinary tract symptoms, when investigated with ACSS/UTISA questionnaire. Approximately 20% of GI patients could be diagnosed with RC, based on the symptoms reported in the questionnaires, with a significant impact on quality of life. However, in our population with RC, we cannot exclude that the alterations of intestinal permeability and gut microbiota may be secondary to concomitant gastrointestinal pathologies. In fact, when patients with RC were investigated by gastroenterologists in our outpatient clinic, most of them could be diagnosed with a definite GI disease: IBD (one patient even had the first diagnosis of Crohn's disease), IBS, lactose intolerance or functional dyspepsia. This would indicate that a significant number of patients with RC might have a misunderstood gastroenterological disease that would predispose them to infection and colonization of bladder. Unfortunately, due to the low number of enrolled patients, our study did not show a significant correlation between RC and specific gastroenterological disease, but the increased prevalence of gastrointestinal diseases in RC patients could highlight a possible common etiology based on dysbiosis and increased gut permeability. However, further studies with a larger cohort of patients are needed to analyze in more depth the specific gut microbiota signature, which could contribute to both RC and different gastrointestinal diseases.

Furthermore, we should take into account that the increasingly massive use of systemic antibiotics for the occurrence of UTIs contributes to the development and spread of antibiotic-resistant pathogens. This also results in the elimination of protective, beneficial microbial species, causing gut and urinary tract dysbiosis, and finally, the recurrence of cystitis itself, which also predisposes patients to other functional gastrointestinal diseases. In this scenario, it is difficult to understand if gastrointestinal disorders in RC patients are primary disorders or they are triggered from antibiotic-induced dysbiosis. Therefore, it is essential to prevent the occurrence of cystitis rather than to just treat it with repeated antibiotic treatment. Several strategies have been suggested in order to prevent the recurrence of cystitis; however, until now, guidelines do not concur on recommendations regarding this topic. Non-antibiotic preventative strategies include the use of cranberry products, despite the low compliance rate among patients, probiotics, phytotherapeutics, or immunotherapies, such as OM-89, which is a bacterial extract from *E. coli* that stimulates the host immune system to produce cytokines and antibodies against several bacteria species due to sharing similar antigenic structures. Vaginal estrogen, methenamine hippurate and replenishment of the glycosaminoglycan (GAG) layers within the bladder urothelium to reduce bacterial adherence, have also been recommended in order to reduce UTIs recurrence but with variable results [42].

Our study showed a strong association between altered intestinal permeability, intestinal dysbiosis, SIBO or other gastroenterological pathologies and the development of recurrent cystitis; this should steer our attention towards new therapeutic strategies for the prevention of RC, such as the reconstitution of the intestinal mucosa integrity or the modulation of gut and urinary microbiota with the use of probiotics or even with fecal microbiota transplantation (FMT). Both these therapeutic strategies should determine the displacement of pathogens by probiotics colonization. Supporting these therapeutic strategies, a pilot study including 11 women with RC compared the incidence of symptomatic, culture-proven, antibiotic-treated UTIs in six months pre-fecal microbiota transplantation with six months post-transplantation. The study showed a decrease in symptomatic UTIs after FMT, though not in a statistically significant way [43]. By modulating the microbiome profiles of recipients, FMT could be an innovative therapeutic strategy for refractory recurrent UTI patients, particularly those with antibiotic resistance. Moreover, lactic acid bacteria seem to interfere with the growth and adhesion of urinary pathogens. Therefore, it is necessary to design new dedicated clinical trials to evaluate, in a deeper way, the efficacy of both probiotics - particularly the most effective candidates *L. crispatus* [44], *L. rhamnosus* GR1 or *reuteri* RC14 [45]-and FMT for the treatment and prevention of RC.

Together with the relatively limited number of patients in this trial, our work has another significant limitation: we have limited information about the nutritional characteristics of the enrolled patients. Given the importance of nutrition in modulating gut microbiota and intestinal permeability, its role in causing urinary infections or improving them should be considered with dedicated trials.

5. Conclusions

Patients with RC showed a high prevalence of gastro-intestinal disorders, increased permeability and associated dysbiosis in the microbiota analysis. These results constitute the rationale for further studies to evaluate the potential clinical effects of active gut microbiota modulation on the recurrence of cystitis.

This pilot study laid the foundations for further investigations, and aimed to understand the role of intestinal barrier integrity in greater depth, as its altered permeability appears to be associated with not only intestinal, but also extra-intestinal diseases. Finally, it should be pointed out that various drugs, such as antibiotics, probiotics, prebiotics, a specific diet and numerous pathological conditions could influence the permeability of the intestine through the modulation of the microbial composition. In this context, the study of the degree of intestinal permeability and the potential role of microbiota modulation using new, reliable, reproducible, non-invasive methods could become a valid diagnostic and therapeutic tool for the clinician, thus allowing the development of new and increasingly personalized therapies.

Supplementary Materials: The following supporting information can be downloaded at: https://www.mdpi.com/article/10.3390/jpm12061005/s1, Supplementary Files: The combined ACSS/UTISA questionnaire.

Author Contributions: Conceptualization, F.S.; Data curation, C.G.; Formal analysis, A.P. (Andrea Poscia), F.D.C., V.M., S.L.M.; Project administration, C.G.; Supervision, A.G.; Validation, L.L., F.D.V., L.M., L.R.L., G.C., D.R. and A.L.; Writing – original draft, L.L., C.T., M.P., N.D.S., S.D., C.R., J.G., S.P., A.P. (Aniello Primiano), F.R.P., L.P., A.U., V.P., F.D.V., L.M., L.R.L., G.C., D.R., A.L. and A.G. All authors have read and agreed to the published version of the manuscript.

Funding: This research received no external funding.

Institutional Review Board Statement: The study was conducted in accordance with the Declaration of Helsinki, and approved by the Institutional Review Board (or Ethics Committee) of Fondazione Policlinico Universitario A. Gemelli IRCCS (Protocol Number 0011046/21 of 03/24/2021).

Informed Consent Statement: Informed consent was obtained from all subjects involved in the study.

Data Availability Statement: Data is contained within the article or Supplementary Material.

Conflicts of Interest: The authors declare no conflict of interest.

References

1. Guglietta, A. Recurrent Urinary Tract Infections in Women: Risk Factors, Etiology, Pathogenesis and Prophylaxis. *Future Microbiol.* **2017**, *12*, 239–246. [CrossRef] [PubMed]
2. Del Popolo, G.; Nelli, F. Recurrent Bacterial Symptomatic Cystitis: A Pilot Study on a New Natural Option for Treatment. *Arch Ital. Urol. Androl.* **2018**, *90*, 101–103. [CrossRef] [PubMed]
3. Scholes, D.; Hooton, T.M.; Roberts, P.L.; Stapleton, A.E.; Gupta, K.; Stamm, W.E. Risk Factors for Recurrent Urinary Tract Infection in Young Women. *J. Infect. Dis.* **2000**, *182*, 1177–1182. [CrossRef] [PubMed]
4. Kinane, D.F.; Blackwell, C.C.; Brettle, R.P.; Weir, D.M.; Winstanley, F.P.; Elton, R.A. ABO Blood Group, Secretor State, and Susceptibility to Recurrent Urinary Tract Infection in Women. *Br. Med. J. (Clin. Res. Ed.)* **1982**, *285*, 7–9. [CrossRef]
5. Tandogdu, Z.; Wagenlehner, F.M.E. Global Epidemiology of Urinary Tract Infections. *Curr. Opin. Infect. Dis.* **2016**, *29*, 73–79. [CrossRef]
6. Scribano, D.; Sarshar, M.; Fettucciari, L.; Ambrosi, C. Urinary Tract Infections: Can We Prevent Uropathogenic Escherichia Coli Infection with Dietary Intervention? *Int. J. Vitam. Nutr. Res.* **2021**, *91*, 391–395. [CrossRef]
7. Meštrović, T.; Matijašić, M.; Perić, M.; Čipčić Paljetak, H.; Barešić, A.; Verbanac, D. The Role of Gut, Vaginal, and Urinary Microbiome in Urinary Tract Infections: From Bench to Bedside. *Diagnostics* **2020**, *11*, 7. [CrossRef]
8. Greenwood-Van Meerveld, B.; Mohammadi, E.; Tyler, K.; Van Gordon, S.; Parker, A.; Towner, R.; Hurst, R. Mechanisms of Visceral Organ Crosstalk: Importance of Alterations in Permeability in Rodent Models. *J. Urol.* **2015**, *194*, 804–811. [CrossRef]
9. Ustinova, E.E.; Fraser, M.O.; Pezzone, M.A. Colonic Irritation in the Rat Sensitizes Urinary Bladder Afferents to Mechanical and Chemical Stimuli: An Afferent Origin of Pelvic Organ Cross-Sensitization. *Am. J. Physiol. Renal Physiol.* **2006**, *290*, F1478–F1487. [CrossRef]
10. Nickel, J.C.; Tripp, D.A.; Pontari, M.; Moldwin, R.; Mayer, R.; Carr, L.K.; Doggweiler, R.; Yang, C.C.; Mishra, N.; Nordling, J. Interstitial Cystitis/Painful Bladder Syndrome and Associated Medical Conditions with an Emphasis on Irritable Bowel Syndrome, Fibromyalgia and Chronic Fatigue Syndrome. *J. Urol.* **2010**, *184*, 1358–1363. [CrossRef]
11. Pezzone, M.A.; Liang, R.; Fraser, M.O. A Model of Neural Cross-Talk and Irritation in the Pelvis: Implications for the Overlap of Chronic Pelvic Pain Disorders. *Gastroenterology* **2005**, *128*, 1953–1964. [CrossRef] [PubMed]
12. Noronha, R.; Akbarali, H.; Malykhina, A.; Foreman, R.D.; Greenwood-Van Meerveld, B. Changes in Urinary Bladder Smooth Muscle Function in Response to Colonic Inflammation. *Am. J. Physiol. Renal Physiol.* **2007**, *293*, F1461–F1467. [CrossRef] [PubMed]
13. Winnard, K.P.; Dmitrieva, N.; Berkley, K.J. Cross-Organ Interactions between Reproductive, Gastrointestinal, and Urinary Tracts: Modulation by Estrous Stage and Involvement of the Hypogastric Nerve. *Am. J. Physiol. Regul. Integr. Comp. Physiol.* **2006**, *291*, R1592–R1601. [CrossRef] [PubMed]
14. Poole, N.M.; Green, S.I.; Rajan, A.; Vela, L.E.; Zeng, X.-L.; Estes, M.K.; Maresso, A.W. Role for FimH in Extraintestinal Pathogenic Escherichia Coli Invasion and Translocation through the Intestinal Epithelium. *Infect. Immun.* **2017**, *85*, e00581-17. [CrossRef]
15. Scaldaferri, F.; Pizzoferrato, M.; Gerardi, V.; Lopetuso, L.; Gasbarrini, A. The Gut Barrier: New Acquisitions and Therapeutic Approaches. *J. Clin. Gastroenterol.* **2012**, *46*, S12–S17. [CrossRef]
16. Graziani, C.; Talocco, C.; De Sire, R.; Petito, V.; Lopetuso, L.R.; Gervasoni, J.; Persichilli, S.; Franceschi, F.; Ojetti, V.; Gasbarrini, A.; et al. Intestinal Permeability in Physiological and Pathological Conditions: Major Determinants and Assessment Modalities. *Eur. Rev. Med. Pharmacol. Sci.* **2019**, *23*, 795–810. [CrossRef]
17. Sturgeon, C.; Fasano, A. Zonulin, a Regulator of Epithelial and Endothelial Barrier Functions, and Its Involvement in Chronic Inflammatory Diseases. *Tissue Barriers* **2016**, *4*, e1251384. [CrossRef]
18. Alidjanov, J.F.; Abdufattaev, U.A.; Makhsudov, S.A.; Pilatz, A.; Akilov, F.A.; Naber, K.G.; Wagenlehner, F.M. New Self-Reporting Questionnaire to Assess Urinary Tract Infections and Differential Diagnosis: Acute Cystitis Symptom Score. *Urol. Int.* **2014**, *92*, 230–236. [CrossRef]
19. Clayson, D.; Wild, D.; Doll, H.; Keating, K.; Gondek, K. Validation of a Patient-Administered Questionnaire to Measure the Severity and Bothersomeness of Lower Urinary Tract Symptoms in Uncomplicated Urinary Tract Infection (UTI): The UTI Symptom Assessment Questionnaire. *BJU Int.* **2005**, *96*, 350–359. [CrossRef]
20. Svedlund, J.; Sjödin, I.; Dotevall, G. GSRS—A Clinical Rating Scale for Gastrointestinal Symptoms in Patients with Irritable Bowel Syndrome and Peptic Ulcer Disease. *Dig. Dis. Sci.* **1988**, *33*, 129–134. [CrossRef]
21. Wild, G.E.; Waschke, K.A.; Bitton, A.; Thomson, A.B.R. The Mechanisms of Prednisone Inhibition of Inflammation in Crohn's Disease Involve Changes in Intestinal Permeability, Mucosal TNFalpha Production and Nuclear Factor Kappa B Expression. *Aliment. Pharmacol. Ther.* **2003**, *18*, 309–317. [CrossRef] [PubMed]
22. Hollander, D. The Intestinal Permeability Barrier. A Hypothesis as to Its Regulation and Involvement in Crohn's Disease. *Scand. J. Gastroenterol.* **1992**, *27*, 721–726. [CrossRef] [PubMed]

23. D'Incà, R.; Di Leo, V.; Corrao, G.; Martines, D.; D'Odorico, A.; Mestriner, C.; Venturi, C.; Longo, G.; Sturniolo, G.C. Intestinal Permeability Test as a Predictor of Clinical Course in Crohn's Disease. *Am. J. Gastroenterol.* **1999**, *94*, 2956–2960. [CrossRef] [PubMed]

24. Schietroma, M.; Pessia, B.; Carlei, F.; Amicucci, G. Intestinal Permeability Changes, Systemic Endotoxemia, Inflammatory Serum Markers and Sepsis after Whipple's Operation for Carcinoma of the Pancreas Head. *Pancreatology* **2017**, *17*, 839–846. [CrossRef] [PubMed]

25. Lostia, A.M.; Lionetto, L.; Principessa, L.; Evangelisti, M.; Gamba, A.; Villa, M.P.; Simmaco, M. A Liquid Chromatography/Mass Spectrometry Method for the Evaluation of Intestinal Permeability. *Clin. Biochem.* **2008**, *41*, 887–892. [CrossRef] [PubMed]

26. Rezaie, A.; Buresi, M.; Lembo, A.; Lin, H.; McCallum, R.; Rao, S.; Schmulson, M.; Valdovinos, M.; Zakko, S.; Pimentel, M. Hydrogen and Methane-Based Breath Testing in Gastrointestinal Disorders: The North American Consensus. *Am. J. Gastroenterol.* **2017**, *112*, 775–784. [CrossRef] [PubMed]

27. Gervasoni, J.; Primiano, A.; Graziani, C.; Scaldaferri, F.; Gasbarrini, A.; Urbani, A.; Persichilli, S. Validation of UPLC-MS/MS Method for Determination of Urinary Lactulose/Mannitol. *Molecules* **2018**, *23*, 2705. [CrossRef]

28. Romani, L.; Del Chierico, F.; Chiriaco, M.; Foligno, S.; Reddel, S.; Salvatori, G.; Cifaldi, C.; Faraci, S.; Finocchi, A.; Rossi, P.; et al. Gut Mucosal and Fecal Microbiota Profiling Combined to Intestinal Immune System in Neonates Affected by Intestinal Ischemic Injuries. *Front. Cell. Infect. Microbiol.* **2020**, *10*, 59. [CrossRef]

29. Bolger, A.M.; Lohse, M.; Usadel, B. Trimmomatic: A Flexible Trimmer for Illumina Sequence Data. *Bioinformatics* **2014**, *30*, 2114–2120. [CrossRef]

30. Caporaso, J.G.; Kuczynski, J.; Stombaugh, J.; Bittinger, K.; Bushman, F.D.; Costello, E.K.; Fierer, N.; Peña, A.G.; Goodrich, J.K.; Gordon, J.I.; et al. QIIME Allows Analysis of High-Throughput Community Sequencing Data. *Nat. Methods* **2010**, *7*, 335–336. [CrossRef]

31. Edgar, R.C. Search and Clustering Orders of Magnitude Faster than BLAST. *Bioinformatics* **2010**, *26*, 2460–2461. [CrossRef]

32. DeSantis, T.Z.; Dubosarskiy, I.; Murray, S.R.; Andersen, G.L. Comprehensive Aligned Sequence Construction for Automated Design of Effective Probes (CASCADE-P) Using 16S RDNA. *Bioinformatics* **2003**, *19*, 1461–1468. [CrossRef] [PubMed]

33. European Association of Urology. *European Association of Urology Pocket Guidelines*; European Association of Urology: Arnhem, The Netherlands, 2021; ISBN 978-94-92671-14-1.

34. Di Vico, T.; Morganti, R.; Cai, T.; Naber, K.G.; Wagenlehner, F.M.E.; Pilatz, A.; Alidjanov, J.; Morelli, G.; Bartoletti, R. Acute Cystitis Symptom Score (ACSS): Clinical Validation of the Italian Version. *Antibiotics* **2020**, *9*, 104. [CrossRef] [PubMed]

35. Chang, S.-J.; Lin, C.-D.; Hsieh, C.-H.; Liu, Y.-B.; Chiang, I.-N.; Yang, S.S.-D. Reliability and Validity of a Chinese Version of Urinary Tract Infection Symptom Assessment Questionnaire. *Int. Braz. J. Urol.* **2015**, *41*, 729–738. [CrossRef] [PubMed]

36. Alidjanov, J.F. Preliminary Clinical Validation of the UK English Version of the Acute Cystitis Symptom Score in UK English-Speaking Female Population of Newcastle, Great Britain. *JOJ Urol. Nephrol.* **2017**, *1*, 555561. [CrossRef]

37. Grigoryan, L.; Mulgirigama, A.; Powell, M.; Schmiemann, G. The emotional impact of urinary tract infections in women: A qualitative analysis. *BMC Women's Health* **2022**, *22*, 182. [CrossRef] [PubMed]

38. Eriksson, I.; Olofsson, B.; Gustafson, Y.; Fagerström, L. Older women's experiences of suffering from urinary tract infections. *J. Clin. Nurs.* **2014**, *23*, 1385–1394. [CrossRef]

39. Foxman, B. Urinary Tract Infection Syndromes: Occurrence, Recurrence, Bacteriology, Risk Factors, and Disease Burden. *Infect. Dis. Clin. N. Am.* **2014**, *28*, 1–13. [CrossRef]

40. Geremia, A.; Biancheri, P.; Allan, P.; Corazza, G.R.; Di Sabatino, A. Innate and Adaptive Immunity in Inflammatory Bowel Disease. *Autoimmun. Rev.* **2014**, *13*, 3–10. [CrossRef]

41. Lopetuso, L.R.; Scaldaferri, F.; Bruno, G.; Petito, V.; Franceschi, F.; Gasbarrini, A. The Therapeutic Management of Gut Barrier Leaking: The Emerging Role for Mucosal Barrier Protectors. *Eur. Rev. Med. Pharmacol. Sci.* **2015**, *19*, 1068–1076.

42. Kwok, M.; McGeorge, S.; Mayer-Coverdale, J.; Graves, B.; Paterson, D.L.; Harris, P.N.A.; Esler, R.; Dowling, C.; Britton, S.; Roberts, M.J. Guideline of guidelines: Management of recurrent urinary tract infections in women. *BJU Int.* **2022**. *ahead of print.* [CrossRef] [PubMed]

43. Jeney, S.E.S.; Lane, F.; Oliver, A.; Whiteson, K.; Dutta, S. Fecal Microbiota transplantation for the treatment of refractory recurrent urinary tract infection. *Obstet. Gynecol.* **2020**, *136*, 771–773. [CrossRef] [PubMed]

44. Sadahira, T.; Wada, K.; Araki, M.; Mitsuhata, R.; Yamamoto, M.; Maruyama, Y.; Iwata, T.; Watanabe, M.; Watanabe, T.; Kariyama, R.; et al. Efficacy of *Lactobacillus* vaginal suppositories for the prevention of recurrent cystitis: A phase II clinical trial. *Int. J. Urol.* **2021**, *28*, 1026–1031. [CrossRef] [PubMed]

45. Ng, Q.X.; Peters, C.; Venkatanarayanan, N.; Goh, Y.Y.; Ho, C.Y.X.; Yeo, W.-S. Use of *Lactobacillus* spp. to prevent recurrent urinary tract infections in females. *Med. Hypotheses* **2018**, *114*, 49–54. [CrossRef]

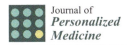

Article

Gut Microbiota as Early Predictor of Infectious Complications before Cardiac Surgery: A Prospective Pilot Study

Ekaterina Chernevskaya [1,*], Evgenii Zuev [1,2], Vera Odintsova [3], Anastasiia Meglei [1] and Natalia Beloborodova [1]

1. Federal Research and Clinical Center of Intensive Care Medicine and Rehabilitology, 25-2 Petrovka Str., 107031 Moscow, Russia; zuev17ev@gmail.com (E.Z.); amegley@fnkcrr.ru (A.M.); nvbeloborodova@yandex.ru (N.B.)
2. N. Pirogov National Medical Surgical Center, 70 Nizhnyaya Pervomayskaya Str., 105203 Moscow, Russia
3. Atlas Biomed Group—Knomics LLC, 31 Malaya Nikitskaya Str., 121069 Moscow, Russia; odintsova@atlas.ru
* Correspondence: echernevskaya@fnkcrr.ru; Tel.: +7-906-792-7041

Abstract: Cardiac surgery remains a field of medicine with a high percentage of postoperative complications, including infectious ones. Modern data indicate a close relationship of infectious disorders with pathological changes in the composition of the gut microbiome; however, the extent of such changes in cardiac surgery patients is not fully clarified. In this prospective, observational, single center, pilot study, 72 patients were included, 12 among them with the infectious complications. We analyzed the features of the fecal microbiota before and in the early postoperative period, as one of the markers for predicting the occurrence of bacterial infection. We also discovered the significant change in microbial composition in the group of patients with infectious complications compared to the non-infectious group before and after cardiac surgery, despite the intra-individual variation in composition of gut microbiome. Our study demonstrated that the group of patients that had a bacterial infection in the early postoperative period already had an altered microbial composition even before the surgery. Further studies will evaluate the clinical significance of the identified proportions of individual taxa of the intestinal microbiota and consider the microbiota as a novel target for reducing the risk of infectious complications.

Keywords: cardiovascular diseases; 16S RNA sequencing; microbiome; biomarkers; critically ill

Citation: Chernevskaya, E.; Zuev, E.; Odintsova, V.; Meglei, A.; Beloborodova, N. Gut Microbiota as Early Predictor of Infectious Complications before Cardiac Surgery: A Prospective Pilot Study. *J. Pers. Med.* **2021**, *11*, 1113. https://doi.org/10.3390/jpm11111113

Academic Editor: Lucrezia Laterza

Received: 10 September 2021
Accepted: 27 October 2021
Published: 29 October 2021

Publisher's Note: MDPI stays neutral with regard to jurisdictional claims in published maps and institutional affiliations.

Copyright: © 2021 by the authors. Licensee MDPI, Basel, Switzerland. This article is an open access article distributed under the terms and conditions of the Creative Commons Attribution (CC BY) license (https://creativecommons.org/licenses/by/4.0/).

1. Introduction

Infections are frequent complications of cardiac surgery [1]. Despite the success in the development of surgical practices, this percentage does not decrease, and ranges from 12.6 to 21%. Among them, a significant portion is postoperative pneumonia and surgical site infections [2–5]. Risk factors include age, chronic lung disease, heart failure, duration of surgery, cardiopulmonary bypass, and others. The state of the microbiota is not taken into the account, although it may be a therapeutic target [6]. Metabolism-dependent and -independent processes are the link between the «gut–heart axis». On the one hand, the gut microbiota acts as an endocrine organ producing bioactive metabolites, including Trimethylamine/trimethylamine N-oxide (TMAO), short chain fatty acids and others. On the other hand, impaired cardiac activity contributes to bowel wall edema, resulting in bacterial translocation with the subsequent pro-inflammatory condition, which also impaired heart function [7,8]. The growing scientific evidence supports the role of the gut microbiota in the pathogenesis of heart failure [9–14]. However, only a very few studies are devoted to the composition of the gut microbiota of elective surgery patients in the intensive care unit [15].

Several studies of gut microbiota dynamics in ICU patients using 16S rRNA gene sequencing indicate a rapid disruption of gut microbiota during ICU stay, and this is associated with a loss of diversity and overgrowth of potentially pathogenic microorganisms [16–19]. The microbial disbalance in the gut may have a clinical relevance and can lead to inflammation and infection [20], also playing a potential role in neurological deficits [21].

More common in cardiac surgery, research is aimed at clarifying and early detection of compromised patients in order to provide customized management strategies that match the patient's molecular and biochemical profile. Along with traditional biomarkers, NT-proBNP, hight-sensitive Troponine T, the use of novel biomarkers, such as microRNAs, mitochondrial peptides, inflammatory cytokines and adhesion molecules are discussed [22].

The aim of the study was to identify the features of changes in the gut microbiota and biomarkers in patients after cardiac surgery and to assess their relationship with postoperative complications. We observed that, despite the large interindividual variability of the microbial composition, the composition of the gut microbiota in patients with infectious complications showed a consistent pattern with the relative predominance of potentially pathogenic species.

2. Materials and Methods

2.1. Study Design

This prospective observational pilot study was performed in the N. Pirogov National Medical Surgical Center, Moscow, Russian Federation. The local Ethics Committee approved the study (no. 04 22.05.2018), which was conducted in accordance with the ethical standards of the Declaration of Helsinki. A formal consent for participation in this study was also obtained from each patient or his/her legal representative.

2.2. Patients and Samples

All patients have received perioperative antibiotic prophylaxis: cefazolin 3 times within 24 h for CABG or vancomycin 4 times within 48 h for valve surgery. The inclusion criteria are as follows: age over 18 years old, planned surgical intervention, patients with the following types of cardiac surgery—heart valve surgery, off-Pump CABG, CABG (Coronary artery bypass grafting), combination surgery—and signed informed consent to participate in the study. Exclusion criteria are as follows: active infectious endocarditis, emergency surgery, previous bacterial infectious diseases in the last three months, antibiotic intake in the last three months, inflammatory bowel disease, and patients refusing to participate in the study.

All stool samples and venous blood samples were collected from each patient before and after 1, 3 and 7 days of cardiac surgery. All samples before surgery were collected prior starting antibiotic prophylaxis. Blood was collected from a venous catheter into an anticoagulant-free test tube. Serum samples were obtained by centrifuging the blood at $1500 \times g$ for 10 min. Serum aliquots (500 µL) were poured into disposable Eppendorf tubes, frozen and stored at $-20\,°C$ until further use. Stool samples were obtained by collecting a small amount of feces as a rectal swab and dissolving it in 1 mL of sterile saline solution; after thorough mixing, it was divided into two Eppendorf tubes and were frozen and stored at $-30\,°C$ prior to analysis.

2.3. Analysis of Serum Biomarkers

Neurological (S100), inflammatory (IL6), cardio (NT-proBNP, hight-sensitive Troponine T (hs-TnT)), "stress" (ACTH, cortisol) and bacterial infection (procalcitonin (PCT)) biomarkers were measured in 200 µL serum samples using reagent kits on automated electrochemiluminescence analyzer Cobas e411 (Roche; Basel, Switzerland). Biomarkers of gut microbiota metabolic activity (Taurine, Trimethylamine N-oxide (TMAO)) were measured using reagent kits by Cloud Clone, Katy, USA, on automated microplate photometer Multiscan (Thermo Scientific; Waltham, MA, USA) which relies on the linked immunosorbent assay.

2.4. Microbiome Sample Preparation

Defrozen fecal solution (200 mL) was placed in the 2.0 mL tube containing 3:1 mix of 0.1 mm and 0.5 mm pre-sterilized glass beads (Sigma, St. Louis, MO, USA). Then 1 mL of a warm 60 °C lysis buffer (500 mM NaCl, 50 mM Tris-HCl, pH 8.0, 50 mM EDTA, 4% SDS) was added. The mixture was vortexed and homogenized with MiniLys (Bertin Technologies S.A.S., Montigny Le Bretonneux, France) for 3 min. The lysate was incubated at 70 °C for 15 min and centrifuged for 20 min at 14,000 rpm. The supernatant (1 mL) was transferred to the sterile tube and put on the ice. The pellet was added to a 1 mL of lysis buffer and the homogenization process was repeated. The supernatants were combined in the 15 mL tubes with the addition of 4 mL of 96% ethanol and 200 μL of 3 M sodium acetate. The mixture was incubated at −20 °C for not less than 1 h. Then the mixture was centrifuged for 15 min at 14,000 rpm at +4 °C, the supernatant was discarded, the DNA pellet was washed twice with 80% ethanol. The pellet was dried at 53 °C for 30–60 min and resuspended in 200 μL of sterilized milliQ water. The mixture was centrifuged and transferred into new tubes. Resulting DNA solution was treated with 10 μL of RNAse A (5 mg/mL) for 1 h at 37 °C, followed by an additional round of chloroform purification. Chloroform was added to the solution in 1:1 ratio, tube was vortexed for 1 min and centrifuged at $5000 \times g$ for 5 min. Aqueous phase was transferred to new sterile tube and used for PCR dilutions. The obtained DNA solution was stored at −20 °C. Amplicon sequencing of V4 variable region of microbial 16S rRNA gene was performed on a MiSeq sequencer (Illumina, San Diego, CA, USA) as described before [23].

2.5. Microbiome Data Processing

Raw microbiome data is available in the Sequence Read Archive (SRA) by the accession number PRJNA688839. The reads were processed using the Knomics-Biota system [23,24] ("16S dada2 Greengenes V4") pipeline based on the DADA2 algorithm and Greengenes database [25,26] as previously described [27]. In the pipeline, the Greengenes database was preprocessed using TaxMan [27,28] based on the F515-R806 primers for V4 region of the 16S rRNA gene. The sequences were clustered with 97% identity using cd-hit software version 4.8.1 [27–29]. The slash ("/") character was used (example: (Blautia/Dorea)), for ambiguous sequences, for which taxonomy could not be resolved based on the used primers. When the sequence could not be resolved at a particular taxonomic rank, the "_u" sign was used (referring to the term "unclassified", example: "Lactobacillus_u"). There were minor changes to the original Knomics-Biota pipeline: the Chao1 index calculated on the level of ASVs (amplicon sequencing variants) after rarefaction to 3000 reads per sample was used to assess the alpha diversity; the beta diversity was estimated using Euclidean distance in Aitchison space [30,31].

2.6. Statistical Analysis

This statistical analysis of microbiome composition was done in R [32]. Only genera that were presented by more than 10 counts in ≥50% of samples were included in the analysis (in total 40 genera). The abundance table was obtained with cmultRepl function from zCompositions library [33,34]. The Aitchison distance was used to estimate beta diversity between samples. Comparison of general proportions in two groups of samples was done in the following way: the independent balances containing 2 or 3 taxa were obtained with DBA-distal method [33], the statistical significance of association between these balances and infectious complications was assessed by linear regression analysis. The Benjamini-Hochberg correction was used to adjust for multiple testing. The adonis function from the vegan library was used for beta-diversity analysis [35]. Changes of microbiome in time were treated separately for subjects with and without complications. Time points were compared pairwise. For each pair of time points, all patients that provided samples in these two days were included in the analysis; patients that did not provide a sample in any of these timepoints were excluded. The analysis of taxa proportions and beta diversity was performed in a similar way. It was done for comparison of samples collected before the surgery, with several changes: subject identifier was included as the "strata" parameter in the adonis function, and as a random effect in a mixed effect model in balances analysis (instead of the linear regression). The lmerTest library was used to fit mixed effect models and estimate significance of its coefficients [36]. The analysis of association between microbiome composition and blood parameters was performed with selbal [37] for the samples collected before the surgery. Only associations that were repeated in at least 50% of iteration of the cross-validation procedure are presented in the Results section. Association of beta-diversity between samples with the difference in blood parameters was analyzed with adonis.

3. Results

3.1. Patients Characteristics

The inclusion of patients and sample collections are shown in Figure 1. Of the 72 patients included in the study, complications developed in 12 cases. For further analysis of the gut microbiota and biomarkers, a group of patients without infectious complications was selected, comparable to infectious group.

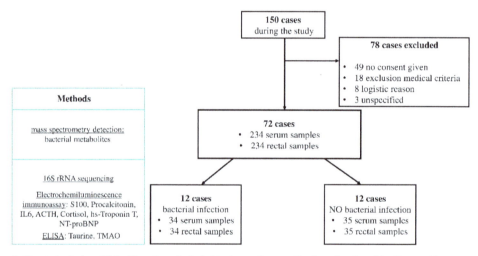

Figure 1. The study design. Of the 72 patients included in the study, complications developed in 12 cases. For comparison, a group of patients without complications was selected, comparable in the number of patients, age, severity of surgery and duration of the extracorporeal circulation.

Patients in both groups were comparable in terms of baseline, risks of surgery, age and duration of the extracorporeal circulation (Table 1).

We revealed significant differences between infectious and non-infectious groups on the SOFA scale and in lactate level on the first day after surgery, on the SOFA scale and WBC—on the 3rd and 7th day after surgery.

Table 1. Patients' baseline characteristics.

Characteristic	Infectious Group	Non-Infectious Group	p
Age	66 (63; 71)	65 (62; 68)	0.378
Ejection Fraction	58 (43; 64)	60 (50; 66)	0.630
EuroScore 2	1.2 (0.7; 1.6)	0.9(0.7; 1.27)	0.318
The total duration of the extracorporeal circulation	90 (83; 107)	85 (66; 138)	0.630
1st day			
WBC (at the end of the 1st day)	17.3 (14.3; 24.8)	14.6 (11.7; 16.3)	0.178
Lactate max, during the 1st day, including EC	7.4 (3.5; 9.4)	4.5 (2.7; 5.9)	0.03
SOFA	6 (5; 9)	5 (2; 6)	0.03
3rd day			
WBC (at the end of the 3rd day)	16.5 (13.3; 22.5)	10.5 (8.7; 13.8)	0.01
SOFA	8 (6; 10)	1 (1; 3)	0.0001
7th day			
WBC (at the end of the 7st day)	11.9 (8.1; 16.3)	7.1 (5.9; 9.7)	0.01
SOFA	3 (1; 6)	0 (0; 0)	0.00001
Length of hospital stay, days	20 (15; 35)	13 (13; 14)	0.001

3.2. The Microbiota Composition

As a first step, we looked for microbiome predictors for the complications. The data obtained by 16S rRNA gene sequencing is known to be compositional [38], which means that ratios between taxa abundances, rather than themselves, should be explored. We used the Aitchison distance to measure the beta-diversity, and the DBA-distal method combined with linear regression analysis to find balances between groups of taxa that differed between subjects with and without complications before the surgery. Analysis of beta-diversity did not show significant difference in microbiome composition between infectious and non-infectious groups (adonis, $p = 0.295$, Figure 2).

The groups differed in individual taxa proportions: the log-ratio of *Staphylococcus* to *Anaerococcus* and *Ruminococcus* to [*Eubacterium*] ($p = 0.038$ for each ratio) and Shannon index were higher in the infectious group (Figure 3) ($p = 0.009$, Welch test).

Beta-diversity analysis shows that for patients without infectious complications, samples (collected in the same time points) were not more similar than samples collected in different time points (adonis, $p = 0.188$). For the subjects with complications, they were more similar ($p = 0.003$). The post hoc pairwise comparison of time points showed that the most significant changes were observed in the period after the surgery (between 3 and 7 days, $p = 0.03125$). Changes (beta-diversity) in case and control groups did not differ significantly. The Shannon index did not change significantly in any of the groups.

Changes in individual taxa proportions are summarized in Table 2. All balances in Table 2 increased with time. An increase in the balance may indicate (1) an increase in the number of bacteria in the numerator, (2) a decrease in the number of bacteria in the denominator, or (3) an increase in the number of bacteria in both the numerator and the denominator, but much more in the numerator.

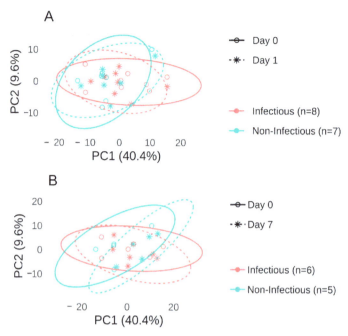

Figure 2. The principal component analysis PCA in ILR-coordinates for comparison of changes between: (**A**) the day before the surgery and the 1st day after it; (**B**) the day before the surgery and the 7th day after it. The principal component analysis was performed using all samples; coordinates on plots A and B are the same.

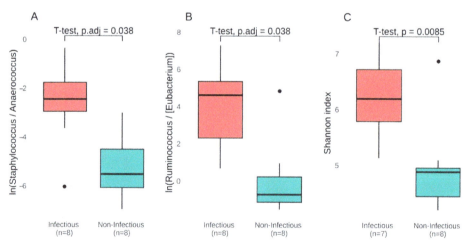

Figure 3. Difference between groups at the baseline. (**A**,**B**) Balances between taxa obtained by discriminative balance analysis and significantly different between groups. (**C**) Shannon index (only samples with total number of reads ≥ 3000 are included).

Table 2. Significant changes in individual taxa proportions after the surgery. The preliminary balances list was obtained by the discriminative balance analysis (DBA). The statistical significance of each balance change was tested by a linear mixed effect model with subject identifier as a random effect. Benjamini-Hochberg method was used to adjust for multiple testing.

		Day 1, Balance (p. adj)	Day 3, Balance (p. adj)	Day 7, Balance (p. adj)
Infectious				
	Day 0	*Prevotella* / *Actinomyces* (0.043)	*Porphyromonas* / *Streptococcus* (0.039) *u_Clostrideacea* / *Blautia* (0.039) *Bacteroides* / *Faecalibacterium* (0.039) *Corynebacterium* / *Peptococcus* (0.039) *Parabacteroides* / *u_Lachnospiraceae* (0.039)	*u_Lachnospiraceae* / [*Eubacterium*] (0.013) *Bacteroides* / *Ruminococcus* (0.013)
	Day 1	-	-	-
	Day 3	-	-	-
Non-Infectious				
	Day 0	-	*u_Lachnospiraceae* / *Faecalibacterium* (0.04) *Dorea* / [*Ruminococcus*] (0.032)	*Clostridium* / *Oscillospira* (0.049) *Bacteroides* / *u_Mogibacteriaceae* (0.049) [*Ruminococcus*] / *Dialister* (0.049)
	Day 1	-	*Lactobacillus* / *u_*[*Mogibacteriaceae*] (0.045) *Finegoldia* / *Peptoniphilus* (0.045) *Porphyromonas* / *Campylobacter* (0.045) *Faecalibacterium* / *Sutterella* (0.009)	*u_Clostridiaceae* / *Oscillospira* (0.029) *Bacteroides* / *u_*[*Mogibacteriaceae*] (0.04) *Collinsella* / *Dialister* (0.029) [*Ruminococcus*] / *Sutterella* (0.018)
	Day 3	-	-	-

We also analyzed association of microbiome composition with biomarkers before the surgery (Figure 4).

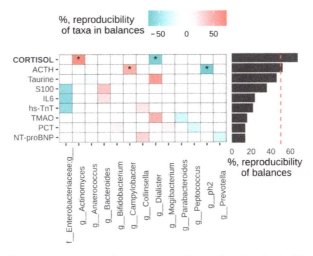

Figure 4. Associations between metabolites in blood and microbiome composition of samples collected day before the surgery. Reproducibility of balances and their components is measured as the proportion of cross-validation iterations in which they were observed. The balances with reproducibility higher than 50% are considered as reproducible; they are signed by *.

Higher cortisol values were associated with increased log-ratio of *Actinomyces* to *Dialister*, higher ACTH—with higher *Campylobacter* to *ph2* log-ratio (genus from family [*Tissierellaceae*]). Significant associations between Aitchison distance and blood parameters were found for cortisol and TMAO ($p = 0.044$ for each of them).

3.3. Biomarkers

The study carried out a comparative assessment of the level of some laboratory markers between groups of patients with infectious complications and without infectious complications (Table A1).

3.3.1. Pro-BNP, HS-Troponin T Levels

Cardiac function was assessed by measuring NT-proBNP and hs-TnT. ProBNP and hs-TnT levels were higher in the group of patients with infectious complications compared to the group without infectious complications, but statistically significant differences between the two groups were found only for proBNP ($p = 0.024$). The pro-BNP level reached its maximum values three days after surgery in both groups (Figure 5a,b).

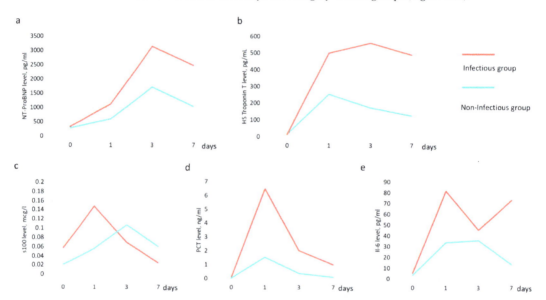

Figure 5. Dynamics of biomarker levels in patients' groups: (**a**)—NT-ProBNP, (**b**)—high-sensetive Troponin T, (**c**)—protein S100, (**d**)-procalcitonin (PCT) and (**e**)—interleukin-6 (IL6).

3.3.2. S100 Level

The degree of involvement in the pathological process of the central nervous system was assessed by the level of S100 in plasma. The maximum values were found on day 1 after surgery and amounted to 0.149 µg/L, with a gradual decrease in the following days (Figure 5c). The S100 level was higher in the infectious group. Clinical neurological features were observed in only four patients and were manifested by short-term delirium. There were no other signs of CNS damage. No association was found between delirium and change in S100 level.

3.3.3. Interleukin—6 (IL), Procalcitonin (PCT) Level

As part of the assessment of the level of inflammation, PCT and IL-6 were investigated. In the group of patients with infectious complications, PCT levels were statistically significantly higher than in patients without infection (Figure 5d). The maximum values were observed on day one after surgery and reached 6.5 ng/mL and 1.54 ng/mL, with a further decrease to 1 ng/mL and 0.09 ng/mL in the infectious and non-infectious groups, respectively. IL-6 levels were also higher in the infectious group, but with no statistical difference (Figure 5e). The IL-6 level in both groups before surgery did not exceed the reference values (no more than 7 pg/mL). The IL-6 level in the non-infectious group did not exceed 35 pg/mL and decreased to 13 pg/mL by the seventh day after surgery. The level of IL-6 in the infectious group remained high, especially on the first and seventh days after surgery, 81.8 pg/mL and 73.4 pg/mL, respectively.

3.3.4. Adrenocorticotropic Hormone (ACTH), Cortisol Level

Stress levels were studied by assessing Cortisol and ACTH levels. Values of Cortisol exceeding the norm were found only in the group of patients with infectious complications on the first day after surgery and amounted to 806.1 nmol/L. They were statistically significantly different from the group of patients with non-infectious complication, median value 197.3 nmol/L at the first day after surgery (Figure 6).

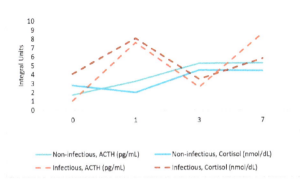

Figure 6. Association between ACTH and cortisol levels in dynamics in patients' groups.

ACTH levels were within the normal range in both groups. In the group with infectious complications, the median values were lower than in the group with non-infectious complications.

3.3.5. Taurine, TMAO Level

The level of intestinal metabolic activity was studied by assessing the levels of Taurine and TMAO. The TMAO values were lower in the infectious group compared with the non-infectious group (Appendix A. Table A1). The level of TMAO in the infectious group decreased on the first and seventh days and reached a maximum on the third day. The TMAO level in the non-infectious group tended to decrease by day three and slightly increase by day seven (Figure 7). This dynamic is similar to the change in the level of Proteobacteria.

We found a positive correlation between Proteobacteria and TMAO in the non-infectious group ($r = -0.38$, $p < 0.05$), and a negative correlation between Firmicutes and Proteobacteria in the infectious group ($r = -0.46$, $p < 0.05$). Taurine levels were not statistically significant between two groups; however, the level of taurine in the group of patients with infectious complications was higher compared to the non-infectious group.

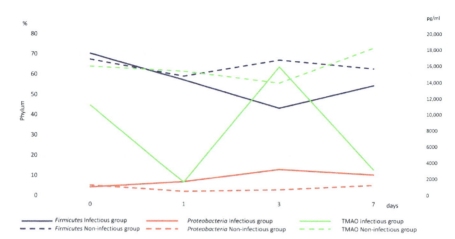

Figure 7. Association between metabolic activity of the gut microbiota by TMAO level (green line) and Phyla (*Firmicutes*—dark blue line, *Proteobacteria*—red line). The group of infectious complications is shown by a solid line, and the group of non-infectious complications is shown by a dotted line.

3.4. Clinical Cases with Microbiological Confirmation of Infection

The dynamics of the gut microbiota composition in groups of patients is shown in Figure 8 and Appendix A. Figure A1. In five patients from the infectious group, microbiological confirmation was obtained with the identification of the pathogen. All these patients needed prolonged treatment with several classes of antibiotics and its correction, based on the obtained microbiological data.

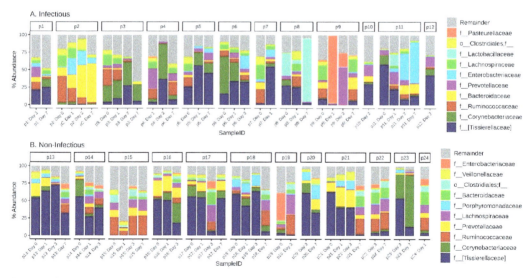

Figure 8. The top 10 families of the gut microbiota composition in both (**A**) infectious and (**B**) non-infectious groups of patients with temporal dynamics.

Patient 4 was admitted after CABG—early postoperative period without complications and with early extubation. He was discharged from the ICU on the second day. However, from the sixth day, leukocytosis, inflammation of the surgical wound (osteomyelitis) with the growth of Enterobacter cloacae, was revealed. In this patient, noticeable overgrowth of Corynebacteriaceae (52%) and [Tissierellaceae] (36.7%) was detected at d3. Anaerobic Gram-negative microorganisms predominated on day seven, belonging to the genera Succinivibrio and Prevotella (11.5 and 11.3, respectively), most of which are pathogenic species. The patient received successful antibiotic therapy and was then discharged home.

Patient 6 was admitted after CABG, extubated in the early hours. Acute postoperative myocardial infarction was developed on the second day. The patient was intubated due to pulmonary edema and unstable hemodynamics. From the third day, signs of lung infection appeared: low P/F, Xray picture, leukocytosis, increased PCT, with the growth of *Staphylococcus aureus*, *Serratia marcescens* and *Candida albicans* in BAL. In this patient, the relative abundance of *Corynebacteriaceae* was 53% at d0 decreasing to 3% by day 3, while at d3 the prevalence of [*Tissierellaceae*] (34%) and *Enterobacteriaceae* (19%) were detected. Clinical improvement was observed after resolution of heart failure and initiation of antibiotic therapy.

Patient 8 was admitted after CABG on pump and suffered an intraoperative myocardial infarction and cardiogenic shock. The multiple organs failure progressed on the second day. Clinical signs of systemic infection were detected as confirmed by positive blood culture on day three with *Enterococcus faecalis*. The gut features are characterized by a relatively high abundance of *Lactobacillaceae* (25%) at d0 up to 90% to d7. The patient received massive antibiotic therapy and was transferred from the ICU in 12 days after stabilization. Length of hospital stay was 21 days.

Patient 9 was admitted after mitral valve replacement. Signs of organ failure were observed on the second day, which required prolonged mechanical ventilation. A picture of exacerbation of COPD, acute purulent bronchitis with the growth of *Haemophilus parainfluenzae biotype I*, *Paenibacillus lactis* and *Streptococcus salivarius* in BAL at d3. This patient, before and after surgery (d7), was prevalently closer to core of gut microbiota genera, such as *Lachnospiraceae*, *Ruminococcaceae*, *Bifidobacteriaceae*, *Bacteroidaceae*. At the same time, on the first day after the surgery, the number of *Pasteurellaceae* (including the genus *Haemophilus*) in the gut was 96%. The relative abundance of this family decreased to 19.5% in d3, with an increase of *Prevotellaceae* (54%) and *Staphylococcaceae* (23%). On the third day, antibacterial therapy was prescribed. Within seven days, the patient's condition stabilized, after which he was discharged from the ICU.

Patient 11 also had nosocomial pneumonia with the growth of Pseudomonas aeruginosa in BAL at d6. The patient was admitted after CABG + aortic valve replacement. On the second day, multiple organ failure (kidneys, lungs, brain) was observed due to postoperative heart failure. Lung infection joined at 4–5 days. In this patient, noticeable overgrowth of [Tissierellaceae] (58%) and Corynebacteriaceae (14%) was detected at d0. The relative abundance of [Tissierellaceae] decreased, 22%, 12% and 8% at d1, d3, d7, respectively, with simultaneous growth of Enterobacteriaceae at d3 - 60% and 38% at d7. The patient spent 21 days in the ICU. His condition stabilized, then he was discharged from the hospital after 16 days.

4. Discussion

The high percentage of postoperative infectious complications in cardiac surgery poses a problem for the search for new markers that allow to identify high-risk patients. One of these markers may be the gut microbiota. In this prospective observational pilot study, we observed that, despite the large interindividual variability of the microbial composition, in patients with infectious complications, it characterized patterns with the relative predominance of potentially pathogenic species.

One of the main findings of our study was that markers of infectious complications can be found in the proportions of individual taxa of the gut microbiota prior to surgery, in particular, by the log-ratio of the *Staphylococcus* to *Anaerococcus* and *Ruminococcus* to [*Eubacterium*]. Among them, *Staphylococcus* is the genus of facultative anaerobic bacteria which frequently colonizes the nares and skin in the healthy population, but in preoperative cardiac patients, carriage is associated with an elevated risk for post-operative surgical site infection and bacteremia [39,40]. *Anaerococcus* have the potential to metabolize peptones and amino acids and to produce short-chain fatty acids (SCFAs), such as butyric acid, but can be associated with skin and soft tissue infections and chronic wounds [41]. *Ruminococcus* and [*Eubacterium*] are usually the part of the resident microflora and also produce SCFAs; in some case, they may be players in the development of inflammation and bloodstream infection [42,43]. The balance on 1st day in infectious group is *Prevotella/Actinomyces*. Several members of [*Eubacterium*], *Actinomyces*, *Prevotella*, are anaerobic flora of the oral cavity and are the cause of infections, including purulent bacterial pericarditis [44]. Moreover, coaggregation was found between *Prevotella intermedia* strains and individual *Actinomyces* species via a protein or glycoprotein on the *Prevotella* strain, which can interact with carbohydrates or carbohydrate-containing molecules on the surface of the *Actinomyces* strain [45]. The predominance of representatives of the oral microbiota as part of the gut microbiota in the infectious group is highlighted by additional studies documenting the effect of patient participation in reducing the risk of postoperative infection by adhering to preoperative oral hygiene regimens [46].

The Shannon Index was low in all patients, which was consistent with previously obtained data on its level, correlating with the heart failure class [47]. Nevertheless, before the surgery, the Shannon Index was higher in the group of infectious complications, but after the surgery this value decreased. While in patients without infectious complications, it increased. This phenomenon can be explained by an increase in the proportion of taxa from the *Proteobacteria* phylum in the patients with infection (Appendix A. Figure A2).

A review of studies showed that changes in taxonomic composition in the infectious group are consistent with earlier studies, where *Streptococcus*, *Blautia*, *Peptococcus*, *Porphyromonas* were associated with infective endocarditis, coronary heart disease, inflammation, sepsis, complications after stroke (Supplementary Table S1).

Assessing the metabolic activity of the microbiota, we compared of the results the study of taurine with the composition of the microbiota of patients using the 16S-sequencing method. This suggests that higher values of taurine in the infectious group may be associated with dysbiotic disorders, towards an increase in species metabolizing taurine, such as *Clostradiales* [48]. It is known that taurine decomposes to hydrogen sulphide under the influence of the intestinal microbiota. High concentrations of hydrogen sulfide can suppress the activity of cytochrome oxidases [49] and, consequently, aerobic respiration, one of the common factors of virulence of microorganisms [50]. Thus, taurine can be not only a nutrient for microbes; it can also stimulate the antimicrobial defense of the body [51] and have positive effects in cardiovascular diseases [52–54].

We found lower serum TMAO levels in patients with infectious complications compared to the group of patients without infectious complications. Serum TMAO levels are genetically determined and also depend on diet [55] and the composition of the intestinal microbiota [56]. Recent studies have reported that several families of bacteria belonging to the type *Firmicutes* and *Proteobacteria* are potential producers of TMA [57,58]. We compared the dynamics of changes in TMAO levels with the levels of *Proteobacteria* and Firmicutes in patients in both groups, using the ratio of *Proteobacteria* and *Firmicutes*. We found that increasing the ratio of *Proteobacteria* and *Firmicutes* associated with elevated levels of TMAO (Figure 7). Previous data indicate that this ratio was a predictor of adverse outcomes in cardiovascular disease [59].

At the same time, biomarker identification to personalize therapy in clinics is more common than microbiota research. Among them, markers of infectious, neurological and cardiac complications are distinguished. Inflammatory biomarkers IL6, PCT, cortisol, ACTH are not always specific for assessing the severity of the infectious process in cardiac surgery patients. Cardiac surgery causes an increase in the PCT level even in the absence of complications, and its level usually does not exceed 5 ng/mL [60,61]. At the same time, in the infectious group, the average value of serum PCT on the first day after surgery was 6.5 ng/mL, which is one of the reliable laboratory criteria for predicting the presence of a bacterial infection. IL-6 levels were also higher in the infectious group, but not statistical different. IL-6 is rarely used in the clinical practice of cardiac surgery due to its lower specificity than PCT [62]. ACTH levels were within the normal range in both groups. There is a direct relationship between an increase in cortisol levels and an increase in ACTH levels, which indicates a central regulation of the level of inflammation despite the administration of exogenous glucocorticosteroids (dexamethasone 80 mg) in high doses before surgery (Figure 6). Only four patients in this case had cortisol values below 149 nmol/L, which may be a sign of adrenal insufficiency, but all four either had no complications after surgery or had minimal complications that did not lengthen the number of days of treatment. Remarkably, among biomarkers and individual taxa, only for high cortisol values and ACTH were found significant association, with increased log-ratio of *Actinomyces* to *Dialister* and with high *Campylobacter* to *ph2* log-ratio (genus from family [*Tissierellaceae*]), respectively.

Endogenous intoxication due to infection can worsen the function of the heart, which can manifest itself both clinically and in a laboratory. In our study, we found higher NT-proBNP values in patients with infectious complications. (Figure 5) NT-proBNP is used in the diagnosis of heart failure. Its values always increase during the first few days after open heart surgery with a further gradual decrease if there are no complications. Typically, NT-proBNP values are higher in more severe patients receiving inotropic therapy. Another promising biomarker to evaluate postoperative complication is high-sensitive Troponin T levels, the release of which should be expected after all CABG procedures. It depends on the procedure, the nature of the cardioplegia and many other factors. According to the Fourth Universal Definition of Myocardial Infarction, CABG-related MI is arbitrarily defined as elevation of troponin values more 10 times the 99th percentile upper-reference limit in patients with normal baseline troponin values in combination with other objective signs of myocardial ischemia [63]. The peak hs-TnT usually occurs within 24 to 48 h after operation [64]. In this study, the level of troponin in the group of infectious complications was significantly higher than in the group of patients without infections. This can be explained by the fact that infectious complications developed more in those patients who had primary cardiac complications in the intraoperative or early postoperative period: myocardial infarction, myocardial injury, severe heart failure. Patients with primary cardiac complications have a greater risk of bacterial infection [65]. However, our findings correlate with data from the study that includes 1318 patients after CABG surgery, with a peak high-sensitivity troponin T level, greater than 400 ng/L measured within 24 h associated with a major adverse cardiac or cerebrovascular event, 30-day mortality, myocardial infection and ICU stay >48 h [66]. Prospectively designed trials may provide further insight into the prognostic value of high-sensitivity troponin T after cardiac surgery.

The S100 as an early marker for damage to the blood–brain barrier and neurons [67] could be used for a risk stratification of cardiac surgical patients for cognitive dysfunction [68] and postoperative delirium [69]. We did not reveal an association between delirium and S100 serum level; at the same time, this marker was higher in the infectious group on the first day after surgery followed by a decline. Studies have shown that the level of serum S100 protein in bacterial infection is significantly higher than that in viral infection [70,71], so it can also be used in combination with other markers to predict infectious complications.

This study has several limitations: a relatively small sample size, due to the impossibility of obtaining stool samples; the widespread use of antibiotics in different combinations in patients with infectious complications and intraoperative complications, which could significantly affect the composition of the microbiota and biomarker levels; and the inclusion multiple valve operations per study group. To exclude bias due to the inclusion of valvular surgeries, we additionally conducted a comparative analysis of patients with valvular surgeries and CABG with each other. Patient groups were similar in all parameters, except for antibiotic prophylaxis and blood loss, but the volume of blood loss during CABG was greater than during valvular procedures (1400 mL vs. 950 mL, respectively, $p = 0.04$). For this reason, the addition of valve surgery in this case is not a significant factor influencing the outcome and the possibility to develop infection, despite the fact that some valve operations are more difficult and time consuming. However, despite these limitations, our project makes it possible to assess the contribution of the taxonomic composition of the microbiota before and in the first days after surgery in dynamics.

5. Conclusions

The adaptation of treatment to the individual characteristics of each patient is the goal of personalized medicine. Clinical signs are faster but are nonspecific tools for this. Specific biomarkers are rapid and make it possible to identify groups of patients compromised with various types of complications. The gut microbiota is a major contributor to the pathophysiological process and may be a potential early biomarker. Predictably, patients with cardiovascular diseases have pronounced imbalances in the taxonomic composition of their gut microbiota. However, even before surgery, markers of subsequent infectious complications can be identified.

Further research is needed to confirm the role of the gut microbiota in the pathogenesis of development of infectious complications in surgical patients. Potentially, microbiota-targeted therapies could significantly improve the effectiveness of cardiac surgery.

Supplementary Materials: The following are available online at https://www.mdpi.com/article/10 .3390/jpm11111113/s1, Table S1. The clinical significance of the found taxa. Data review.

Author Contributions: E.C. and N.B. designed the study. E.Z. worked with patients. E.C., E.Z., A.M. and V.O. performed the data analysis, contributed to the interpretation, E.C., E.Z., V.O., A.M. and N.B. wrote the manuscript. All authors have read and agreed to the published version of the manuscript.

Funding: This research received no external funding.

Institutional Review Board Statement: The study was conducted according to the guidelines of the Declaration of Helsinki, and approved by the local Ethics Committee of N. Pirogov National Medical Surgical Center, Moscow, Russian Federation (no. 04 22.05.2018).

Informed Consent Statement: Informed consent was obtained from all subjects involved in the study.

Data Availability Statement: Raw microbiome data are available in the Sequence Read Archive (SRA) by the accession number PRJNA762260.

Acknowledgments: The authors thank all of the study participants and the clinical and research staff from N. Pirogov National Medical Surgical Center for their contributions to this study.

Conflicts of Interest: The authors declare no conflict of interest.

Appendix A

Table A1. Levels of biomarkers in groups of patients with infectious complications and without infectious complications. Data are presented as median and interquartile range (IQR).

Biomarkers	Patients (Median [IQR 25–75%])				
	Infectious Group		Non-Infectious Group		p-Level
ACTH, pg/mL	2.59	(1.26–8.7)	3.47	(1.4–7.3)	1
* Cortisol, nmol/L	473.2	(344.1–805.5)	384.25	(209.8–482.6)	0.037
IL-6, pg/mL	41.84	(7.7–83.03)	19.57	(7.04–37.7)	0.127
* PCT, ng/mL	0.924	(0.27–5.76)	0.183	(0.025–0.65)	0.002
* pro-BNP, pg/mL	1679	(674.25–4315.5)	908	(462.5–1378)	0.024
Troponin T-HS, pg/mL	279.4	(18.87–628.5)	126.9	(19.69–253)	0.369
S100, µg/L	0.084	(0.036–0.1375)	0.053	(0.031–0.136)	0.657
TMAO, pg/mL	9764	(1675–19,300)	15,848	(11,127–19,844)	0.052
Taurine, pg/mL	694	(379–769)	455	(325–720)	0.101

* Statistically significant differences.

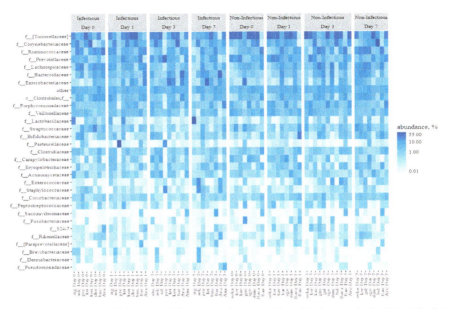

Figure A1. Heatmap of the temporal dynamics of the taxonomic composition of the intestinal microbiota in both infectious and non-infectious patient groups.

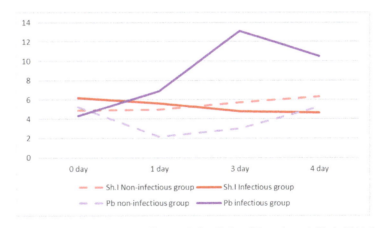

Figure A2. Association between Shannon Index (Sh.I) and Proteobacteria Phyla (Pb) in both Infectious and Non-infectious groups of patients with temporal dynamics. Decrease in Proteobacteria by 1 day in patients in the non-infectious group, most likely with surgical antimicrobial prophylaxis.

References

1. Vesteinsdottir, E.; Helgason, K.O.; Sverrisson, K.O.; Gudlaugsson, O.; Karason, S. Infections and outcomes after cardiac surgery-The impact of outbreaks traced to transesophageal echocardiography probes. *Acta Anaesthesiol. Scand.* **2019**, *63*, 871–878. [CrossRef] [PubMed]
2. Gelijns, A.C.; Moskowitz, A.J.; Acker, M.A.; Argenziano, M.; Geller, N.L.; Puskas, J.D.; Perrault, L.P.; Smith, P.K.; Kron, I.L.; Michler, R.E.; et al. Management practices and major infections after cardiac surgery. *J. Am. Coll. Cardiol.* **2014**, *64*, 372–381. [CrossRef]
3. Hamouda, K.; Oezkur, M.; Sinha, B.; Hain, J.; Menkel, H.; Leistner, M.; Leyh, R.; Schimmer, C. Different duration strategies of perioperative antibiotic prophylaxis in adult patients undergoing cardiac surgery: An observational study. *J. Cardiothorac. Surg.* **2015**, *10*, 25. [CrossRef] [PubMed]

4. Dixon, L.K.; Di Tommaso, E.; Dimagli, A.; Sinha, S.; Sandhu, M.; Benedetto, U.; Angelini, G.D. Impact of sex on outcomes after cardiac surgery: A systematic review and meta-analysis. *Int. J. Cardiol.* **2021**, *15*, 27–34. [CrossRef]
5. O'Keefe, S.; Williams, K.; Legare, J.-F. Hospital-Acquired Infections after Cardiac Surgery and Current Physician Practices: A Retrospective Cohort Study. *J. Clin. Med. Res.* **2017**, *9*, 10–16. [CrossRef] [PubMed]
6. Li, Q.; Gao, B.; Siqin, B.; He, Q.; Zhang, R.; Meng, X.; Naiheng, Z.; Zhang, N.; Li, M. Gut Microbiota: A Novel Regulator of Cardiovascular Disease and Key Factor in the Therapeutic Effects of Flavonoids. *Front. Pharmacol.* **2021**, *12*, 651926. [CrossRef] [PubMed]
7. Tang, W.H.W.; Kitai, T.; Hazen, S.L. Gut Microbiota in Cardiovascular Health and Disease. *Circ. Res.* **2017**, *120*, 1183–1196. [CrossRef]
8. Piccioni, A.; Saviano, A.; Cicchinelli, S.; Franza, L.; Rosa, F.; Zanza, C.; Rosa, F.; Zanza, C.; Santoro, M.C.; Candelli, M.; et al. Microbiota and Myopericarditis: The New Frontier in the Car-Diological Field to Prevent or Treat Inflammatory Cardiomyo-Pathies in COVID-19 Outbreak. *Biomedicines* **2021**, *9*, 1234. [CrossRef]
9. Yamashita, T.; Emoto, T.; Sasaki, N.; Hirata, K.-I. Gut Microbiota and Coronary Artery Disease. *Int. Heart J.* **2016**, *57*, 663–671. [CrossRef]
10. Xu, H.; Wang, X.; Feng, W.; Liu, Q.; Zhou, S.; Liu, Q.; Cai, L. The gut microbiota and its interactions with cardiovascular disease. *Microb. Biotechnol.* **2020**, *13*, 637–656. [CrossRef]
11. Suslov, A.V.; Chairkina, E.; Shepetovskaya, M.D.; Suslova, I.S.; Khotina, V.A.; Kirichenko, T.V.; Postnov, A.Y. The neuroimmune role of intestinal Microbiota in the pathogenesis of cardiovascular disease. *J. Clin. Med. Res.* **2021**, *10*, 1995.
12. Chen, X.; Li, H.-Y.; Hu, X.-M.; Zhang, Y.; Zhang, S.-Y. Current understanding of gut microbiota alterations and related therapeutic intervention strategies in heart failure. *Chin. Med. J.* **2019**, *132*, 1843–1855. [CrossRef]
13. Jia, Q.; Li, H.; Zhou, H.; Zhang, X.; Zhang, A.; Xie, Y.; Li, Y.; Lv, S.; Zhang, J. Role and Effective Therapeutic Target of Gut Microbiota in Heart Failure. *Cardiovasc. Ther.* **2019**, *2019*, 5164298. [CrossRef] [PubMed]
14. Piccioni, A.; de Cunzo, T.; Valletta, F.; Covino, M.; Rinninella, E.; Raoul, P.; Zanza, C.; Mele, M.C.; Franceschi, F. Gut Microbiota and Environment in Coronary Artery Disease. *Int. J. Environ. Res. Public Health* **2021**, *18*, 4242. [CrossRef]
15. Aardema, H.; Lisotto, P.; Kurilshikov, A.; Diepeveen, J.R.J.; Friedrich, A.W.; Sinha, B.; de Smet, A.M.G.A.; Harmsen, H.J.M. Marked Changes in Gut Microbiota in Cardio-Surgical Intensive Care Patients: A Longitudinal Cohort Study. *Front. Cell Infect. Microbiol.* **2019**, *9*, 467. [CrossRef]
16. Iapichino, G.; Callegari, M.L.; Marzorati, S.; Cigada, M.; Corbella, D.; Ferrari, S.; Morelli, M. Impact of antibiotics on the gut microbiota of critically ill patients. *J. Med. Microbiol.* **2008**, *57*, 1007–1014. [CrossRef]
17. McDonald, D.; Ackermann, G.; Khailova, L.; Baird, C.; Heyland, D.; Kozar, R.; Lemieux, M.; Derenski, K.; King, J.; Vis-Kampen, C.; et al. Extreme Dysbiosis of the Microbiome in Critical Illness. *Msphere* **2016**, *1*. [CrossRef]
18. Ojima, M.; Motooka, D.; Shimizu, K.; Gotoh, K.; Shintani, A.; Yoshiya, K.; Nakamura, S.; Ogura, H.; Iida, D.; Shimazu, T. Metagenomic Analysis Reveals Dynamic Changes of Whole Gut Microbiota in the Acute Phase of Intensive Care Unit Patients. *Dig. Dis. Sci.* **2016**, *61*, 1628–1634. [CrossRef] [PubMed]
19. Chernevskaya, E.; Beloborodova, N.; Klimenko, N.; Pautova, A.; Shilkin, D.; Gusarov, V.; Tyakht, A. Serum and fecal profiles of aromatic microbial metabolites reflect gut microbiota disruption in critically ill patients: A prospective observational pilot study. *Crit. Care* **2020**, *24*, 312. [CrossRef]
20. Sekirov, I.; Russell, S.L.; Antunes, L.C.M.; Finlay, B.B. Gut microbiota in health and disease. *Physiol. Rev.* **2010**, *90*, 859–904. [CrossRef]
21. Chernevskaya, E.; Klimenko, N.; Pautova, A.; Buyakova, I.; Tyakht, A.; Beloborodova, N. Host-Microbiome Interactions Mediated by Phenolic Metabolites in Chronically Critically Ill Patients. *Metabolites* **2021**, *11*, 122. [CrossRef]
22. Piccioni, A.; Valletta, F.; Zanza, C.; Esperide, A.; Franceschi, F. Novel biomarkers to assess the risk for acute coronary syndrome: Beyond troponins. *Intern. Emerg. Med.* **2020**, *15*, 1193–1199. [CrossRef] [PubMed]
23. Klimenko, N.; Tyakht, A.; Popenko, A.; Vasiliev, A.; Altukhov, I.; Ischenko, D.; Shashkova, T.I.; Efimova, D.A.; Nikogosov, D.A.; Osipenko, D.A.; et al. Microbiome Responses to an Uncontrolled Short-Term Diet Intervention in the Frame of the Citizen Science Project. *Nutrients* **2018**, *10*, 576. [CrossRef]
24. Efimova, D.; Tyakht, A.; Popenko, A.; Vasilyev, A.; Altukhov, I.; Dovidchenko, N.; Odintsova, V.; Klimenko, N.; Loshkarev, R.; Pashkova, M.; et al. Knomics-Biota—A system for exploratory analysis of human gut microbiota data. *BioData Min.* **2018**, *11*, 25. [CrossRef] [PubMed]
25. Callahan, B.J.; McMurdie, P.J.; Rosen, M.J.; Han, A.W.; Johnson, A.J.A.; Holmes, S.P. DADA2: High-resolution sample inference from Illumina amplicon data. *Nat. Methods* **2016**, *13*, 581–583. [CrossRef]
26. DeSantis, T.Z.; Hugenholtz, P.; Larsen, N.; Rojas, M.; Brodie, E.L.; Keller, K.; Huber, T.; Dalevi, D.; Hu, P.; Andersen, G.L. Greengenes, a chimera-checked 16S rRNA gene database and workbench compatible with ARB. *Appl. Environ. Microbiol.* **2006**, *72*, 5069–5072. [CrossRef] [PubMed]
27. Andrianova, N.V.; Popkov, V.A.; Klimenko, N.S.; Tyakht, A.V.; Baydakova, G.V.; Frolova, O.Y.; Zorova, L.D.; Pevzner, I.P.; Zorov, D.B.; Plotnikov, E.Y. Microbiome-Metabolome Signature of Acute Kidney Injury. *Metabolites* **2020**, *10*, 142. [CrossRef]
28. Brandt, B.W.; Bonder, M.J.; Huse, S.M.; Zaura, E. TaxMan: A server to trim rRNA reference databases and inspect taxonomic coverage. *Nucleic Acids Res.* **2012**, *40*, W82–W87. [CrossRef]

29. Fu, L.; Niu, B.; Zhu, Z.; Wu, S.; Li, W. CD-HIT: Accelerated for clustering the next-generation sequencing data. *Bioinformatics* **2012**, *28*, 3150–3152. [CrossRef]
30. Shen, S.-M. *The Statistical Analysis of Compositional Data*; Open Dissertation Press: Pokfulam, Kong Kong, 2017.
31. Aitchison, J. The Statistical Analysis of Compositional Data. *J. R. Stat. Soc.* **1986**, *44*, 139–177. [CrossRef]
32. R Core Team. *R: A Language and Environment for Statistical Computing*; R Foundation for Statistical Computing: Vienna, Austria, 2020.
33. Quinn, T.P.; Erb, I. Interpretable Log Contrasts for the Classification of Health Biomarkers: A New Approach to Balance Selection. *Msystems* **2020**, *5*. [CrossRef]
34. Palarea-Albaladejo, J.; Martín-Fernández, J.A. zCompositions—R package for multivariate imputation of left-censored data under a compositional approach. *Chemom. Intell. Lab. Systems.* **2015**, *143*, 85–96. [CrossRef]
35. Dixon, P. VEGAN, a package of R functions for community ecology. *J. Veg. Sci.* **2003**, 927–930. [CrossRef]
36. Kuznetsova, A.; Brockhoff, P.B.; Christensen, R.H.B. lmerTest Package: Tests in Linear Mixed Effects Models. *J. Stat. Softw.* **2017**, *82*. [CrossRef]
37. Rivera-Pinto, J.; Egozcue, J.J.; Pawlowsky-Glahn, V.; Paredes, R.; Noguera-Julian, M.; Calle, M.L. Balances: A New Perspective for Microbiome Analysis. *Msystems* **2018**, *3*. [CrossRef] [PubMed]
38. Gloor, G.B.; Macklaim, J.M.; Pawlowsky-Glahn, V.; Egozcue, J.J. Microbiome Datasets Are Compositional: And This Is Not Optional. *Front. Microbiol.* **2017**, *8*, 2224. [CrossRef] [PubMed]
39. Kanafani, Z.A.; Arduino, J.M.; Muhlbaier, L.H.; Kaye, K.S.; Allen, K.B.; Carmeli, Y.; Corey, G.R.; Cosgrove, S.E.; Fraser, T.G.; Harris, A.D.; et al. Incidence of and preoperative risk factors for Staphylococcus aureus bacteremia and chest wound infection after cardiac surgery. *Infect. Control. Hosp. Epidemiol.* **2009**, *30*, 242–248. [CrossRef]
40. Paling, F.P.; Olsen, K.; Ohneberg, K.; Wolkewitz, M.; Fowler, V.G., Jr.; DiNubile, M.J.; Jafri, H.S.; Sifakis, F.; Bonten, M.J.M.; Harbarth, S.J.; et al. Risk prediction for Staphylococcus aureus surgical site infection following cardiothoracic surgery; A secondary analysis of the V710-P003 trial. *PLoS ONE* **2018**, *13*, e0193445. [CrossRef] [PubMed]
41. Dunyach-Remy, C.; Salipante, F.; Lavigne, J.-P.; Brunaud, M.; Demattei, C.; Yahiaoui-Martinez, A.; Bastide, S.; Palayer, C.; Sotto, A.; Gélis, A. Pressure ulcers microbiota dynamics and wound evolution. *Sci. Rep.* **2021**, *11*, 18506. [CrossRef]
42. Fan, X.; Chen, Y.; Liu, Y.; Hu, L. First Case of Bloodstream Infection Caused by Ruminococcus gnavus in an 85 Year Old Man in China. *Lab. Med.* **2021**, e0–e4. [CrossRef]
43. Yamakawa, H.; Hagiwara, E.; Hayashi, M.; Katano, T.; Isomoto, K.; Otoshi, R.; Shintani, R.; Ikeda, S.; Tanaka, K.; Ogura, T. A case of relapsed lung abscess caused by infection following an initial diagnosis of pulmonary actinomycosis. *Respir. Med. Case Rep.* **2017**, *22*, 171–174. [CrossRef]
44. Kanwal, A.; Avgeropoulos, D.; Kaplan, J.G.; Saini, A. Idiopathic Purulent Pericarditis: A Rare Diagnosis. *Am. J. Case Rep.* **2020**, *21*, e921633. [CrossRef]
45. Nesbitt, W.E.; Fukushima, H.; Leung, K.P.; Clark, W.B. Coaggregation of Prevotella intermedia with oral Actinomyces species. *Infect. Immun.* **1993**, *61*, 2011–2014. [CrossRef] [PubMed]
46. Pedersen, P.U.; Tracey, A.; Sindby, J.E.; Bjerrum, M. Preoperative oral hygiene recommendation before open-heart surgery: Patients' adherence and reduction of infections: A quality improvement study. *BMJ Open Qual.* **2019**, *8*, e000512. [CrossRef]
47. Yuzefpolskaya, M.; Bohn, B.; Nasiri, M.; Zuver, A.M.; Onat, D.D.; Royzman, E.A.; Nwokocha, J.; Mabasa, M.; Pinsino, A.; Brunjes, D.; et al. Gut microbiota, endotoxemia, inflammation, and oxidative stress in patients with heart failure, left ventricular assist device, and transplant. *J. Heart Lung Transplant.* **2020**, *39*, 880–890. [CrossRef] [PubMed]
48. Stacy, A.; Andrade-Oliveira, V.; McCulloch, J.A.; Hild, B.; Oh, J.H.; Perez-Chaparro, P.J.; Sim, C.K.; Lim, A.I.; Link, V.M.; Enamorado, M.; et al. Infection trains the host for microbiota-enhanced resistance to pathogens. *Cell* **2021**, *184*, 615–627. [CrossRef]
49. Forte, E.; Borisov, V.B.; Falabella, M.; Colaço, H.G.; Tinajero-Trejo, M.; Poole, R.K.; Vicente, J.B.; Sarti, P.; Giuffrèet, A. The Terminal Oxidase Cytochrome bd Promotes Sulfide-resistant Bacterial Respiration and Growth. *Sci. Rep.* **2016**, *6*, 23788. [CrossRef] [PubMed]
50. Neumann-Schaal, M.; Jahn, D.; Schmidt-Hohagen, K. Metabolism the Difficile Way: The Key to the Success of the Pathogen. *Front. Microbiol.* **2019**, *10*, 219. [CrossRef]
51. Levy, M.; Thaiss, C.A.; Zeevi, D.; Dohnalová, L.; Zilberman-Schapira, G.; Mahdi, J.A.; David, E.; Savidor, A.; Korem, T.; Herzig, Y.; et al. Microbiota-Modulated Metabolites Shape the Intestinal Microenvironment by Regulating NLRP6 Inflammasome Signaling. *Cell* **2015**, *163*, 1428–1443. [CrossRef] [PubMed]
52. Xu, S.; Ilyas, I.; Little, P.J.; Li, H.; Kamato, D.; Zheng, X.; Luo, S.; Li, Z.; Liu, P.; Han, J.; et al. Endothelial Dysfunction in Atherosclerotic Cardiovascular Diseases and Beyond: From Mechanism to Pharmacotherapies. *Pharmacol. Rev.* **2021**, *73*, 924–967. [CrossRef] [PubMed]
53. Abebe, W.; Mozaffari, M.S. Role of taurine in the vasculature: An overview of experimental and human studies. *Am. J. Cardiovasc. Dis.* **2011**, *1*, 293–311.
54. Bkaily, G.; Jazzar, A.; Normand, A.; Simon, Y.; Al-Khoury, J.; Jacques, D. Taurine and cardiac disease: State of the art and perspectives. *Can. J. Physiol. Pharmacol.* **2020**, *98*, 67–73. [CrossRef] [PubMed]
55. Manor, O.; Zubair, N.; Conomos, M.P.; Xu, X.; Rohwer, J.E.; Krafft, C.E.; Lovejoy, J.C.; Magis, A.T. A Multi-omic Association Study of Trimethylamine N-Oxide. *Cell Rep.* **2018**, *24*, 935–946. [CrossRef]

56. Cho, C.E.; Taesuwan, S.; Malysheva, O.V.; Bender, E.; Tulchinsky, N.F.; Yan, J.; Sutter, J.L.; Caudill, M.A. Trimethylamine-N-oxide (TMAO) response to animal source foods varies among healthy young men and is influenced by their gut microbiota composition: A randomized controlled trial. *Mol. Nutr. Food Res.* **2017**, *61*. [CrossRef]
57. Romano, K.A.; Vivas, E.; Amador-Noguez, D.; Rey, F.E. Intestinal Microbiota Composition Modulates Choline Bioavailability from Diet and Accumulation of the Proatherogenic Metabolite Trimethylamine-N-Oxide. *Mbio* **2015**, *6*, e02481. [CrossRef]
58. Rath, S.; Heidrich, B.; Pieper, D.H.; Vital, M. Uncovering the trimethylamine-producing bacteria of the human gut microbiota. *Microbiome* **2017**, *5*, 54. [CrossRef]
59. Tang, T.W.H.; Chen, H.-C.; Chen, C.-Y.; Yen, C.Y.T.; Lin, C.-J.; Prajnamitra, R.P.; Chen, L.L.; Ruan, S.C.; Lin, J.H.; Lin, P.J.; et al. Loss of Gut Microbiota Alters Immune System Composition and Cripples Postinfarction Cardiac Repair. *Circulation* **2019**, *139*, 647–659. [CrossRef] [PubMed]
60. Sponholz, C.; Sakr, Y.; Reinhart, K.; Brunkhorst, F. Diagnostic value and prognostic implications of serum procalcitonin after cardiac surgery: A systematic review of the literature. *Crit. Care* **2006**, *10*, R145. [CrossRef]
61. Jiao, J.; Wang, M.; Zhang, J.; Shen, K.; Liao, X.; Zhou, X. Procalcitonin as a diagnostic marker of ventilator-associated pneumonia in cardiac surgery patients. *Exp. Ther. Med.* **2015**, 1051–1057. [CrossRef] [PubMed]
62. Sander, M.; von Heymann, C.; von Dossow, V.; Spaethe, C.; Konertz, W.F.; Jain, U.; Spies, C.D. Increased interleukin-6 after cardiac surgery predicts infection. *Anesth. Analg.* **2006**, *102*, 1623–1629. [CrossRef]
63. Thygesen, K.; Alpert, J.S.; Jaffe, A.S.; Chaitman, B.R.; Bax, J.J.; Morrow, D.A.; White, H.D. Fourth Universal Definition of Myocardial Infarction. *Circulation* **2018**, *138*, e618–e651. [CrossRef]
64. Gu, Y.; Shan, L.; Liu, B.; Lv, M.; Chen, X.; Yan, T.; Shi, Y.; Chen, J.; Li, Z.; Zhang, Y. Release Profile of Cardiac Troponin T and Risk Factors of Postoperative Myocardial Injury in Patients Undergoing CABG. *Int. J. Gen. Med.* **2021**, *14*, 2541–2551. [CrossRef]
65. Singh, N.; Anchan, R.K.; Besser, S.A.; Belkin, M.N.; Cruz, M.D.; Lee, L.; Yu, D.; Mehta, N.; Nguyen, A.B.; Alenghat, F.J. High sensitivity Troponin-T for prediction of adverse events in patients with COVID-19. *Biomarkers* **2020**, *25*, 626–633. [CrossRef] [PubMed]
66. Nellipudi, J.A.; Baker, R.A.; Dykes, L.; Krieg, B.M.; Bennetts, J.S. Prognostic Value of High-Sensitivity Troponin T After On-Pump Coronary Artery Bypass Graft Surgery. *Heart Lung Circ.* **2021**, *30*, 1562–1569. [CrossRef]
67. Janigro, D.; Bailey, D.M.; Lehmann, S.; Badaut, J.; O'Flynn, R.; Hirtz, C.; Marchi, N. Peripheral Blood and Salivary Biomarkers of Blood-Brain Barrier Permeability and Neuronal Damage: Clinical and Applied Concepts. *Front. Neurol.* **2020**, *11*, 577312. [CrossRef] [PubMed]
68. Silva, F.P.; Schmidt, A.P.; Valentin, L.S.; Pinto, K.O.; Zeferino, S.P.; Oses, J.P.; Wiener, C.D.; Otsuki, D.A.; Tort, A.B.L.; Portela, L.V.; et al. S100B protein and neuron-specific enolase as predictors of cognitive dysfunction after coronary artery bypass graft surgery: A prospective observational study. *Eur. J. Anaesthesiol.* **2016**, *33*, 681–689. [CrossRef] [PubMed]
69. Al Tmimi, L.; van de Velde, M.; Meyns, B.; Meuris, B.; Sergeant, P.; Milisen, K.; Pottel, H.; Poesen, K.; Rex, S. Serum protein S100 as marker of postoperative delirium after off-pump coronary artery bypass surgery: Secondary analysis of two prospective randomized controlled trials. *Clin. Chem. Lab. Med.* **2016**, *54*, 1671–1680. [CrossRef]
70. Wang, J.; Wu, X.; Tian, Y.; Li, X.; Zhao, X.; Zhang, M. Dynamic changes and diagnostic and prognostic significance of serum PCT, hs-CRP and s-100 protein in central nervous system infection. *Exp. Ther. Med.* **2018**, *16*, 5156–5160. [CrossRef]
71. Wu, L.; Feng, Q.; Ai, M.-L.; Deng, S.-Y.; Liu, Z.-Y.; Huang, L.; Ai, Y.H.; Zhang, L. The dynamic change of serum S100B levels from day 1 to day 3 is more associated with sepsis-associated encephalopathy. *Sci. Rep.* **2020**, *10*, 7718. [CrossRef]

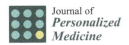

Article

Sphingomonas and *Phenylobacterium* as Major Microbiota in Thymic Epithelial Tumors

Rumi Higuchi [1,†], Taichiro Goto [1,*,†], Yosuke Hirotsu [2], Sotaro Otake [1], Toshio Oyama [3], Kenji Amemiya [2], Hiroshi Ohyama [2], Hitoshi Mochizuki [2] and Masao Omata [2,4]

1. Lung Cancer and Respiratory Disease Center, Yamanashi Central Hospital, Yamanashi 400-8506, Japan; r-higuchi1504@ych.pref.yamanashi.jp (R.H.); ootake.sotaro.gx@mail.hosp.go.jp (S.O.)
2. Genome Analysis Center, Yamanashi Central Hospital, Yamanashi 400-8506, Japan; hirotsu-bdyu@ych.pref.yamanashi.jp (Y.H.); amemiya-bdcd@ych.pref.yamanashi.jp (K.A.); ooyama-bdcx@ych.pref.yamanashi.jp (H.O.); h-mochiduki2a@ych.pref.yamanashi.jp (H.M.); m-omata0901@ych.pref.yamanashi.jp (M.O.)
3. Department of Pathology, Yamanashi Central Hospital, Yamanashi 400-8506, Japan; t-oyama@ych.pref.yamanashi.jp
4. Department of Gastroenterology, The University of Tokyo Hospital, Tokyo 113-8655, Japan
* Correspondence: taichiro@1997.jukuin.keio.ac.jp; Tel.: +81-55-253-7111
† These authors contributed equally to this work.

Simple Summary: In this study, we evaluated the microbiota in resected thymoma samples and identified *Sphingomonas* and *Phenylobacterium* as the dominant genera in thymomas. This is the first study that evaluated the microbiota in thymoma and that identified bacterial genera specific to thymoma. Furthermore, our study indicates a potential approach for preventing the development of thymoma as a new "precision medicine".

Abstract: The microbiota has been reported to be closely associated with carcinogenesis and cancer progression. However, its involvement in the pathology of thymoma remains unknown. In this study, we aimed to identify thymoma-specific microbiota using resected thymoma samples. Nineteen thymoma tissue samples were analyzed through polymerase chain reaction amplification and 16S rRNA gene sequencing. The subjects were grouped according to histology, driver mutation status in the *GTF2I* gene, PD-L1 status, and smoking habits. To identify the taxa composition of each sample, the operational taxonomic units (OTUs) were classified on the effective tags with 97% identity. The Shannon Index of the 97% identity OTUs was calculated to evaluate the alpha diversity. The linear discriminant analysis effect size (LEfSe) method was used to compare the relative abundances of all the bacterial taxa. We identified 107 OTUs in the tumor tissues, which were classified into 26 genera. *Sphingomonas* and *Phenylobacterium* were identified as abundant genera in almost all the samples. No significant difference was determined in the alpha diversity within these groups; however, type A thymoma tended to exhibit a higher bacterial diversity than type B thymoma. Through the LEfSe analysis, we identified the following differentially abundant taxa: Bacilli, Firmicutes, and Lactobacillales in type A thymoma; Proteobacteria in type B thymoma; Gammaproteobacteria in tumors harboring the *GTF2I* mutation; and Alphaproteobacteria in tumors without the *GTF2I* mutation. In conclusion, *Sphingomonas* and *Phenylobacterium* were identified as dominant genera in thymic epithelial tumors. These genera appear to comprise the thymoma-specific microbiota.

Keywords: thymoma; microbiome; 16S RNA sequencing; genera; driver mutation

Citation: Higuchi, R.; Goto, T.; Hirotsu, Y.; Otake, S.; Oyama, T.; Amemiya, K.; Ohyama, H.; Mochizuki, H.; Omata, M. *Sphingomonas* and *Phenylobacterium* as Major Microbiota in Thymic Epithelial Tumors. *J. Pers. Med.* **2021**, *11*, 1092. https://doi.org/10.3390/jpm11111092

Academic Editor: Lucrezia Laterza

Received: 19 August 2021
Accepted: 23 October 2021
Published: 26 October 2021

Publisher's Note: MDPI stays neutral with regard to jurisdictional claims in published maps and institutional affiliations.

Copyright: © 2021 by the authors. Licensee MDPI, Basel, Switzerland. This article is an open access article distributed under the terms and conditions of the Creative Commons Attribution (CC BY) license (https://creativecommons.org/licenses/by/4.0/).

1. Introduction

Early microbiome research focused primarily on gastrointestinal diseases, such as pseudomembranous enterocolitis, inflammatory bowel disease, and irritable colitis [1]. Recently, the human intestinal microbiota has been reported to be involved in carcinogenesis and cancer progression, and this phenomenon has been attracting attention [2,3]. In addition, the microbiota has been identified in tissues of the pancreatic, lung, and breast cancers through advanced sequencing technology [4–8].

Thymoma is a relatively rare mediastinal tumor with malignant potential that is difficult to treat [9,10]. According to the histological classification by the World Health Organization, thymomas can be categorized into types A, AB, B1, B2, and B3, depending on the tumor cell morphology and proportion of coexisting lymphocytes [11]. Type A thymomas are the least aggressive with the best prognosis; the extent of the aggressiveness increases and the prognosis worsens according to the following order: type A, AB, B1, B2, and B3 [12,13]. Thymoma has been reported to commonly occur in people aged 40–60 years [14]. The development of thymoma is not associated with smoking habits or sex; its causes are unknown [15]. However, thymoma coexists in approximately 20% of patients with myasthenia gravis [16,17]. Owing to the absence of an effective treatment other than surgical resection, there is an urgent need to elucidate the pathology and establish preventive measures and new treatment strategies for thymoma [18–21].

Although recent reports have indicated an association between the microbiome and colorectal, oral, pancreatic, lung, and other cancers [22–27], there is no report on the microbiome in thymoma. Unlike oral, gastrointestinal, and respiratory cancers, which have been previously reported, thymoma is anatomically located in the anterior mediastinum, and it does not communicate with the outer environment. Since the tumor environment of thymoma has been theoretically assumed to be sterile, microbiome research has not been conducted in the past. Consequently, little progress has been made in research on the involvement of the microbiota in the pathology of thymoma.

In this study, we performed a polymerase chain reaction (PCR) to amplify the 16S ribosomal RNA (rRNA) region in the bacterial genome in resected thymoma samples. Subsequently, we performed 16S rRNA sequencing and metagenomic analyses using next-generation sequencing to investigate the composition and diversity of the microbiota and to identify thymoma-specific microbiota. On the basis of the results from these analyses, we presented a predictive model of pathogenesis and evaluated its potential for the prevention and control of the development of thymoma.

2. Results

2.1. Patient Characteristics

Nineteen consecutive patients with thymomas who underwent surgery at our hospital between January 2014 and August 2020 were enrolled without bias. In three patients with type AB thymomas, the type A and B portions were microdissected and examined separately. Thus, in total, 22 tissue samples were analyzed for microbiota. The clinico-pathologic characteristics of the patients are summarized in Table 1. The 19 patients were divided into groups by the following characteristics: 11 males, 8 females; 12 smokers, 7 nonsmokers; histological type A (five), AB (three), B1 (five), B2 (four), or B3 (two); and Masaoka stage I (seven), II (nine), III (two), or IV (one). The diameter of the tumor was between 20 and 95 mm, with a mean tumor diameter of 43.6 ± 22.8 mm. Patients' ages at the time of surgery were between 42 and 81 years (68.2 ± 12.9 years). One patient with type B2 thymoma (Case 20; Figure 1) had a comorbidity of myasthenia gravis.

Table 1. Patient characteristics.

Parameter		Number of Patients	Overall Percentage
Total number		19	
Age, median (range)		68 (42–81)	
Sex			
	Male	11	57.9%
	Female	8	42.1%
Histology			
	Type A	5	26.3%
	Type AB	3	15.8%
	Type B1	5	26.3%
	Type B2	4	21.1%
	Type B3	2	10.5%
Tumor size (cm)			
	≤3	7	36.8%
	3 < size ≤ 5	8	42.1%
	>5	4	21.1%
Masaoka Stage			
	I	7	36.8%
	II	9	47.4%
	III	2	10.5%
	IV	1	5.3%
Smoking Status (Pack year)			
	0	7	36.8%
	0 < PY ≤ 30	8	42.1%
	>30	4	21.1%
Myasthenia gravis			
	present	1	5.3%
	absent	18	94.7%

No.	1	2	3	4	5	6	7	8	9	10	11	12	13	14	15	16	17	18	19	20	21	22	MEAN	±SD
Type	A	A	A	A	A	AB_A	AB_A	AB_A	AB_B	AB_B	AB_B	B1	B1	B1	B1	B1	B2	B2	B2	B2	B3	B3		
Stage	II	I	III	I	I	I	II	I	I	I	I	II	II	II	II	II	IV	II	I	I	I	II		
Pack Year	0	2	0	1	2	1	1	0	1	1	0	1	0	2	0	0	1	0	1	1	2	1		
GTF2I	+	+	+	+	+	+	+	+	+	+	+	−	−	+	−	+	−	+	−	−	−	−		
PD-L1	−	+	−	−	+	−	−	−	−	+	+	+	−	+	−	+	+	+	+	+	+	+		
Acinetobacter	0.8%						0.2%				0.8%												0.1%	0.2%
Anoxybacillus		4.8%																					0.2%	1.0%
Bradyrhizobium													0.7%										0.0%	0.1%
Phenylobacterium	10.4%	22.6%	24.4%	24.7%	21.3%	24.7%	26.6%	30.9%	28.4%	32.2%	37.5%	23.7%	43.2%	28.9%	27.9%	26.8%	31.8%		22.6%	32.4%	29.5%	21.9%	26.0%	8.7%
Tepidimonas	0.3%																						0.0%	0.1%
Phyllobacterium	2.2%	2.9%	3.6%	1.6%	2.2%	4.2%	2.9%	3.4%	3.0%	2.5%	0.4%	0.8%	6.9%	2.1%	2.4%	3.3%				2.7%	2.6%		2.2%	1.7%
Sphingomonas	44.4%	56.7%	64.9%	73.6%	74.0%	71.1%	66.3%	64.8%	68.6%	65.0%	60.8%	73.0%	48.6%	68.4%	67.6%	69.9%	68.2%	100.0%	77.4%	64.0%	68.0%	57.2%	66.9%	10.8%
Staphylococcus		1.0%					0.6%					1.1%											0.1%	0.3%
Bifidobacterium	1.6%																						0.1%	0.3%
Bacillus	1.2%	3.1%																					0.2%	0.7%
Haemophilus					1.2%																		0.1%	0.3%
Finegoldia					0.6%																		0.0%	0.1%
Gemella														0.3%									0.0%	0.1%
Chryseobacterium	1.2%																						0.1%	0.3%
Corynebacterium	11.2%		1.3%																			19.4%	1.5%	4.7%
Streptococcus			1.1%				2.6%							0.3%									0.2%	0.6%
Thermicanus	2.9%	2.0%																					0.2%	0.7%
Isoptericola	1.1%																						0.0%	0.2%
Geobacillus	2.3%																						0.1%	0.5%
Burkholderia							0.1%																0.0%	0.0%
Enterococcus	6.1%	5.9%																					0.5%	1.8%
Pseudoxanthomonas			0.9%																				0.0%	0.2%
Methyloversatilis							0.2%																0.0%	0.0%
Methylobacterium	1.5%		2.8%		0.7%	0.5%	0.9%		0.3%	0.4%	1.6%	0.4%			2.1%				0.9%			1.4%	0.6%	0.8%
Nocardioides	0.4%																						0.0%	0.1%
Cloacibacterium	12.5%	2.0%																					0.7%	2.7%

Figure 1. Composition and abundance of the dominant genera in all the samples. In total, 26 genera were identified. The heatmap visualizes the abundance of the detected genera. PY (pack-year) 0 represents nonsmokers; PY1, smokers with >0 to ≤30 packs/year history; and PY2, smokers with >30 packs/year history.

2.2. OTU Analyses

A total of 136 OTUs were identified in the 22 samples, while no OTU was found in the negative control samples (without any tissue). The dominant (>1% average relative abundance) classifiable OTUs belonged to four families: namely, Sphingomonadaceae (abundance: 62.0 ± 12.2%), Caulobacteraceae (abundance: 23.9 ± 7.6%), Bradyrhizobiaceae (abundance: 6.7% ± 5.3%), and Phyllobacteriaceae (abundance: 2.0% ± 1.4%) (Supplementary Materials Figure S1). We identified 107 genera (>1% average relative abundance); the predominant genera are presented in Figure 1. The top two genera with a high abundance and composition were *Sphingomonas* (abundance: 66.9 ± 10.8%) and *Phenylobacterium* (abundance: 26.0 ± 8.7%). *Sphingomonas* was detected in all the samples, and *Phenylobacterium* was detected in all the samples except in case 18. Both bacterial genera were significantly more abundant than the others (Supplementary Materials Figure S2).

2.3. Differences in Microbiota between Thymomas and Pancreatic Cancers

To identify the thymoma-specific microbiota, we compared the microbiota between thymoma and pancreatic cancer (Supplementary Materials Table S1). In the thymoma samples, compared with the pancreatic cancer samples, *Phenylobacterium*, *Phyllobacterium*, and *Sphingomonas* were significantly more abundant (Figure 2). Since *Phenylobacterium*, *Phyllobacterium*, and *Sphingomonas* were detected only in four, three, and eight of the 30 pancreatic cancer samples, respectively, the composition of these genera in the 22 thymoma samples (detected in 21, 18, and 22 samples, respectively) was significantly higher.

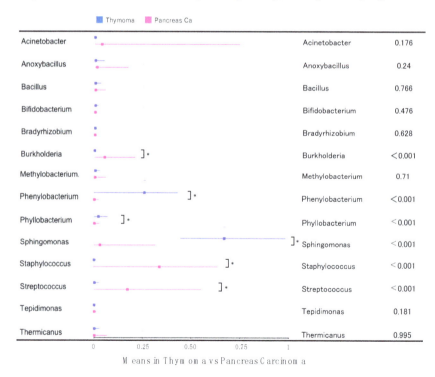

Figure 2. Microbiome differences between thymoma and pancreatic cancer samples. * $p < 0.05$.

2.4. Analysis of Microbial Diversity within Groups

The Shannon Index was calculated to evaluate the bacterial diversity within the different groups. No significant differences were observed in terms of the histology, presence or absence of the *GTF2I* mutation, PD-L1 expression, and smoking habits (Figure 3). However, the type A samples exhibited a tendency toward increased microbiome diversity compared with the type B samples (p = 0.059, Figure 3A).

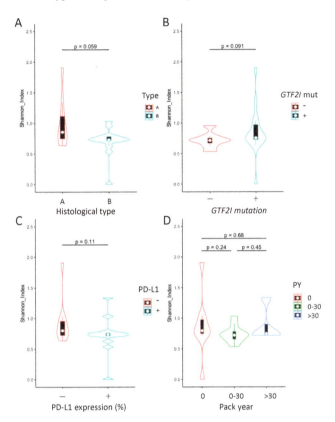

Figure 3. Taxonomic alpha diversity of thymoma microbiomes within samples in different groups. (**A**) Comparison of the Shannon Index between type A and B histology groups. (**B**) Comparison of the Shannon Index between tumors exhibiting the presence and those exhibiting an absence of the *GTF2I* driver mutation. (**C**) Comparison of the Shannon Index between tumors exhibiting the presence and those exhibiting an absence of PD-L1 expression on tumor cells. (**D**) Comparison of the Shannon Index among nonsmokers, light smokers, and heavy smokers. No significant difference was found among these groups.

2.5. Analysis of Differentially Abundant Taxa

To further identify the specific species in every group, we used the LEfSe method to identify the differentially abundant taxa at each level. First, in the type A and B histological groups, we identified four differential bacterial taxa, including two phyla, Firmicutes and Proteobacteria; one class, Bacilli; and one order, Lactobacillales (Figure 4A). The differential features were Firmicutes, Bacilli, and Lactobacillales in type A thymomas and Proteobacteria in type B thymomas (Figure 4B). Alphaproteobacteria was dominant in thymomas without the *GTF2I* mutation, while Gammaproteobacteria was dominant in thymomas harboring the *GTF2I* mutation (Figure 4C,D). No differential bacterial composition and abundance were observed in association with the stage, PD-L1 expression, or smoking habits.

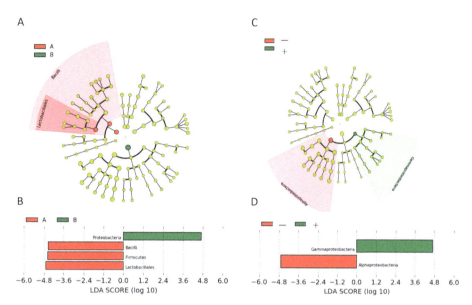

Figure 4. Differential taxa in the histology and driver mutation groups. (**A**) Cladogram of differential taxa between Types A and B histology. Dominant taxa are indicated in red for the type A group and in green for the type B group. (**B**) Kruskal–Wallis test results on the relative abundance between type A and type B histology. Type A is presented in the red column and type B in the green column. * $p < 0.05$. (**C**) The results of the LEfSe analysis between tumors exhibiting the presence and those exhibiting the absence of the *GTF2I* driver mutation. (**D**) Kruskal–Wallis test results for the relative abundance between tumors exhibiting the presence and those exhibiting the absence of the *GTF2I* driver mutation. * $p < 0.05$.

3. Discussion

In this study, the sequencing of microbiota in resected thymoma samples identified two genera, *Sphingomonas* and *Phenylobacterium*, in almost all the thymoma samples; the bacterial composition and abundance of these genera were markedly high. We separately analyzed type AB thymoma for type A and type B components and detected *Sphingomonas* and *Phenylobacterium* in both components. Although the oral microbiome is likely to affect and contaminate the lung microbiome, thymoma is anatomically unlikely to be affected by the oral microbiome [28,29]. The composition and abundance of these two genera were significantly higher in the microbiota of thymoma tissues than in the microbiota of pancreatic cancer tissues. Our results suggest that these two genera are thymoma-specific microbiota. In addition, we chose pancreatic cancer as control because the pancreatic cancer and thymoma tissue samples were analyzed in the same process at the genome analysis center of our hospital during the same period. There is also a factor common to both the pancreatic cancer and thymoma: they do not communicate directly with outer environment. This analysis suggested that the presence of the two genera was not a result of contamination during the analysis process. In contrast, *Sphingomonas* and *Phenylobacterium* have not been detected in lung cancer tissues according to recent reviews on the microbiota in patients with lung cancer [4,30–32]. In this study, because these two genera were detected in almost all the thymoma samples, it was suggested that *Sphingomonas* and *Phenylobacterium* may represent differential microbiome functions in thymoma development.

Sphingomonas is a bacterial genus that was subclassified from *Pseudomonas* approximately 30 years ago. Members of the former are Gram-negative bacteria; however, they do not contain lipopolysaccharides specific to Gram-negative bacteria [33]. Instead, these bacteria contain glycosphingolipids, which are found in eukaryotic cells [33]. They are common microorganisms inhabiting various environments, such as water environments (e.g., freshwater and seawater), soil, and plant root systems. The wide ecological distribution of these bacteria is attributed to their ability to use diverse organic compounds and their strong vitality, allowing them to survive in nutrient-poor environments [34]. Although several bacteria in the genus *Sphingomonas* were isolated in relatively clean environments, certain bacterial species were isolated in contaminated environments containing toxic organic compounds, such as polychlorinated biphenyl, creosote, and pentachlorophenol [35]. Subsequent studies revealed that these bacteria take up certain organic contaminants and use them as energy sources [36]. On the basis of these findings, progress has been made in elucidating the mechanism through which *Sphingomonas* metabolizes organic contaminants. Furthermore, several attempts have been made worldwide for applying this mechanism in environmental cleanup (bioremediation). Meanwhile, with respect to the microbiome, *Sphingomonas* has been reported to be enriched as blood microbiota in the serum of healthy patients and patients with breast cancer who exhibit a favorable prognosis [37,38].

Species within the genus *Phenylobacterium* are capable of degrading xenobiotic compounds with a phenyl moiety such as chloridazon, antipyrine, pyramidon, or their analogs [39]. Additionally, these bacteria can degrade polycyclic aromatic hydrocarbons [40]. *Phenylobacterium* has now been used in the bioremediation of a petroleum-contaminated soil to degrade polycyclic aromatic hydrocarbons and their analogs [41]. Unlike *Sphingomonas*, there has been no report of the detection of *Phenylobacterium* as blood microbiota. Future studies are expected to elucidate how *Sphingomonas* and *Phenylobacterium*, which are two genera of environmentally indigenous bacteria used for bioremediation, coexist in thymoma and how they are involved in the carcinogenic mechanism of thymoma.

Several indigenous microorganisms exist in the epithelium of the whole human body (e.g., the mouth, ear, nasal cavity, respiratory organs, digestive tract, skin, and reproductive organs); form microbiota; play various roles in the body; and form a symbiotic relationship with humans [1,2]. In recent years, it has been considered that disturbance in the microbiota composition (dysbiosis) may alter the risk of disease development, and there is a growing number of reports on the association between intestinal microbiota and several diseases, such as allergy, cancer, multiple sclerosis, Parkinson's disease, depression, inflammatory bowel disease, and rheumatism [30]. Furthermore, sterilization and specific pathogen-free breeding have been reported to alleviate or cure these diseases in pathological mouse models [42]. Improvement of the microbiota may additionally prevent the development of diseases in humans [43]. If one or several species of bacteria cause a disease, they can be potential therapeutic targets. For example, the eradication of *Helicobacter pylori* is the standard of care for the prevention of gastric cancer in infected patients at present [44]. This study indicates that the microbiota may be associated with thymoma. The clinical application of this finding may pave the way for the prevention of thymoma through controlling the growth of the bacterial genera *Sphingomonas* and *Phenylobacterium*. Patients with myasthenia gravis are at a high risk of developing thymoma [16,17], and the prevention of thymoma is important for their long-term survival. In this study, case 20 involved a patient with thymoma complicated by myasthenia gravis (Figure 1); this patient was positive for *Sphingomonas* and *Phenylobacterium*, which were abundant. The development of probiotic models for antibiotics, vaccines, and other therapies targeting these genera identified in this study may be important for the prevention of thymoma.

The bacterial diversity tends to be higher in type A thymoma (less aggressive type) than in type B (more aggressive type). A study comparing the microbiota between tumor and normal peritumoral tissues in lung cancer demonstrated that the bacterial diversity was significantly higher in normal peritumoral tissues [6]. According to these data, cancer aggressiveness and alpha diversity are negatively correlated. Since the cancer microenvironment is more perturbed, dysbiosis might be enhanced; consequently, the bacterial diversity might decrease. In addition, because the lymphocyte counts in the tissues are higher in type B thymoma than in type A thymoma, the immunity against these bacteria may fundamentally differ between these types.

Using a LEfSe analysis, we identified variations in specific species between type A and B tumors and between tumors with and without the *GTF2I* mutation, indicating the differential microbiome functions in the development of each type of tumor [45]. We determined that Firmicutes, Bacilli, and Lactobacillales were common Gram-positive bacteria in type A thymoma, and Proteobacteria were common Gram-negative bacteria in type B thymoma. When the *p*-value based on the Kruskal–Wallis test was increased from 0.05 to 0.1 (Supplementary Materials Figure S3), 15 out of 20 bacteria that were significantly detected in the microbiota of type A thymoma were Gram-positive bacteria, and all four bacteria significantly detected in the microbiota of type B thymoma were Gram-negative bacteria. Although these findings indicated a correlation between the histological types (types A and B) and Gram-staining results for the microbiota, the biological significance of this correlation is unknown. Since Gram-negative bacteria are generally more pathogenic than Gram-positive bacteria, the former may be involved in carcinogenesis in type B thymoma, which is the more aggressive phenotype. Additionally, it is unclear from our observational study whether the identified bacterial differences are causally related to carcinogenesis or merely reflective of the disease process in thymoma. It is also difficult to practically prove how the microbiota colonized the thymoma tissue, which has no direct communication with the outside. In the future, detailed studies with a larger sample size may be needed.

We previously reported that the *GTF2I* mutation is a driver mutation in thymoma [46]. In the present study, specific species were identified between tumors with and without a *GTF2I* mutation. While Alphaproteobacteria were detected in a significantly high number of cases without the driver mutation in the *GTF2I* gene, a clear pathway involved in the oncological development of thymoma without a driver mutation remains to be demonstrated. Additionally, the mechanisms through which the microbiota in general contributes to carcinogenesis need to be examined in detail using a large sample size in the future.

This study is associated with some limitations. First, the patient cohort was relatively small owing to the rarity of the tumor. Second, patient survival could not be analyzed, as no patients have shown recurrence in the cohort. Third, no blood samples were analyzed for the microbiota containing the two genera, *Sphingomonas* and *Phenylobacterium*. An analysis of blood samples might have elucidated the reasons for the presence of the microbiota in the sterile anterior mediastinal environment [47]. In addition, the higher abundance of *Sphingomonas* and *Phenylobacterium* may be related to the impaired immunity of the tumor microenvironment, which may cause proliferation of these bacteria in the blood. Thus, they may be clinically applicable as serum biomarkers for thymoma. Fourth, a control thymus tissue should have been obtained to show that *Sphingomonas* and *Phenylobacterium* are microbiota associated with cancer progression. However, normal thymic tissue is known to rapidly atrophy and to be replaced with adipose tissue after puberty in the teens, and thymoma is presumed to be derived from atrophied residual thymic tissue. Therefore, even if a surgical specimen of adipose tissue in the anterior mediastinal of an age-matched population was obtained, thymic tissue is usually not left behind and cannot be analyzed. In addition, surgical specimens of the anterior mediastinal tissue of young individuals are extremely difficult to obtain, and it is ethically problematic to collect the functional thymic tissue of young individuals. Thus, it was not possible to compare microbiota between thymoma and normal thymic tissue in this study. In this context, a larger series of studies needs to be performed for evaluating the microbiome landscape of thymomas more comprehensively and elucidate the associations with clinical parameters through a more exhaustive multivariate analysis. Nevertheless, since the major aim of this preliminary analysis was identification of the thymoma-specific microbiota that should be prioritized for clinical development, the modestly sized samples provided useful insight.

4. Methods

4.1. Patients and Sample Preparation

In this study, we enrolled 19 patients in an unbiased manner who underwent surgical resection for thymoma at our hospital between January 2014 and August 2020. Since antibiotics would affect the microbiome, patients who had used oral or systematic antibiotics in the past 3 months were not included in this study. We obtained written informed consent for genetic research from all the patients in accordance with the protocols approved by the Institutional Review Board at Yamanashi Central Hospital. The specimens were categorized histologically according to the classification guidelines by the World Health Organization [48,49] and staged according to the Masaoka Staging System [19,50,51]. Sections of formalin-fixed and paraffin-embedded (FFPE) tissues were stained with hematoxylin–eosin and microdissected using the ArcturusXT laser-capture microdissection system (Thermo Fisher Scientific, Waltham, MA, USA), as previously reported [52–57]. For type AB thymomas, the type A and B portions were microdissected and examined separately. A thymoma is an encapsulated tumor, and the tumor tissue and surrounding fat are clearly separated by a fibrous capsule. In this study, DNA was extracted from the tumor tissue of the FFPE specimen of thymoma with laser-capture microdissection, so contamination of the adipose tissue around the tumor was unlikely.

We analyzed 22 samples obtained from all 19 patients, including three patients with type AB thymomas. The GeneRead DNA FFPE Kit (Qiagen, Hilden, Germany) was used according to the manufacturer's instructions, and the DNA quality was evaluated using primers against ribonuclease P, as previously reported [58]. In the same manner, tumor DNA was extracted from FFPE samples obtained from patients with pancreatic cancer in our hospital ($n = 30$) and used as a control. As the preliminary experiment, PCR amplification of the 16S rDNA V4 region was attempted using distilled water, and a DNA elution buffer was used in the experiment for the samples, but DNA amplification was not obtained (below the detection sensitivity).

4.2. 16S rRNA Amplification and Targeted Sequencing

Although there is no hypervariable region of the 16S gene that allows an accurate classification of all bacterial strains at the domain to the species level, there is a known region that allows the near-perfect prediction at a specific taxonomic level [59]. In many studies on microbiome analyses, a commonly selected region is the V4 hypervariable region that allows a strain analysis at the phylum level with accuracy similar to that of the analysis of the complete 16S rRNA gene. The 16S rDNA V4 region was amplified using PCR and sequenced as described previously with minor modifications [7]. FFPE DNA was amplified using Platinum PCR SuperMix High Fidelity (Thermo Fisher Scientific) with the forward primer 5'-GTGYCAGCMGCCGCGGTAA-3' (16S_rRNA_V4_515F) and reverse primer 5'-GGACTACNVGGGTWTCTAAT-3' (16S_rRNA_V4_806R). The PCR products were confirmed using agarose gel electrophoresis and purified using Agencourt AMPure XP reagents (Beckman Coulter, Brea, CA, USA). End repair and barcode adaptors were ligated with the Ion Plus Fragment Library Kit (Thermo Fisher Scientific), in accordance with the manufacturer's instructions, to construct the libraries. The library concentration was determined using an Ion Library Quantitation Kit (Thermo Fisher Scientific), and the same number of libraries was pooled for one sequence. Emulsion PCR and chip loading was performed on Ion Chef with the Ion PGM Hi-Q View Chef Kit; sequencing was performed on an Ion PGM Sequencer (Thermo Fisher Scientific). Sequence data were transferred to the IonReporter local server using the IonReporterUploader plugin. The coverage of the sequencing was 329.2 (Supplementary Table S2). Data was analyzed using the Metagenomics Research application using a custom primer set. The analytical parameters were set as the default. The control paraffin block without any tissue was processed similarly.

4.3. Data Analysis

The original raw tags were obtained through splicing the reads using FLASH (v 1.2.7) and subsequently filtered to acquire clean tags using QIIME (Version 1.9.1). To identify the taxa composition of each sample, the operational taxonomic units (OTUs) were classified on the effective tags with 97% identity using Usearch (Uparse v 7.0.1001) software. The presentative sequence of each OTU was annotated using the RDP classifier against the SILVA (SSU123)16S rRNA database using a confidence threshold of 80%, obtaining taxonomic classification at the phylum, class, order, family, genus, and species levels. Multiple sequence alignment was performed using MUSCLE3.6 (Version 3.8.31) to further explore the phylogenetic relationships among the different OTUs. The Shannon Index was performed using QIIME to determine the alpha diversity. Linear discriminant analysis (LDA) effect size (LEfSe) analyses were performed using the online LEfSe tool (http://huttenhower.sph.harvard.edu/lefse/ (accessed on 12 October 2020)). The LDA (linear discriminant analysis) threshold score was set at 2.

4.4. Targeted Deep Sequencing of GTF2I Mutation

In this study, the presence of a point mutation in the *GTF2I* gene was investigated in thymomas using targeted sequencing coupled with molecular barcoding, as we previously reported [47].

4.5. Immunohistochemistry for PD-L1

Specimens from the 19 patients were fixed using 10% buffered formalin. The formalin-fixed paraffin-embedded tissues were cut into 5-μm sections, deparaffinized, rehydrated, and stained in an automated system (Ventana Benchmark ULTRA system; Roche, Tucson, AZ, USA) using commercially available detection kits and antibodies against PD-L1 (28–8, ab205921; Abcam, Cambridge, MA, USA). PD-L1 was primarily localized to the cell membranes of the tumor cells, and its expression was determined quantitatively by two pathologists on the basis of the proportion of PD-L1-positive tumor cells. Cells were considered PD-L1-positive based on $\geq$1% PD-L1 expression.

4.6. Statistics

Continuous variables were presented as the mean $\pm$ standard deviation (SD) and compared using unpaired Student's t-tests. One-way analysis of variance and the Tukey–Kramer multiple comparison test were used to detect significant differences between groups. p-values less than 0.05 in the two-tailed analyses were considered to denote statistical significance.

5. Conclusions

This is the first study that examined the microbiota in thymomas and revealed two genera specific to thymomas: *Sphingomonas* and *Phenylobacterium*.

Supplementary Materials: The following are available online at https://www.mdpi.com/article/10.3390/jpm11111092/s1: Figure S1: Composition and abundance of the dominant families in all the samples. Figure S2: Comparison of the abundance of the detected genera. Figure S3: LEfSe analysis between type A and B histology. Table S1: Characteristics of the patients with pancreatic cancer. Table S2: Read depths of the sequencing.

Author Contributions: T.G., Y.H. and R.H. wrote the manuscript. T.G., R.H. and S.O. performed the surgery. T.O., K.A. and R.H. carried out the pathological examination. Y.H., K.A., T.G., H.O., H.M., R.H., S.O. and M.O. participated in the genomic analyses. M.O. and T.G. edited the final manuscript. All authors have read and agreed to the published version of the manuscript.

Funding: This study was supported by a Grant-in-Aid for Genome Research Project from Yamanashi Prefecture (to Y.H. and M.O.).

Institutional Review Board Statement: The study was conducted in accordance with the guidelines of the Declaration of Helsinki and approved by the Institutional Review Board at Yamanashi Central Hospital (protocol code GenomeH26-14).

Informed Consent Statement: Informed consent was obtained from all subjects involved in the study.

Acknowledgments: The authors greatly appreciate Yumiko Kakizaki, Toshiharu Tsutsui, and Yoshihiro Miyashita for their helpful scientific discussions.

Conflicts of Interest: The authors declare no conflict of interest. The funder had no role in the design of the study; in the collection, analyses, or interpretation of the data; in the writing of the manuscript; or in the decision to publish the results.

References

1. Power, S.E.; O'Toole, P.W.; Stanton, C.; Ross, R.P.; Fitzgerald, G.F. Intestinal microbiota, diet and health. *Br. J. Nutr.* **2014**, *111*, 387–402. [CrossRef] [PubMed]
2. Kovaleva, O.V.; Romashin, D.; Zborovskaya, I.B.; Davydov, M.M.; Shogenov, M.S.; Gratchev, A. Human lung microbiome on the way to cancer. *J. Immunol. Res.* **2019**, *2019*, 1394191. [PubMed]
3. Mao, Q.; Jiang, F.; Yin, R.; Wang, J.; Xia, W.; Dong, G.; Ma, W.; Yang, Y.; Xu, L.; Hu, J. Interplay between the lung microbiome and lung cancer. *Cancer Lett.* **2018**, *415*, 40–48. [CrossRef] [PubMed]
4. Goto, T. Airway microbiota as a modulator of lung cancer. *Int. J. Mol. Sci.* **2020**, *21*, 3044. [CrossRef] [PubMed]
5. Laborda-Illanes, A.; Sanchez-Alcoholado, L.; Dominguez-Recio, M.E.; Jimenez-Rodriguez, B.; Lavado, R.; Comino-Méndez, I.; Alba, E.; Queipo-Ortuño, M.I. Breast and gut microbiota action mechanisms in breast cancer pathogenesis and treatment. *Cancers* **2020**, *12*, 2465. [CrossRef]
6. Peters, B.A.; Hayes, R.B.; Goparaju, C.; Reid, C.; Pass, H.I.; Ahn, J. The microbiome in lung cancer tissue and recurrence-free survival. *Cancer Epidemiol. Biomarkers Prev.* **2019**, *28*, 731–740. [CrossRef]
7. Riquelme, E.; Zhang, Y.; Zhang, L.; Montiel, M.; Zoltan, M.; Dong, W.; Quesada, P.; Sahin, I.; Chandra, V.; San Lucas, A.; et al. Tumor microbiome diversity and composition influence pancreatic cancer outcomes. *Cell* **2019**, *178*, 795–806.e12. [CrossRef] [PubMed]
8. Wei, M.Y.; Shi, S.; Liang, C.; Meng, Q.C.; Hua, J.; Zhang, Y.Y.; Liu, J.; Zhang, B.; Xu, J.; Yu, X.J. The microbiota and microbiome in pancreatic cancer: More influential than expected. *Mol. Cancer* **2019**, *18*, 97. [CrossRef] [PubMed]
9. Engels, E.A. Epidemiology of thymoma and associated malignancies. *J. Thorac. Oncol.* **2010**, *5* (Suppl. S4), S260–S265. [CrossRef]
10. Venuta, F.; Anile, M.; Diso, D.; Vitolo, D.; Rendina, E.A.; De Giacomo, T.; Francioni, F.; Coloni, G.F. Thymoma and thymic carcinoma. *Eur. J. Cardiothorac. Surg.* **2010**, *37*, 13–25. [CrossRef] [PubMed]
11. Marx, A.; Chan, J.K.; Coindre, J.M.; Detterbeck, F.; Girard, N.; Harris, N.L.; Jaffe, E.S.; Kurrer, M.O.; Marom, E.M.; Moreira, A.L.; et al. The 2015 world health organization classification of tumors of the thymus: Continuity and changes. *J. Thorac. Oncol.* **2015**, *10*, 1383–1395. [CrossRef] [PubMed]
12. Marx, A.; Strobel, P.; Badve, S.S.; Chalabreysse, L.; Chan, J.K.; Chen, G.; de Leval, L.; Detterbeck, F.; Girard, N.; Huang, J.; et al. ITMIG consensus statement on the use of the WHO histological classification of thymoma and thymic carcinoma: Refined definitions, histological criteria, and reporting. *J. Thorac. Oncol.* **2014**, *9*, 596–611. [CrossRef] [PubMed]
13. Moon, J.W.; Lee, K.S.; Shin, M.H.; Kim, S.; Woo, S.Y.; Lee, G.; Han, J.; Shim, Y.M.; Choi, Y.S. Thymic epithelial tumors: Prognostic determinants among clinical, histopathologic, and computed tomography findings. *Ann. Thorac. Surg.* **2015**, *99*, 462–470. [CrossRef] [PubMed]
14. Thomas, C.R.; Wright, C.D.; Loehrer, P.J. Thymoma: State of the art. *J. Clin. Oncol.* **1999**, *17*, 2280–2289. [CrossRef] [PubMed]
15. Conforti, F.; Pala, L.; Giaccone, G.; De Pas, T. Thymic epithelial tumors: From biology to treatment. *Cancer Treat Rev.* **2020**, *86*, 102014. [CrossRef] [PubMed]
16. Kumar, R. Myasthenia gravis and thymic neoplasms: A brief review. *World J. Clin. Cases* **2015**, *3*, 980–983. [CrossRef] [PubMed]
17. Romi, F. Thymoma in myasthenia gravis: From diagnosis to treatment. *Autoimmune Dis.* **2011**, *2011*, 474512. [CrossRef]
18. Girard, N.; Lal, R.; Wakelee, H.; Riely, G.J.; Loehrer, P.J. Chemotherapy definitions and policies for thymic malignancies. *J. Thorac. Oncol.* **2011**, *6* (Suppl. S3), S1749–S1755. [CrossRef] [PubMed]
19. Litvak, A.M.; Woo, K.; Hayes, S.; Huang, J.; Rimner, A.; Sima, C.S.; Moreira, A.L.; Tsukazan, M.; Riely, G.J. Clinical characteristics and outcomes for patients with thymic carcinoma: Evaluation of Masaoka staging. *J. Thorac. Oncol.* **2014**, *9*, 1810–1815. [CrossRef]
20. Schmitt, J.; Loehrer, P.J., Sr. The role of chemotherapy in advanced thymoma. *J. Thorac. Oncol.* **2010**, *5* (Suppl. S4), S357–S360. [CrossRef] [PubMed]
21. Zhao, Y.; Shi, J.; Fan, L.; Hu, D.; Yang, J.; Zhao, H. Surgical treatment of thymoma: An 11-year experience with 761 patients. *Eur. J. Cardiothorac. Surg.* **2016**, *49*, 1144–1149. [CrossRef] [PubMed]
22. Castellarin, M.; Warren, R.L.; Freeman, J.D.; Dreolini, L.; Krzywinski, M.; Strauss, J.; Barnes, R.; Watson, P.; Allen-Vercoe, E.; Moore, R.A.; et al. Fusobacterium nucleatum infection is prevalent in human colorectal carcinoma. *Genome Res.* **2012**, *22*, 299–306. [CrossRef] [PubMed]

23. Gethings-Behncke, C.; Coleman, H.G.; Jordao, H.W.T.; Longley, D.B.; Crawford, N.; Murray, L.J.; Kunzmann, A.T. Fusobacterium nucleatum in the colorectum and its association with cancer risk and survival: A systematic review and meta-analysis. *Cancer Epidemiol. Biomarkers Prev.* **2020**, *29*, 539–548. [CrossRef] [PubMed]
24. Gur, C.; Ibrahim, Y.; Isaacson, B.; Yamin, R.; Abed, J.; Gamliel, M.; Enk, J.; Bar-On, Y.; Stanietsky-Kaynan, N.; Coppenhagen-Glazer, S.; et al. Binding of the Fap2 protein of Fusobacterium nucleatum to human inhibitory receptor TIGIT protects tumors from immune cell attack. *Immunity* **2015**, *42*, 344–355. [CrossRef]
25. Kostic, A.D.; Chun, E.; Robertson, L.; Glickman, J.N.; Gallini, C.A.; Michaud, M.; Clancy, T.E.; Chung, D.C.; Lochhead, P.; Hold, G.L.; et al. Fusobacterium nucleatum potentiates intestinal tumorigenesis and modulates the tumor-immune microenvironment. *Cell Host Microbe* **2013**, *14*, 207–215. [CrossRef] [PubMed]
26. Kostic, A.D.; Gevers, D.; Pedamallu, C.S.; Michaud, M.; Duke, F.; Earl, A.M.; Ojesina, A.I.; Jung, J.; Bass, A.J.; Tabernero, J.; et al. Genomic analysis identifies association of Fusobacterium with colorectal carcinoma. *Genome Res.* **2012**, *22*, 292–298. [CrossRef]
27. Rubinstein, M.R.; Wang, X.; Liu, W.; Hao, Y.; Cai, G.; Han, Y.W. Fusobacterium nucleatum promotes colorectal carcinogenesis by modulating E-cadherin/beta-catenin signaling via its FadA adhesin. *Cell Host Microbe* **2013**, *14*, 195–206. [CrossRef] [PubMed]
28. Hujoel, P.P.; Drangsholt, M.; Spiekerman, C.; Weiss, N.S. An exploration of the periodontitis-cancer association. *Ann. Epidemiol.* **2003**, *13*, 312–316. [CrossRef]
29. Yang, J.; Mu, X.; Wang, Y.; Zhu, D.; Zhang, J.; Liang, C.; Chen, B.; Wang, J.; Zhao, C.; Zuo, Z.; et al. Dysbiosis of the salivary microbiome is associated with non-smoking female lung cancer and correlated with immunocytochemistry markers. *Front. Oncol.* **2018**, *8*, 520. [CrossRef] [PubMed]
30. Maddi, A.; Sabharwal, A.; Violante, T.; Manuballa, S.; Genco, R.; Patnaik, S.; Yendamuri, S. The microbiome and lung cancer. *J. Thorac. Dis.* **2019**, *11*, 280–291. [CrossRef] [PubMed]
31. Ramirez-Labrada, A.G.; Isla, D.; Artal, A.; Arias, M.; Rezusta, A.; Pardo, J.; Galvez, E.M. The influence of lung microbiota on lung carcinogenesis, immunity, and immunotherapy. *Trends Cancer* **2020**, *6*, 86–97. [CrossRef] [PubMed]
32. Xu, N.; Wang, L.; Li, C.; Ding, C.; Li, C.; Fan, W.; Cheng, C.; Gu, B. Microbiota dysbiosis in lung cancer: Evidence of association and potential mechanisms. *Transl. Lung Cancer Res.* **2020**, *9*, 1554–1568. [CrossRef]
33. Stolz, A. Molecular characteristics of xenobiotic-degrading sphingomonads. *Appl. Microbiol. Biotechnol.* **2009**, *81*, 793–811. [CrossRef] [PubMed]
34. Aso, Y.; Miyamoto, Y.; Harada, K.M.; Momma, K.; Kawai, S.; Hashimoto, W.; Mikami, B.; Murata, K. Engineered membrane superchannel improves bioremediation potential of dioxin-degrading bacteria. *Nat. Biotechnol.* **2006**, *24*, 188–189. [CrossRef]
35. Miller, T.R.; Delcher, A.L.; Salzberg, S.L.; Saunders, E.; Detter, J.C.; Halden, R.U. Genome sequence of the dioxin-mineralizing bacterium Sphingomonas wittichii RW1. *J. Bacteriol.* **2010**, *192*, 6101–6102. [CrossRef]
36. Asaf, S.; Numan, M.; Khan, A.L.; Al-Harrasi, A. Sphingomonas: From diversity and genomics to functional role in environmental remediation and plant growth. *Crit. Rev. Biotechnol.* **2020**, *40*, 138–152. [CrossRef]
37. Dong, Z.; Chen, B.; Pan, H.; Wang, D.; Liu, M.; Yang, Y.; Zou, M.; Yang, J.; Xiao, K.; Zhao, R.; et al. Detection of microbial 16S rRNA gene in the serum of patients with gastric cancer. *Front. Oncol.* **2019**, *9*, 608. [CrossRef] [PubMed]
38. Huang, Y.F.; Chen, Y.J.; Fan, T.C.; Chang, N.C.; Chen, Y.J.; Midha, M.K.; Chen, T.H.; Yang, H.H.; Wang, Y.T.; Yu, A.L.; et al. Analysis of microbial sequences in plasma cell-free DNA for early-onset breast cancer patients and healthy females. *BMC Med. Genom.* **2018**, *11* (Suppl. S1), 16. [CrossRef] [PubMed]
39. Li, X.; Yu, Y.; Choi, L.; Song, Y.; Wu, M.; Wang, G.; Li, M. Phenylobacterium soli sp. nov., isolated from arsenic and cadmium contaminated farmland soil. *Int. J. Syst. Evol. Microbiol.* **2019**, *69*, 1398–1403. [CrossRef] [PubMed]
40. Yang, S.; Wen, X.; Zhao, L.; Shi, Y.; Jin, H. Crude oil treatment leads to shift of bacterial communities in soils from the deep active layer and upper permafrost along the China-Russia Crude Oil Pipeline route. *PLoS ONE* **2014**, *9*, e96552. [CrossRef]
41. Huang, Y.; Pan, H.; Wang, Q.; Ge, Y.; Liu, W.; Christie, P. Enrichment of the soil microbial community in the bioremediation of a petroleum-contaminated soil amended with rice straw or sawdust. *Chemosphere* **2019**, *224*, 265–271. [CrossRef] [PubMed]
42. Aron-Wisnewsky, J.; Warmbrunn, M.V.; Nieuwdorp, M.; Clément, K. Metabolism and metabolic disorders and the microbiome: The intestinal microbiota associated with obesity, lipid metabolism and metabolic health: Pathophysiology and therapeutic strategies. *Gastroenterology* **2021**, *160*, 573–599. [CrossRef] [PubMed]
43. Sommariva, M.; Le Noci, V.; Bianchi, F.; Camelliti, S.; Balsari, A.; Tagliabue, E.; Sfondrini, L. The lung microbiota: Role in maintaining pulmonary immune homeostasis and its implications in cancer development and therapy. *Cell. Mol. Life Sci.* **2020**, *77*, 2739–2749. [CrossRef] [PubMed]
44. Liou, J.M.; Malfertheiner, P.; Lee, Y.C.; Sheu, B.S.; Sugano, K.; Cheng, H.C.; Yeoh, K.G.; Hsu, P.I.; Goh, K.L.; Mahachai, V.; et al. Screening and eradication of *Helicobacter pylori* for gastric cancer prevention: The Taipei global consensus. *Gut* **2020**, *69*, 2093–2112. [CrossRef] [PubMed]
45. Yu, G.; Gail, M.H.; Consonni, D.; Carugno, M.; Humphrys, M.; Pesatori, A.C.; Caporaso, N.E.; Goedert, J.J.; Ravel, J.; Landi, M.T. Characterizing human lung tissue microbiota and its relationship to epidemiological and clinical features. *Genome Biol.* **2016**, *17*, 163. [CrossRef] [PubMed]
46. Higuchi, R.; Goto, T.; Hirotsu, Y.; Yokoyama, Y.; Nakagomi, T.; Otake, S.; Amemiya, K.; Oyama, T.; Mochizuki, H.; Omata, M. Primary driver mutations in *GTF2I* specific to the development of thymomas. *Cancers* **2020**, *12*, 2032. [CrossRef] [PubMed]

47. Loessner, H.; Endmann, A.; Leschner, S.; Westphal, K.; Rohde, M.; Miloud, T.; Hämmerling, G.; Neuhaus, K.; Weiss, S. Remote control of tumour-targeted Salmonella enterica serovar Typhimurium by the use of L-arabinose as inducer of bacterial gene expression in vivo. *Cell. Microbiol.* **2007**, *9*, 1529–1537. [CrossRef] [PubMed]
48. Gibbs, A.R.; Thunnissen, F.B. Histological typing of lung and pleural tumours: Third edition. *J. Clin. Pathol.* **2001**, *54*, 498–499. [CrossRef]
49. Travis, W.D.; Brambilla, E.; Nicholson, A.G.; Yatabe, Y.; Austin, J.H.M.; Beasley, M.B.; Chirieac, L.R.; Dacic, S.; Duhig, E.; Flieder, D.B.; et al. The 2015 World Health Organization classification of lung tumors: Impact of genetic, clinical and radiologic advances since the 2004 classification. *J. Thorac. Oncol.* **2015**, *10*, 1243–1260. [CrossRef] [PubMed]
50. Chansky, K.; Detterbeck, F.C.; Nicholson, A.G.; Rusch, V.W.; Vallieres, E.; Groome, P.; Kennedy, C.; Krasnik, M.; Peake, M.; Shemanski, L.; et al. The IASLC lung cancer staging project: External validation of the revision of the TNM Stage groupings in the eighth edition of the TNM classification of lung cancer. *J. Thorac. Oncol.* **2017**, *12*, 1109–1121. [CrossRef] [PubMed]
51. Ruffini, E.; Fang, W.; Guerrera, F.; Huang, J.; Okumura, M.; Kim, D.K.; Girard, N.; Bille, A.; Boubia, S.; Cangir, A.K.; et al. The international association for the study of lung cancer thymic tumors staging project: The impact of the Eighth edition of the Union for international cancer control and american joint committee on cancer TNM stage classification of thymic tumors. *J. Thorac. Oncol.* **2020**, *15*, 436–447. [CrossRef] [PubMed]
52. Amemiya, K.; Hirotsu, Y.; Goto, T.; Nakagomi, H.; Mochizuki, H.; Oyama, T.; Omata, M. Touch imprint cytology with massively parallel sequencing (TIC-seq): A simple and rapid method to snapshot genetic alterations in tumors. *Cancer Med.* **2016**, *5*, 3436–3436. [CrossRef] [PubMed]
53. Goto, T.; Hirotsu, Y.; Amemiya, K.; Nakagomi, T.; Shikata, D.; Yokoyama, Y.; Okimoto, K.; Oyama, T.; Mochizuki, H.; Omata, M. Distribution of circulating tumor DNA in lung cancer: Analysis of the primary lung and bone marrow along with the pulmonary venous and peripheral blood. *Oncotarget* **2017**, *8*, 59268–59281. [CrossRef] [PubMed]
54. Higuchi, R.; Nakagomi, T.; Goto, T.; Hirotsu, Y.; Shikata, D.; Yokoyama, Y.; Otake, S.; Amemiya, K.; Oyama, T.; Mochizuki, H.; et al. Identification of clonality through genomic profile analysis in multiple lung cancers. *J. Clin. Med.* **2020**, *9*, 573. [CrossRef] [PubMed]
55. Nakagomi, T.; Goto, T.; Hirotsu, Y.; Shikata, D.; Yokoyama, Y.; Higuchi, R.; Otake, S.; Amemiya, K.; Oyama, T.; Mochizuki, H.; et al. Genomic characteristics of invasive mucinous adenocarcinomas of the lung and potential therapeutic targets of B7-H3. *Cancers* **2018**, *10*, 478. [CrossRef] [PubMed]
56. Nakagomi, T.; Hirotsu, Y.; Goto, T.; Shikata, D.; Yokoyama, Y.; Higuchi, R.; Otake, S.; Amemiya, K.; Oyama, T.; Mochizuki, H.; et al. Clinical implications of noncoding indels in the surfactant-encoding genes in lung cancer. *Cancers* **2019**, *11*, 552. [CrossRef]
57. Oyama, T.; Goto, T.; Amemiya, K.; Hirotsu, Y.; Omata, M. Squamous cell carcinoma of the lung with micropapillary pattern. *J. Thorac. Oncol.* **2020**, *15*, 1541–1544. [CrossRef] [PubMed]
58. Goto, T.; Hirotsu, Y.; Oyama, T.; Amemiya, K.; Omata, M. Analysis of tumor-derived DNA in plasma and bone marrow fluid in lung cancer patients. *Med. Oncol.* **2016**, *33*, 29. [CrossRef] [PubMed]
59. Yang, B.; Wang, Y.; Qian, P.Y. Sensitivity and correlation of hypervariable regions in 16S rRNA genes in phylogenetic analysis. *BMC Bioinform.* **2016**, *17*, 135. [CrossRef]

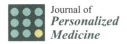

Article

Lipid and Energy Metabolism of the Gut Microbiota Is Associated with the Response to Probiotic *Bifidobacterium breve* Strain for Anxiety and Depressive Symptoms in Schizophrenia

Ryodai Yamamura [1], Ryo Okubo [2,*], Noriko Katsumata [3], Toshitaka Odamaki [3], Naoki Hashimoto [4], Ichiro Kusumi [4], Jinzhong Xiao [3] and Yutaka J. Matsuoka [5]

1. Division of Biomedical Oncology, Institute for Genetic Medicine, Hokkaido University, Sapporo 060-0815, Japan; ryamamura@igm.hokudai.ac.jp
2. Department of Clinical Epidemiology, Translational Medical Center, National Center of Neurology and Psychiatry, Tokyo 187-8551, Japan
3. Next Generation Science Institute, Morinaga Milk Industry Co. Ltd., Zama 252-8583, Japan; n_katumt@morinagamilk.co.jp (N.K.); t-odamak@morinagamilk.co.jp (T.O.); j_xiao@morinagamilk.co.jp (J.X.)
4. Department of Psychiatry, Hokkaido University Graduate School of Medicine, Sapporo 060-8638, Japan; hashinao@med.hokudai.ac.jp (N.H.); ikusumi@med.hokudai.ac.jp (I.K.)
5. Division of Health Care Research, Center for Public Health Sciences, National Cancer Center Japan, Tokyo 104-0045, Japan; yumatsuo@ncc.go.jp
* Correspondence: ryo-okubo@ncnp.go.jp; Tel.: +81-42-341-2712

Abstract: A recent meta-analysis found that probiotics have moderate-to-large beneficial effects on depressive symptoms in patients with psychiatric disorders. However, it remains unclear how the baseline gut microbiota before probiotic administration influences the host's response to probiotics. Therefore, we aimed to determine whether the predicted functional profile of the gut microbiota influences the effectiveness of probiotic treatment in patients with schizophrenia. A total of 29 patients with schizophrenia consumed *Bifidobacterium breve* A-1 (synonym *B. breve* MCC1274) for 4 weeks. We considered patients who showed a 25% or more reduction in the Hospital Anxiety and Depression Scale total score at 4 weeks from baseline to be "responders" and those who did not to be "non-responders". We predicted the gut microbial functional genes based on 16S rRNA gene sequences and applied the linear discriminant analysis effect size method to determine the gut microbial functional genes most likely to explain the differences between responders and non-responders at baseline. The results showed that lipid and energy metabolism was elevated at baseline in responders ($n = 12$) compared to non-responders ($n = 17$). These findings highlight the importance of assessing the gut microbial functional genes at baseline before probiotic therapy initiation in patients with psychiatric disorders.

Keywords: gut microbiota; schizophrenia; depression; anxiety; probiotics; functional genes

1. Introduction

The close relationship between the gut and the brain, termed the gut–brain axis, is supported by numerous basic and clinical studies showing that the gut microbiota influences the host's mental state [1]. Probiotics, defined as "live microorganisms which when administered in adequate amounts confer a health benefit on the host", have been attracting attention as a novel treatment for mental disorders. Probiotics such as *Bifidobacterium* and *Lactobacillus* were determined in a recent meta-analysis to have mild beneficial effects on depressive symptoms in patients with mental disorders [2]. In line with the results of this meta-analysis, we also reported the beneficial effects of *Bifidobacterium breve* A-1 on anxiety and depressive symptoms in patients with schizophrenia [3].

While probiotics are attracting attention, some researchers have focused on the influence of the gut microbiota on the host response to pharmacotherapy [4]. For example, the efficacy of immune checkpoint inhibitors for cancer depends on the patient's gut microbiota [5]. Their anticancer effects are related to the relative abundance of *Bifidobacterium*, acting via augmented immune activity [6] and the amounts of metabolites produced by gut microbiota [7]. However, to our knowledge, it remains unclear how the baseline gut microbiota before probiotic administration influences the host's response to probiotic therapy. In this context, using data from our previous interventional study [3], we sought to determine which predicted functional profiles of the gut microbiota at baseline are associated with improvement of anxiety and depressive symptoms. This functional gene profiling approach allowed us to clarify the function of the gut microbiota as a whole.

2. Materials and Methods

2.1. Study Design and Procedure

Our previous interventional study was conducted from November 2017 to May 2018 [3]. We recruited participants among consecutive outpatients with schizophrenia based on the following inclusion and exclusion criteria. The inclusion criteria were as follows: outpatients, aged 20 years or older, not hospitalized for at least 6 months since last discharge, and anxiety and depressive symptoms rated by doctors as ≥ 10 points on the Brief Psychiatric Rating Scale anxiety and depressive subscale (items 1, 2, 5 and 9).

The exclusion criteria were as follows: uncontrolled disease or untreatable malignancy; cognitive impairment or disorientation; severe suicidal ideation or symptoms requiring urgent treatment; desire to take medication for anxiety or depressive symptoms; antidepressant medication in the past month; daily consumption of foods or supplements containing Bifidobacterium; heavy alcohol consumption (>500 mL of beer/day); psychiatric disorders other than schizophrenia, mood disorders, or anxiety disorders; any other conditions deemed inappropriate by the physician in charge.

For the first 4 weeks, the participants consumed two 2-g sachets of freeze-dried *Bifidobacterium breve* A-1 (synonym *B. breve* MCC1274) per day, each containing 5.0×10^{10} colony-forming units. Fecal samples were collected from each patient prior to probiotic administration, and subjective anxiety and depressive symptoms were assessed using the self-administered Hospital Anxiety and Depression Scale (HADS) [8] every 4 weeks. Participants showing a 25% or more reduction in the HADS total score at 4 weeks from baseline were regarded as displaying a clinical response. Participants showing a clinical response were defined as "responders" and those not showing a response were defined as "non-responders".

2.2. Bacterial DNA Extraction and Sequencing

Fecal bacterial DNA was extracted and purified as described previously [9]. We then amplified the V3–V4 region of bacterial 16S rRNA and sequenced it using the Illumina MiSeq platform (Illumina, San Diego, CA, USA) according to a previously described method [10].

2.3. Bioinformatics and Statistical Analysis

From trimming of the paired-end read FASTQ files obtained by 16S rRNA amplicon sequencing to analysis of gut microbiota diversity, all steps were carried out using QIIME 2. First, we demultiplexed the raw sequence results and used the Deblur algorithm to identify microbial operational taxonomic units (OTUs). The output feature table was diluted to 9000 sequences per sample. We then taxonomically classified the OTUs into 5 taxonomic rank categories—phylum, order, class, family, and genus—by using the SILVA 132 reference database at 99% similarity.

Phylogenetic Investigation of Communities by Reconstruction of Unobserved States 2 (PICRUSt2) was used to predict the gut microbial functional genes based on the 16S rRNA gene sequences with default settings. We then applied the linear discriminant analysis effect size (LEfSe) method with default settings to determine the gut microbial functional genes most likely to explain the differences between responders and non-responders at baseline. All statistical analyses were performed using R version 4.0.3 (R Core Team,

Vienna, Austria) [11], the ggplot2 [12] and the dplyr [13] packages. *p*-values less than 0.05 were considered statistically significant.

3. Results

3.1. Characteristics of the Study Participants

There were 12 responders and 17 non-responders. All were prescribed anti-psychotic medication, and none had their antipsychotic dosage changed during the study period. In addition, none of the participants used antibiotics, took diets or supplements containing *Bifidobacterium*, or consumed a high amount of alcohol during the study period. The median age of the responders was 46 years (interquartile range, 16 years) and that of the non-responders was 41 years (interquartile range, 16 years). There were no significant differences in age between the groups (*p* = 0.49). There were 8 women (66.7%) among the 12 responders and 9 women (52.9%) among the 17 non-responders (*p* = 0.290; data not shown). The proportion of the responders and the non-responders with comorbidity of physical disease was 41.7% and 29.4%, respectively (*p* = 0.490; data not shown). Furthermore, the mean (standard deviation (SD)) of the body mass index (BMI) of the responders and the non-responders was 26.5 (6.4) and 23.6 (5.1), respectively (*p* = 0.240; data not shown). Finally, the proportion of smokers among the responders and the non-responders was 41.7% and 35.3%, respectively (*p* = 0.730; data not shown).

3.2. Functional Gene Compositions of the Gut Microbiota at Baseline

The gut microbial functional genes whose relative abundances were significantly different between responders and non-responders at baseline in LEfSe analysis are shown in Figure 1. Compared with non-responders, responders showed higher relative abundances of 5 functional genes included in the Kyoto Encyclopedia of Genes and Genomes (KEGG) pathway "Metabolism" (Energy metabolism, glycosyltransferases, lipid metabolism, retinol metabolism, and penicillin and cephalosporin biosynthesis), one in "Genetic Information Processing" (Protein processing in endoplasmic reticulum), and one in "Organismal Systems" (Insulin signaling pathway) (Figure 1A,B). In contrast, non-responders showed higher relative abundances of 2 functional genes included in the KEGG pathway "Metabolism" (Nucleotide metabolism and glycerophospholipid metabolism) and 2 in "Genetic Information Processing" (RNA transport and base excision repair) (Figure 1). In addition, as shown in Figure 2, we compared 14 functional genes at the same level (KEGG pathway Level 2) included in "Metabolism". The relative abundances of the functional genes related to energy metabolism and lipid metabolism were higher in responders than in non-responders. In contrast, the relative abundances of the functional genes related to nucleotide metabolism were higher in non-responders than in responders.

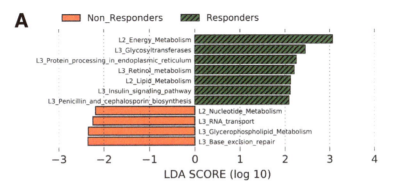

Figure 1. *Cont.*

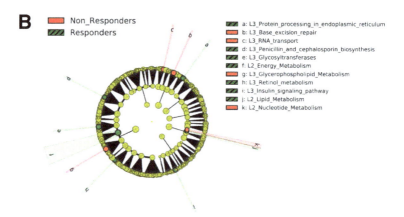

Figure 1. LDA scores calculated from features of the gut microbial functional genes found to exhibit different abundances between non-responders and responders at baseline. The criterion for feature selection was a $\log_{10}$ LDA score > 2.0. (**A**), Plot of pathways discovered by LEfSe ranked according to their effect size. (**B**), Cladogram representing the LEfSe results on the hierarchy. Abbreviations: L2, KEGG pathway Level 2; L3, KEGG pathway Level 3; LDA, linear discriminant analysis.

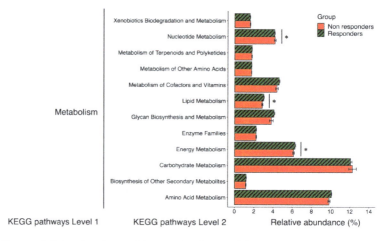

Figure 2. Relative abundances of functional pathways of the gut microbiota involved in metabolism. Error bars: standard error. * $p < 0.05$ on linear discriminant analysis effect size analysis (see Figure 1). KEGG, Kyoto Encyclopedia of Genes and Genomes.

4. Discussion

This is the first study examining the impact of the predicted functional profile of the gut microbiota at baseline on the therapeutic effects of probiotics using an interventional study in patients with mental disorder. Our results suggest that an elevated lipid and energy metabolism at baseline might be associated with the effects of probiotics on anxiety and depressive symptoms. As one potential mechanism, the end-products of lipid and energy metabolism by the gut microbiota may contribute to the maintenance of a healthy gut environment and influence anxiety and depressive symptoms associated with systemic inflammation in the host. These findings highlight the importance of assessing functional genes in the gut microbiota at baseline before probiotic therapy initiation for patients with mental disorders.

Among 11 bacterial functional genes found to have significantly different levels between responders and non-responders, "Lipid metabolism" and "Energy metabolism" are known to affect host metabolism and immune activity through their metabolites [14]. On the other hand, the other 9 bacterial functional genes play unknown roles in host metabolism and immune activity or are known to be housekeeping genes that are essential for maintaining functions in bacteria according to the KEGG. For example, glycerophospholipids are a major component of the bilayer envelope of Gram-negative bacteria and glycosyltransferases are involved in the biosynthesis of bacterial cell walls [15]. "Protein processing in endoplasmic reticulum" refers to the processing pathway in which proteins are glycosylated and folded in the endoplasmic reticulum within the bacteria, whereas "Insulin signaling pathway" is also involved in the insulin signaling pathway within bacteria. "RNA transport" is the pathway responsible for RNA transport from the bacterial nucleus to the cytoplasm, and "Base excision repair" is the major DNA damage repair pathway for processing small base lesions produced by oxidative and alkylation damage. These pathways are thus important for the maintenance of bacterial, not host, function. Therefore, of the pathways whose expression levels differed between the two groups in this study, all but Energy and Lipid metabolism are unlikely to be related to host homeostasis. Further in vitro and in vivo studies are needed to determine how these functional genes that play unknown roles in host metabolism and immune activity or that are known to be housekeeping genes influence the therapeutic response to probiotics.

The relative abundances of the functional pathways of "Lipid metabolism" and "Energy metabolism" of the gut microbiota at baseline were significantly higher in responders than in non-responders. These results might imply that the effects of *B. breve* A-1 on anxiety and depressive symptoms require sufficient lipid and energy metabolic function of the gut microbiota at baseline, although additional animal experiments and detailed mechanistic analysis are needed. The lipid and energy metabolic function of the gut microbiota has been linked to its ability to produce short-chain fatty acids (SCFAs). Gut bacteria consume and metabolize indigestible foods such as dietary fiber and mainly synthesize SCFAs as the final metabolites [16]. Gut bacteria also produce gases (CO_2, CH_4, H_2) and heat, but the gross energy of SCFAs is considerably higher than that of gases and heat [17]. High production of SCFAs prevents host obesity and maintains a healthy gut environment, which could affect anxiety-depression symptoms related to systemic inflammation in the host. SCFAs are sensed by G protein-coupled receptors expressed in adipose tissue as an indicator of energy status, preventing excessive fat deposition in adipose tissue and promoting fat utilization in other tissues [18]. SCFAs have are also a major energy source for intestinal epithelial cells and to play a key role in inhibiting the growth of bad bacteria and promoting the establishment of good bacteria by lowering intestinal pH [16].

Interestingly, *Bifidobacterium* has been reported to influence the metabolism of lipids with anti-inflammatory properties, such as SCFAs and polyunsaturated fatty acids (PUFAs). Administration of *Bifidobacterium* increases the production of the SCFA butyrate by altering the relative abundance of other microbiota involved in lipid metabolism [19]. Elevated butyrate in the gut has been reported to activate regulatory T cells and thereby reduce the host's systemic inflammation [20]. Furthermore, a higher relative abundance of *Bifidobacterium* is associated with higher levels of the PUFA docosahexaenoic acid, which is known to have anti-inflammatory properties [21]. Taken together, our results and those of these studies suggest that lipid metabolism could play an important role in the anti-inflammatory effects underlying the impact of *Bifidobacterium* on anxiety and depressive symptoms.

Evaluation and modification of the bacterial species and functional gene composition of the microbiota prior to therapy initiation may become an essential step in clinical practice to achieve maximum therapeutic efficacy. Indeed, technology for modifying the microbiota using the CRISPR-Cas system has already been established [22], and the application of this technology to clinical practice will be one of the cornerstones in the development of personalized medicine. In the field of psychiatry, where the response to treatment varies greatly from patient to patient, there are growing expectations for the evaluation of gut microbiota before therapeutic interventions and its modification.

We acknowledge that this study is subject to several important limitations. First, the functional gene analysis was performed not with shotgun metagenomic sequences, but with 16S rRNA gene sequences. One of the limitations of PICRUSt2 is that it predicts genes at the genomic level, not the transcriptional level. Therefore, what PICRUSt2 builds is not a profile of predicted functional activity, but rather a "potential" for predicted function, which needs to be interpreted with care. However, PICRUSt2, which we used to predict functional genes in the microbiota, can rigorously predict the abundance of pathways present based on a huge database of reference genomes and gene families, and the accuracy of metagenomic inference is sufficiently high [23]. Second, we did not conduct a detailed analysis of the differences in lipid and energy in particular. In the future, we would like to use metabolome analysis to measure SCFAs and lipid levels in the intestine gut and further investigate the role of SCFAs and lipid metabolism in the effects of probiotics. Third, it is unclear whether the present results can be extrapolated to depressive symptoms in patients with depression or to psychological distress in individuals without mental disorders because the study was focused on anxiety and depression in patients with schizophrenia. However, studies of gut bacteria in mental disorders have reported differences by symptom domain, regardless of differences by disease [24]. There may be a cross-disease relationship between gut bacteria and anxiety and depression, and further studies focusing on this aspect are needed.

5. Conclusions

In conclusion, our results indicate that elevated lipid and energy metabolism at baseline might be associated with the effects of probiotic treatment with *B. breve* A-1 on anxiety and depressive symptoms. The effect of probiotics on anxiety and depressive symptoms may require sufficient metabolic function of the gut microbiota at baseline. These findings highlight the importance of assessing functional genes in the gut microbiota at baseline before the initiation of probiotic therapy in patients with mental disorders. We believe that clinical application of the results of this study will lead to the realization of personalized medicine that maximizes the therapeutic effect on patients with mental disorders through gut microbiota analysis in the future.

Author Contributions: R.O., N.K., N.H., I.K., J.X. and Y.J.M. significantly contributed to making the protocol of this study. N.K., T.O. and J.X., who are the employee of Morinaga Milk Industry Co., Ltd., provided the test samples (*Bifidobacterium breve* A-1) and conducted analyses of the gut microbiome. R.O., N.H. and I.K. significantly contributed to the data collection. R.O. and R.Y. significantly contributed to the interpretation of our data and writing the manuscript. All authors have read and agreed to the published version of the manuscript.

Funding: Morinaga Milk Industry Co., Ltd. provided the test samples (*Bifidobacterium breve* A-1) and conducted analyses of the gut microbiome. A Japan Society for the Promotion of Science KAKENHI Grant-in-Aid for Young Scientists (Grant No. 19K20171), which Okubo has received, was used for manuscript writing and editing. Kusumi has received honoraria from Daiichi Sankyo, Dainippon Sumitomo Pharma, Eisai, Eli Lilly, Janssen Pharmaceutical, Lundbeck, Meiji Seika Pharma, Mochida Pharmaceutical, MSD, Mylan, Novartis Pharma, Ono Pharmaceutical, Otsuka Pharmaceutical, Pfizer, Shionogi, Shire, Taisho Toyama Pharmaceutical, Takeda Pharmaceutical, Tsumura, and Yoshito-miyakuhin outside the submitted work, and has received research/grant support from Asahi Kasei Pharma, Astellas, Daiichi Sankyo, Dainippon Sumitomo Pharma, Eisai, Eli Lilly, Mochida Pharmaceutical, Novartis Pharma, Otsuka Pharmaceutical, Pfizer, Shionogi, Takeda Pharmaceutical and Tanabe Mitsubishi Pharma outside the submitted work. Hashimoto received personal fees from Janssen Pharmaceutical, Yoshitomiyakuhin, Otsuka Pharmaceutical, Dainippon Sumitomo Pharma, Novartis Pharma, and Meiji Seika Pharma, outside the submitted work. Matsuoka has received speaker fees from Suntory Wellness, Pfizer, Mochida, Eli Lilly, Morinaga Milk outside the submitted work, and Cimic and is conducting collaborative research with SUSMED outside the submitted work.

Institutional Review Board Statement: The study was conducted according to the Declaration of Helsinki and approved by the Ethics Committee of Hokkaido University Hospital.

Informed Consent Statement: Informed consent was obtained from all subjects involved in the study.

Data Availability Statement: This study was registered in the University Hospital Medical Information Network Clinical Trials Registry (A study examining the effect of consuming foods containing probiotics on anxiety and depressive symptoms: a non-randomized and open trial, https://upload.umin.ac.jp/cgi-open-bin/ctr/ctr_view.cgi?recptno=R000029257 (accessed 29 September 2021), UMIN000025417).

Acknowledgments: We thank Asami Wada for managing the data collection schedule, and Koki Ito, Yuki Kako, Rie Kameyama, and Kuniyoshi Toyoshima for data collection.

Conflicts of Interest: Yamamura has nothing to disclose. Okubo reports grants from A Japan Society for the Promotion of Science, during the conduct of the study. Katsumata and Odamaki has nothing to disclose and are employees of Morinaga Milk Industry Co., Ltd. Hashimoto reports personal fees from Janssen Pharmaceutical, personal fees from Yoshitomiyakuhin, personal fees from Otsuka Pharmaceutical, personal fees from Dainippon Sumitomo Pharma, personal fees from Novartis Pharma, personal fees from Meiji Seika Pharma, outside the submitted work. Kusumi reports personal fees from Janssen Pharmaceutical, personal fees from Yoshitomiyakuhin, personal fees from Otsuka Pharmaceutical, personal fees from Dainippon Sumitomo Pharma, personal fees from Novartis Pharma, personal fees from Meiji Seika Pharma, personal fees from Daiichi Sankyo, personal fees from Eisai, personal fees from Eli Lilly, personal fees from Lundbeck, personal fees from Mochida Pharmaceutical, personal fees from MSD, personal fees from Mylan, personal fees from Ono Pharmaceutical, personal fees from Pfizer, personal fees from Shionogi, personal fees from Shire, personal fees from Taisho Toyama Pharmaceutical, personal fees from Takeda Pharmaceutical, personal fees from Tsumura, grants from Asahi Kasei Pharma, grants from Astellas, grants from Daiichi Sankyo, grants from Dainippon Sumitomo Pharma, grants from Eisai, grants from Eli Lilly, grants from Mochida Pharmaceutica, grants from Novartis Pharma, grants from Otsuka Pharmaceutical, grants from Pfizer, grants from Shionogi, grants from Takeda Pharmaceutical, grants from Tanabe Mitsubishi Pharma, outside the submitted work. Xiao has nothing to disclose and is an employee of Morinaga Milk Industry Co., Ltd. Matsuoka reports personal fees from Suntory Wellness, personal fees from Pfizer, personal fees from Mochida, personal fees from Eli Lilly, personal fees from Morinaga Milk, personal fees from Cimic, other from SUSMED, outside the submitted work. The funders had no role in the design of the study; in the collection, analyses, or interpreting of data; in the writing of the manuscript, or in the decision to publish the results.

References

1. Carabotti, M.; Scirocco, A.; Maselli, M.A.; Severi, C. The gut-brain axis: Interactions between enteric microbiota, central and enteric nervous systems. *Ann. Gastroenterol.* **2015**, *28*, 203–209. [PubMed]
2. Liu, R.T.; Walsh, R.F.L.; Sheehan, A.E. Prebiotics and probiotics for depression and anxiety: A systematic review and meta-analysis of controlled clinical trials. *Neurosci. Biobehav. Rev.* **2019**, *102*, 13–23. [CrossRef] [PubMed]
3. Okubo, R.; Koga, M.; Katsumata, N.; Odamaki, T.; Matsuyama, S.; Oka, M.; Narita, H.; Hashimoto, N.; Kusumi, I.; Xiao, J. Effect of bifidobacterium breve A-1 on anxiety and depressive symptoms in schizophrenia: A proof-of-concept study. *J. Affect. Disord.* **2019**, *245*, 377–385. [CrossRef] [PubMed]
4. Flowers, S.A.; Ward, K.M.; Clark, C.T. The Gut Microbiome in Bipolar Disorder and Pharmacotherapy Management. *Neuropsychobiology* **2020**, *79*, 43–49. [CrossRef]
5. Yan, X.; Zhang, S.; Deng, Y.; Wang, P.; Hou, Q.; Xu, H. Prognostic Factors for Checkpoint Inhibitor Based Immunotherapy: An Update With New Evidences. *Front. Pharmacol.* **2018**, *9*, 1050. [CrossRef]
6. Sivan, A.; Corrales, L.; Hubert, N.; Williams, J.B.; Aquino-Michaels, K.; Earley, Z.M.; Benyamin, F.W.; Lei, Y.M.; Jabri, B.; Alegre, M.-L. Commensal Bifidobacterium promotes antitumor immunity and facilitates anti–PD-L1 efficacy. *Science* **2015**, *350*, 1084–1089. [CrossRef]
7. Frankel, A.E.; Coughlin, L.A.; Kim, J.; Froehlich, T.W.; Xie, Y.; Frenkel, E.P.; Koh, A.Y. Metagenomic shotgun sequencing and unbiased metabolomic profiling identify specific human gut microbiota and metabolites associated with immune checkpoint therapy efficacy in melanoma patients. *Neoplasia* **2017**, *19*, 848–855. [CrossRef]
8. Kugaya, A.; Akechi, T.; Okuyama, T.; Okamura, H.; Uchitomi, Y. Screening for psychological distress in Japanese cancer patients. *Jpn. J. Clin. Oncol.* **1998**, *28*, 333–338. [CrossRef]
9. Odamaki, T.; Kato, K.; Sugahara, H.; Hashikura, N.; Takahashi, S.; Xiao, J.Z.; Abe, F.; Osawa, R. Age-related changes in gut icrobiota composition from newborn to centenarian: A cross-sectional study. *BMC Microbiol.* **2016**, *16*, 90. [CrossRef]
10. Kato, K.; Ishida, S.; Tanaka, M.; Mitsuyama, E.; Xiao, J.-Z.; Odamaki, T. Association between functional lactase variants and a high abundance of Bifidobacterium in the gut of healthy Japanese people. *PLoS ONE* **2018**, *13*, e0206189. [CrossRef]
11. R Core Team. *R: A Language and Environment for Statistical Computing*; R Foundation for Statistical Computing: Vienna, Austria, 2017.

12. Villanueva, R.A.M.; Chen, Z.J. ggplot2: Elegant Graphics for Data Analysis (2nd ed.). *Meas. Interdiscip. Res. Perspect.* **2019**, *17*, 160–167. [CrossRef]
13. Wickham, H.; François, R. Dplyr: A Grammar of Data Manipulation. Available online: https://CRAN.R-project.org/package= dplyr (accessed on 29 September 2021).
14. Heiss, C.N.; Olofsson, L.E. Gut Microbiota-Dependent Modulation of Energy Metabolism. *J. Innate Immun.* **2018**, *10*, 163–171. [CrossRef] [PubMed]
15. Dalebroux, Z.D. Cues from the Membrane: Bacterial Glycerophospholipids. *J. Bacteriol.* **2017**, *199*, e00136-17. [CrossRef] [PubMed]
16. Yamamura, R.; Nakamura, K.; Kitada, N.; Aizawa, T.; Shimizu, Y.; Nakamura, K.; Ayabe, T.; Kimura, T.; Tamakoshi, A. Associations of gut microbiota, dietary intake, and serum short-chain fatty acids with fecal short-chain fatty acids. *Biosci. Microbiota Food Health* **2020**, *39*, 11–17. [CrossRef] [PubMed]
17. Wong, J.M.; de Souza, R.; Kendall, C.W.; Emam, A.; Jenkins, D.J. Colonic health: Fermentation and short chain fatty acids. *J. Clin. Gastroenterol.* **2006**, *40*, 235–243. [CrossRef] [PubMed]
18. Kimura, I.; Inoue, D.; Maeda, T.; Hara, T.; Ichimura, A.; Miyauchi, S.; Kobayashi, M.; Hirasawa, A.; Tsujimoto, G. Short-chain fatty acids and ketones directly regulate sympathetic nervous system via G protein-coupled receptor 41 (GPR41). *Proc. Natl. Acad. Sci. USA* **2011**, *108*, 8030–8035. [CrossRef] [PubMed]
19. Sugahara, H.; Odamaki, T.; Fukuda, S.; Kato, T.; Xiao, J.-Z.; Abe, F.; Kikuchi, J.; Ohno, H. Probiotic Bifidobacterium longum alters gut luminal metabolism through modification of the gut microbial community. *Sci. Rep.* **2015**, *5*, 13548. [CrossRef] [PubMed]
20. Furusawa, Y.; Obata, Y.; Fukuda, S.; Endo, T.A.; Nakato, G.; Takahashi, D.; Nakanishi, Y.; Uetake, C.; Kato, K.; Kato, T.; et al. Commensal microbe-derived butyrate induces the differentiation of colonic regulatory T cells. *Nature* **2013**, *504*, 446–450. [CrossRef]
21. Horigome, A.; Okubo, R.; Hamazaki, K.; Kinoshita, T.; Katsumata, N.; Uezono, Y.; Xiao, J.Z.; Matsuoka, Y.J. Association between blood omega-3 polyunsaturated fatty acids and the gut microbiota among breast cancer survivors. *Benef Microbes* **2019**, *10*, 751–758. [CrossRef]
22. Ramachandran, G.; Bikard, D. Editing the microbiome the CRISPR way. *Philos. Trans. R. Soc. B* **2019**, *374*, 20180103. [CrossRef]
23. Douglas, G.M.; Maffei, V.J.; Zaneveld, J.R.; Yurgel, S.N.; Brown, J.R.; Taylor, C.M.; Huttenhower, C.; Langille, M.G.I. PICRUSt2 for prediction of metagenome functions. *Nat. Biotechnol.* **2020**, *38*, 685–688. [CrossRef] [PubMed]
24. Nguyen, T.T.; Kosciolek, T.; Maldonado, Y.; Daly, R.E.; Martin, A.S.; McDonald, D.; Knight, R.; Jeste, D.V. Differences in gut microbiome composition between persons with chronic schizophrenia and healthy comparison subjects. *Schizophr. Res.* **2019**, *204*, 23–29. [CrossRef] [PubMed]

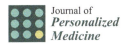

Review

Gut and Endometrial Microbiome Dysbiosis: A New Emergent Risk Factor for Endometrial Cancer

Soukaina Boutriq [1,2,3], Alicia González-González [1,2], Isaac Plaza-Andrades [1,2], Aurora Laborda-Illanes [1,2,3], Lidia Sánchez-Alcoholado [1,2,3], Jesús Peralta-Linero [1,2], María Emilia Domínguez-Recio [1], María José Bermejo-Pérez [1], Rocío Lavado-Valenzuela [2,*], Emilio Alba [1,4,*] and María Isabel Queipo-Ortuño [1,2,4]

[1] Unidad de Gestión Clínica Intercentros de Oncología Médica, Hospitales Universitarios Regional y Virgen de la Victoria, Instituto de Investigación Biomédica de Málaga (IBIMA)-CIMES-UMA, 29010 Málaga, Spain; soukaina@ibima.eu (S.B.); alicia.gonzalez@ibima.eu (A.G.-G.); isaac.plaza.andrades@ibima.eu (I.P.-A.); aurora.laborda@ibima.eu (A.L.-I.); l.sanchez.alcoholado@ibima.eu (L.S.-A.); jesus.peralta@ibima.eu (J.P.-L.); emilia.dominguez@ibima.eu (M.E.D.-R.); cheberpe@gmail.com (M.J.B.-P.); maribel.queipo@ibima.eu (M.I.Q.-O.)
[2] Instituto de Investigación Biomédica de Málaga (IBIMA), Campus de Teatinos s/n, 29071 Málaga, Spain
[3] Facultad de Medicina, Universidad de Málaga, 29071 Málaga, Spain
[4] Centro de Investigación Biomédica en Red de Cáncer (Ciberonc CB16/12/00481), 28029 Madrid, Spain
* Correspondence: rocio.lavado@ibima.eu (R.L.-V.); ealbac@uma.es (E.A.)

Abstract: Endometrial cancer is one of the most common gynaecological malignancies worldwide. Histologically, two types of endometrial cancer with morphological and molecular differences and also therapeutic implications have been identified. Type I endometrial cancer has an endometrioid morphology and is estrogen-dependent, while Type II appears with non-endometrioid differentiation and follows an estrogen-unrelated pathway. Understanding the molecular biology and genetics of endometrial cancer is crucial for its prognosis and the development of novel therapies for its treatment. However, until now, scant attention has been paid to environmental components like the microbiome. Recently, due to emerging evidence that the uterus is not a sterile cavity, some studies have begun to investigate the composition of the endometrial microbiome and its role in endometrial cancer. In this review, we summarize the current state of this line of investigation, focusing on the relationship between gut and endometrial microbiome and inflammation, estrogen metabolism, and different endometrial cancer therapies.

Keywords: endometrial cancer; endometrial microbiome; gut microbiome; dysbiosis; estrogen metabolism; estrobolome; inflammation; antitumour treatment; prebiotics; probiotics

1. Introduction

The endometrium is a very dynamic tissue that undergoes proliferation and differentiation processes during the menstrual cycle in response to variations in the levels of steroid sex hormones (estrogen and progesterone) produced in the ovaries, and the release of local factors [1].

Endometrial cancer is the sixth most common malignancy in women, and the fifteenth most common cancer [2]. It accounts for nearly 5% of total cancer cases and more than 2% of cancer deaths among women worldwide [3]. In the United States and some European countries, the incidence of endometrial cancer is higher than in other developed countries, being the fourth most common cancer in women, accounting for approximately 6% of new cancer cases and 3% of cancer deaths each year [4].

This high incidence in the United States and Europe compared to other countries may be due to high rates of obesity, as well as other important risk factors such as advanced age, early menarche, late menopause, nulliparity, and post-menopausal estrogen therapy [5]. Endometrial cancer occurs more frequently after menopause and is generally associated with a good prognosis [6].

Whereas high parity, late age at last birth, physical activity, the use of combined oral contraceptives and tabacco consumption are considered factors with a protective role against endometrial cancer [7], there are other several factors that increase the risk of endometrial cancer, such as obesity, the use of hormone replacement therapy (HRT) to treat menopausal symptoms, and a family history of cancers such as Lynch syndrome (an autosomal dominant disorder characterized by juvenile onset of malignant tumours and colorectal cancer). Women with Lynch syndrome have an increased endometrial cancer risk as well as an increased risk for other types of cancer such us colorectal cancer [8]. This syndrome is caused by a loss-of-function germline mutation in one of four genes (human mutL homolog 1 (*MLH1*), *MSH2*, *MSH6*, and *PMS1* Homolog 2 (*PMS2*)) involved in mismatch-pair recognition and initiation of repair [9]. *MLH1* and *MSH2* mutations are more frequent (60–80%) in patients with lynch syndrome compared to *MSH6* and *PMS2* mutations. Mutation in epithelial cellular adhesion molecule (*EPCAM*) (gene located in *MSH2* gene promoter and that lead to its epigenetic inactivation) is also identificated in lynch syndrome. The mismatch repair genes inactivation induces accumulation of different gene mutations, leading to cancer development with microsatellite instability phenotype [10].

Bokhman was the first to classify endometrial cancer into two different histological types in 1983 [11]. This classification, into Type I and Type II endometrial cancer, has revealed the existence of differences in molecular characteristics, which consequently translate into differences in prognosis and treatment [12]. In Bokhman's study, the frequency of the first pathological type (Type I) in the group of women studied was 65%, while the frequency of the second type (Type II) was 35% [13].

Endometrioid, or Type I endometrial cancer generally originates in a hyperplastic endometrial context [14], expressing estrogen and progesterone receptors, and is therefore typically associated with hormonal disorders [15]. In addition to phosphatase and tensin homolog (*PTEN*) and phosphatidylinositol 3-kinase (*PIK3CA*) mutations, which are the most common in Type I endometrial cancer, other mutations have been identified in *KRAS* and cadherin associated protein (*β-catenin*) genes [16]. In some Type I endometrial cancers, mutations that inactivate *MSH6* have been identified as being associated with microsatellite instability [17] (Figure 1).

Non-endometrioid, or Type II endometrial cancer, is less common, accounting for approximately 10–20% of endometrial cancer cases [18]. Type II endometrial cancer develops in an atrophic endometrial context, histologically poorly differentiated, with a tendency towards a deep invasion into the myometrium, and a high frequency of metastasis [19]. Type II endometrial cancer is characterized by a high number of tumour suppressor *p53* mutations [20], and other low-frequency genomic alterations such as tumour suppressor cyclin-dependent kinase inhibitor 2A (*p16*) inactivation and Erb-B2 receptor tyrosine kinase 2 (*HER-2/neu*) over-activation [17]. Type II endometrial carcinoma includes carcinosarcomas, serous and clear cell carcinomas, and mixed Mullerian tumours [21] (Figure 1).

However, genetic alterations alone are not enough to explain the origins of endometrial cancer; other environmental factors such as hormones, obesity, and diabetes also have an influence, as does the microbiome, which comprises an important part of the uterine microenvironment [22]. Nevertheless, the molecular mechanisms involved in the interaction between microbiome and endometrial cancer still need further elucidation.

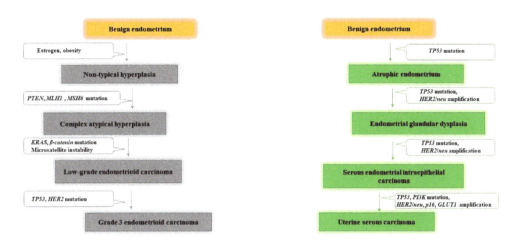

Figure 1. Commonly altered genes in endometrial carcinogenesis. Endometrioid carcinoma is estrogen dependent, and obesity is associated with an elevated endometrioid cancer risk and mortality. Several mutations can lead to initiation and development of endometrioid carcinoma, such as *PTEN*, *KRAS* and *β-catenin* mutations, wheras non-endometrioid carcinoma more often harbours mutations in *TP53*. PTEN: phosphatase and tensin homolog. MLH1: human mutL homolog 1, involved in DNA mismatch repair. MSH6: human mutS homolog 6, involvedd in DNA mismatch repair. KRAS: KRAS proto-oncogene, GTPase. β-catenin: CTNNB gene (cadherin associated protein) a signaling molecule involved in the control of cell growth and differentiation. TP53: tumour protein p53, tumour supressor. HER2/neu: Erb-B2 receptor tyrosine kinase 2, proto-oncogen. PI3K: phosphatidylinositol 3-kinase, proto-oncogen. P16: cyclin-dependent kinase inhibitor 2A gene, tumour supressor. Glut1: glucose transporter 1.

2. Endometrial Microbiome

Previously, it had long been thought that the human uterus was a sterile environment free of microorganisms. However, recent studies using molecular techniques have confirmed the existence of microbiota in the endometrium, playing an important role in the proper functioning of the endometrium and in the development of pregnancy under normal conditions [23].

In the vagina, the microbiota has an important preventive role against various urogenital diseases, such as bacterial vaginosis, fungal infections, sexually transmitted infections, urinary tract infections, and HIV. This protective role is mainly due to the production of lactic acid by *Lactobacillus* species (spp.), which are commonly associated with a healthy vagina, and which produce several bacteriostatic and bactericidal components that help to lower the pH of the vaginal microenvironment and promote competitive exclusion [24]. However, the composition of vaginal microbiota varies between the different phases of menopause (pre-, peri-, and post-menopause) and also in pathological conditions such as vaginal atrophy in which the abundance of *Lactobacillus* decreases while *Anaerococcus*, *Peptoniphilus*, and *Prevotella* levels increase [25].

Until now, few studies have been devoted to investigating the composition of endometrial microbiota, so it is a subject that remains quite obscure today.

Many of the studies done have confirmed that, as in the vagina, *Lactobacillus* is the dominant genus in the endometrium. In fact, Mitchell et al. compared vaginal microbiota with uterine microbiota and found that the endometrium is characterized by the presence of *Lactobacillus*, being the most abundant genus, followed by *Gardnerella*, *Prevotella*, *Atopobium*, and *Sneathia* [26]. Fang et al. compared the bacterial composition of the vagina with that of the endometrium, and also compared endometrial microbiome composition between patients in different situations including healthy women, patients with endometrial polyps, and patients with chronic endometritis. They found that Proteobacteria, Firmicutes, and Actinobacteria dominated the intrauterine microbiome in all the studied groups. Furthermore, although they found significant differences between the vaginal and the endometrial microbiome, at the genus level, *Lactobacillus*, *Gardnerella*, *Bifidobacterium*, *Streptococcus*, and *Alteromonas* were significantly higher in the healthy group when compared with the others [27].

However, in contrast to these studies, others have suggested that non-*Lactobacillus* species are more common in the endometrium. In 2016, Verstraelen et al. found that 90% of the women included in their study had an endometrial microbiota profile dominated by *Bacteroides* (*Bacteroides xylanisolvens*, *Bacteroides thetaiotaomicron*, and *Bacteroides fragilis*) and *Pelomonas* [28]. Chen et al. confirmed the existence of different bacterial communities throughout the female reproductive system, with a continuous change from the vagina to the ovaries, with *Pseudomonas*, *Acinetobacter*, *Vagococcus*, and *Sphingobium* being the most abundant in the endometrium [29]. Winters et al. also sequenced endometrial samples from 25 women who underwent total hysterectomy for fibroids or endometrial hyperplasia, and found that the most abundant genera in their endometria were *Acinetobacter*, *Pseudomonas*, *Comamonadaceae*, and *Cloacibacterium* [30]. Finally, in a more recent study, Lu et al. also suggested that *Lactobacillus* is not the predominant genus in the endometrium, observing a greater abundance of *Rhodococcus*, *Phyllobacterium*, *Sphingomonas*, *Bacteroides*, and *Bifidobacterium* [31] (Table 1).

Table 1. Endometrial microbiome characterization studies.

Author	Year	Sample Size	Sample Type	Methods	Finding
Mitchell et al.	2018	Women underwent hysteroctomy for benign disease without cancer indications (n = 58).	Vaginal and endometrial swabs.	Bacterial 16S rRNA sequencing.	↑*Lactobacillus iners* (45%), *Lactobacillus crispatus* (33%), *Gardnerella vaginalis*, *Prevotella* spp., *Atopobium vaginae*, and *Sneathia*.
Fang et al.	2016	-Patients with only endometrial polyps (n = 10). -Patients with both endometrial polyps and chronic endometritis (n = 10). -Healthy women (n = 10).	Vaginal and endometrial swabs.	Bacterial 16S rRNA genes sequencing.	↑*Lactobacillus*, *Gardnerella*, *Bifidobacterium*, *Streptococcus*, and *Alteromonas* in healthy group compared to endometrial polyps and chronic endometriosis group.
Verstraelen et al.	2016	Women with various reproductive conditions, without uterine anomalies (n = 90).	Endometrial biopsy: tissue and mucus.	16S rRNA gene V1–2 region	Uterine microbiome dominated by *Bacteroides* (*B. xylanisolvens*, *B. thetaiotaomicron*, and *B. fragilis*) and *Pelomonas*.
Chen et al.	2017	Reproductive age women operated for conditions not known to involve infection (n = 95).	Endometrial swab and tissue.	16S rRNA amplicon sequencing	↑*Pseudomonas*, *Acinetobacter*, *Vagococcus*, and *Sphingobium* in the endometrium
Winters et al.	2019	Women (n = 25) underwent a hysterectomy for fibroids (23) and endometrial hyperplasia (2).	Endometrial swab.	Sequencing of the 16S rRNA gene.	↑*Acinetobacter*, *Pseudomonas*, Comamonadaceae, and *Cloacibacterium* in endometrium.
Lu et al.	2020	Women undergone a hysterectomy for benign disease and any stage of endometrial cancer (n = 50).	Endometrial tissue.	16S rRNA gene sequencing for bacterial communities.	↑*Rhodococcus*, *Phyllobacterium*, *Sphingomonas*, *Bacteroides*, and *Bifidobacterium*.

3. Microbiome and Endometrial Cancer

Currently, there is abundant evidence demonstrating the involvement of bacteria in the development and expansion of various pathologies, including different types of cancers [32]. Many of the bacteria that colonize the human body establish beneficial relationships with their host. Notwithstanding, dysbiosis promotes the development of various diseases [33].

For example, in the stomach, *Helicobacter pylori* is one of the most common human infectious agents that produces several virulence factors linked to significant disorders in the host's intracellular signalling pathways, favouring the appearance of neoplastic transformations. Consequently, infection by this bacterium is considered to be an important risk factor for gastrointestinal cancer [34]. Furthermore, in cervical (cervix) cancer, human papillomavirus is a known cause of the disease [35].

It is known that the pathogenesis of endometrial cancer involves mainly an excess of estrogen levels, and there is also evidence that the composition of the microbiota may be an important risk factor, given the inflammatory profile in endometrial cancer. However, the composition of endometrial microbiota in endometrial cancer remains poorly studied.

Accordingly, Walther-Antónuio et al. identified the differences in the composition of endometrial microbiota in different diseases. In women with abnormal bleeding and endometritis they found *Shigella* and *Barnesiella* to be the most dominant genera in their endometria. They also observed that there is a difference in the composition of the endometrial microbiota under normal conditions as compared with hyperplasia, which suggests a role for microbiota in the early phases of cell transformation, since hyperplasia is considered to be a precancerous transformation of the endometrium. To test this hypothesis, they compared the microbiota of patients with endometrial hyperplasia and those with endometrial cancer, and found no significant differences. Furthermore, as a result of sequencing samples from endometrial cancer patients, they saw that the taxa Firmicutes (*Anaerostipes*, *ph2*, *Dialister*, *Peptoniphilus*, *1–68*, *Ruminococcus*, and *Anaerotruncus*), Spirochaetes (*Treponema*), Actinobacteria (*Atopobium*), Bacteroidetes (*Bacteroides* and *Porphyromonas*), and Proteobacteria (*Arthrospira*) were enriched. However, the most prevalent result they obtained is the close correlation between the species *Atopobium vaginae* and *Porphyromonas sp.* and endometrial cancer, especially when the vaginal pH is high (>4.5) [22]. *Porphyromonas gingivalis* is considered to be a biomarker of death risk from aerodigestive cancer, independent of periodontal diseases [36]. Based on the relationship between this bacteria and various pathologies, Walther-Antónuio et al. predicted the possible involvement of *Porphyromonas* spp. in the progression of the processes leading to the development of endometrial cancer. Furthermore, knowing that *Atopobium vaginae* is associated with bacterial vaginosis, they hypothesized that it may be involved in creating chronic inflammation that leads to local immune dysregulation, thus facilitating intracellular infection by *Porphyromonas* species [22]. Moreover, *Porphyromonas* spp. combined with high pH in the vagina could be a promising biomarker for endometrial cancer [37].

Lu et al. demonstrated that there is a difference in the composition of endometrial microbiota between patients with endometrial cancer and patients with benign uterine lesions. In the results they obtained, a decrease in the local diversity of the microbiota was observed in the group of patients with endometrial cancer compared to patients with benign uterine lesions. This decrease in the diversity of microorganisms led to the overgrowth of the few remaining species and a decrease in resilience. Furthermore, in this study, *Pseudomoramibacter_Eubacterium*, *Rhodobacter*, *Vogesella*, *Bilophila*, *Rheinheimera*, and *Megamonas* were enriched in patients with benign uterine lesions, while *Micrococcus* was associated with an inflammatory profile in endometrial cancer [31].

With the aim of studying the possible differences in bacterial, archaea, and viral transcript (BAVT) in different gynaecological cancers and in normal fallopian tubes, Gonzalez-Bosquet et al. carried out a metagenomic analysis of high-grade serous carcinoma (HGSC) and endometrioid endometrial carcinoma (EEC), and compared them with normal fallopian tubes. They found that there were 93 BAVTs differentially expressed between HGSC and EEC. However, 12 BAVT species were independently expressed in all the samples, and 6 of them were also significantly expressed (*Pusillimonas* sp. *ye³*, *Riemerella anatipestifer*, *Salinibacter ruber*, *Bacillus tropicus*, *Nostocales cyanobacterium HT-58-2*, and *Corynebacterium pseudotuberculosis*). Nevertheless, in normal samples these BAVT species were the highest, while they were decreased in EEC, and even more so in HGSC samples.

Gonzalez-Bosquet et al. also investigated the origins of these BAVTs, and they saw some human loci that harbour genetic material from these microorganisms; more exactly BAVTs were located within or close to genes or lncRNAS [38].

Walsh et al., like Walther et al., identified *Porphyromonas somerae* as the most abundant organism in patients with endometrial cancer. They also found that in addition to obesity and postmenopause, a high vaginal pH is considered an additional risk factor for endometrial cancer. In that study, they confirmed that *Porphyromonas somerae* is not associated with postmenopause; it is, however, related to four other microorganisms (*Anaerococcus tetradius*, *Anaerococcus lactolyticus*, *Peptoniphilus coxii*, and *Campylobacter ureolyticus*) which are associated with postmenopause, suggesting that they could be first-colonizers to facilitate the subsequent colonization by *Porphyromonas somerae* and others. *Porphyromonas somerae* was found in 100% of samples from patients with Type II endometrial cancer and in 57% of patients with endometrial hyperplasia. Therefore, *Porphyromonas somerae* is considered to be a biomarker of the disease.

In contrast to the results obtained by Lu et al. which affirm that the diversity of the local microbiota decreases in endometrial cancer, Walsh et al. observed that the risk factors for endometrial cancer (postmenopause, obesity, and high vaginal pH) increase the diversity of endometrial microbiota. Walsh et al. identified seventeen enriched taxa in patients with endometrial cancer, eight of which were enriched by menopause. Because of the prominence of postmenopause as a risk factor for endometrial cancer, it could be considered as one of the main conditions that favour the disease state [39]. In postmenopausal women, the production of ovarian estrogens ceases, leading to a decrease in glycogen levels, which induces a decrease in colonization by *Lactobacillus*, basifying the pH of the medium. Under normal conditions, *Lactobacillus* produces lactic acid that contributes to the maintenance of the low pH of the vagina, so it can act as a selective barrier to the rest of the reproductive system, avoiding its colonization by pathogens and helping to maintain the microbiota specific to each part of the reproductive system [40].

According to circumstances, species favoured by menopause are not directly involved in endometrial cancer, but they are probably facilitating colonization by other species associated with endometrial cancer [39]. *Atopobium vaginae* is a characteristic pathogen of bacterial vaginosis [41]. It is conceivable that some women with endometrial cancer may have been previously diagnosed with bacterial vaginosis, which could explain the association of this bacteria with endometrial cancer [39] (Table 2).

Table 2. Studies of intratumoural microbiota in endometrial cancer patients.

Author	Year	Simple Size	Sample Type	Methods	Finding
Walther-António et al.	2016	-Patients with endometrial cancer ($n = 17$). -Patients with endometrial hyperplasia ($n = 4$). -Patients with benign uterine conditions ($n = 10$).	Endometrial swab and scrabe.	16S rRNA sequencing of V3-V5 region.	Patients with endometrial cancer: ↑Firmicutes (*Anaerostipes*, *ph2*, *Dialister*, *Peptoniphilus*, *1–68*, *Ruminococcus*, and *Anaerotruncus*), Spirochaetes (*Treponema*), Actinobacteria (*Atopobium*), Bacteroidetes (*Bacteroides* and *Porphyromonas*), and Proteobacteria (*Arthrospira*). Close correlation between *Atopobium vaginae* and *Porphyromonas* spp. and endometrial cancer, especially when the vaginal pH is high (>4.5).
Lu et al.	2020	Patients undergone a hysterectomy for benign disease and any stage of endometrial cancer ($n = 50$).	Endometrial cancer tissue.	16S rRNA gene sequencing for bacterial communities.	↓Local microbiome diversity in patients with endomatrial cancer. ↑*Micrococcus* associated with an inflammatory profile in endometrial cancer patients.
Gonzalez-Bosquet et al.	2021	-Patients with high grade serous ovarian cancer (HGSC) ($n = 112$). -Patients with endometrioid endometrial cancer (EEC) ($n = 62$). -Women with normal fallopian tubes, and no risk factors for cancer ($n = 12$).	Frozen ovarian and endometrial tumour tissue.	16S rRNA gene sequencing.	-93 bacterial, archaea, and viral transcripts (BAVTs) were differentially expressed between HGSC and EEC. -The diversity of BAVT species decreased in EEC, and even more in HGSC compared to normal samples.
Walsh et al.	2019	Patients with a variety of uterine conditions ($n = 148$): -Patients without endometrial cancer ($n = 75$). -Patients with Type I endometrial cancer ($n = 56$). -Patients with Type II endometrial cancer ($n = 10$). -Patients with complex atypical hyperplasia ($n = 7$).	Uterine, fallopian and ovarian samples (swabs and scrapes)	-Amplification and sequencing of V3-V5 region of the 16S rRNA gene.	In endometrial cancer patients: ↑*Porphyromonas somerae*. ↑*Anaerococcus tetradius*, *Anaerococcus lactolyticus*, *Peptoniphilus coxii*, and *Campylobacter ureolyticus* related to postmenopause status, facilitating the subsequent colonization by *Porphyromonas somerae*.

4. Estrogen Metabolism, Gut Microbiota, and Endometrial Cancer

Estrogens play a major role in modulating the growth of the endometrium by inducing proliferation at the end of the proliferative phase of the menstrual cycle [42]. However, after ovulation, in the luteal phase, the increase in estrogen levels induces the production of progesterone which inhibits the proliferation of the endometrium, and promotes its transition to a receptive state, preparing it for the implantation of a blastocyst. An increase in estrogen levels leads to an imbalance between the production of estrogens and progesterone, favouring the appearance and development of endometrial cancer [43].

Endometrioid carcinoma accounts for 80% of all endometrial cancer cases. This type of endometrial cancer is fundamentally caused by excessive exposure to estrogens which, in the absence of the counteractive effects of progesterone, induces endometrial proliferation and therefore endometrial hyperplasia and ultimately cancer [44].

Estrogens are produced in the ovaries and are then transported to the organs, including the uterus and breasts, where they have different functions. Later, they are transported to the liver where they are metabolized to facilitate their elimination from the body. The estrogenic hormones, estrone (E1) and estradiol (E2), undergo irreversible hydroxylation at the C-2, C-4, or C-16 carbon of the steroid ring. Estrogen metabolites are conjugated by sulfonation or glucuronidation, producing changes in their structure and bioavailability. Conjugated estrogens are excreted in urine or bile. Finally, the inactive conjugated estrogens excreted in the bile are transported to the distal part of the intestine to be eliminated through faeces [45].

However, inactive estrogens in the intestine are occasionally activated by deconjugation and are reabsorbed through the intestinal mucosa and enter the bloodstream via the portal vein (Figure 2). It has been established that the intestinal microbiota is involved in the reactivation of estrogens and, therefore, in the regulation of estrogen levels [46]. Estrobolome was defined for the first time in 2011 as an aggregate of genes from enteric bacteria, whose products are capable of metabolizing estrogens, specifically, bacteria with β-glucuronidase activity, an enzyme involved in the deconjugation of estrogens [47].

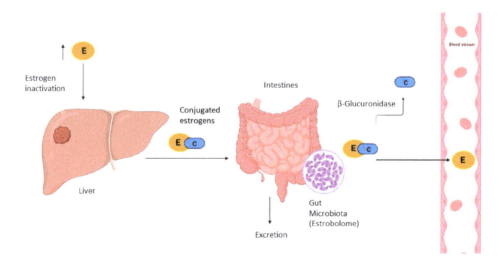

Figure 2. Estrogen metabolism involving gut microbiota (estrobolome). Estrogens are inactivated in liver through conjugation for further excretion. However, some of inactivated estrogens are reabsorbed into the bloodstream across activation in intestines by estrobolome. E: estrogen; C: conjugation with glucuronide acid binding.

β-glucuronidase activity plays a significant role in the generation of toxic and carcinogenic metabolites in the intestine, and also in the reabsorption of various compounds into the circulatory system, such as estrogens [48]. β-glucuronidase facilitates binding to estrogen receptors, and the activation of these receptors increases the number of cells in the G0/G1 phase of the cell cycle, promoting proliferation, a process well described in breast cancer, highlighting the relationship existing between gut microbiota and estrogen levels in breast cancer.

Like breast cancer, endometrial cancer is also considered to be hormone-dependent, in which the intestinal microbiota is involved, especially in obese patients. There is a possibility that the composition and diversity of the microbiota favours bacteria capable of metabolizing estrogens, which allows greater reabsorption of estrogens and increased binding to receptors, contributing to the development of endometrial hyperplasia and endometrial cancer [49].

An active estrobolome is capable of modulating endogenous estrogen metabolism by β-glucuronidase and β-glucosidase enzymatic activity, thereby controlling circulating and excreted estrogen levels. In the gastrointestinal tract, the most important genes encoding β-glucuronidase enzyme activity are the β-glucuronidase (*GUS*) genes (Figure 2). Recently, an atlas for the characterization of the β-glucuronidase of the human intestinal microbiota was compiled. Approximately 112 new *GUS* genes were identified and grouped into six classes expressed in four bacterial phyla, denominated as Bacteroidetes, Firmicutes, Verrucomicrobia, and Proteobacteria. Within them, the phylum Bacteroidetes presents a greater abundance and diversity of *GUS* enzymes [50]. β-glucuronidase activity is modulated by diet and the microbiota. A diet rich in fat or protein has been associated with high faecal levels of β-glucuronidase, while a fibre-based diet decreases the activity of this enzyme. Furthermore, the β-glucuronidase activity of *Escherichia coli* cultures is controlled by population density, suggesting the involvement of quorum sensing in the control of enzyme activity. Although it remains to be determined how β-glucuronidase and β-glucosidase contribute to breast and endometrial cancer, there is ample evidence which suggests that both play an important role [51].

In one of their studies, Flores et al. found that in postmenopausal women and in men, non-ovarian estrogen levels were closely associated with the amount and diversity of faecal microbiota, with the taxa Clostridia within Firmicutes being the most related, in addition to three genera of the Ruminococcaceae family. Furthermore, the activity of β-glucuronidase has been associated with the levels of estrone, but not estrogen, in urine, whereas in pre-menopausal women, estrogen levels are not influenced by the microbiota or by β-glucuronidase activity [46].

Therefore, estrobolome can modulate circulating estrogen levels, which can alter vaginal microbial communities. In accordance with this concept, previous studies have established that gut microbiome is indirectly involved in endometrial carcinogenesis through its altering of genital microbial communities [52]. Thus, more attention is being paid to the study of gut microbiome modulation methods to treat estrogen-dependent diseases, including endometrial cancer, through bariatric surgery, faecal bacteria transfer, the use of pharmaceutical (Metformin) and nutraceutical (Genistein) methods, which in several studies have shown favourable results in treating the metabolic aspects of the disease [49].

5. Microbiome, Inflammation, and Endometrial Cancer

In 1863, Rudolf Virchow discovered the existence of leukocytes in neoplastic tissues, and established a correlation between inflammation and cancer. Since then, many studies have relied on Virchow's hypothesis to investigate cancer prevention and treatment methods [53]. There are many examples that support this hypothesis, such as hepatitis and liver cancer, or colitis and colorectal cancer. In addition, the use of non-steroidal anti-inflammatory drugs has been shown to reduce the risk of various cancers.

Even though the mechanisms by which local inflammation facilitates cancer development are unknown, the production of cytokines, such as tumour necrosis factor α (TNF-α) by local tissue and infiltrated inflammatory cells, seems to play a key role [54]. Chronic inflammation promotes angiogenesis, cell proliferation, and the production of free radicals that cause DNA damage and facilitate tumour initiation and development [55].

After menopause, when estrogen production comes to an end, most of the circulating estrogens are produced in adipose tissue through the conversion of androgens by the enzyme Aromatase [56]. IL-6 has been shown to stimulate aromatase activity in adipose tissue and in endometrial cancer stromal cells, which then increases estrogen levels [57]. Patients with endometrial cancer have high levels of IL-6 and nuclear factor-kB (NF-kB), a cellular transcription factor that activates several genes involved in the inflammatory and immune response [55]. The activation of NF-kB leads to the expression of COX-2, which induces the production of prostaglandin E2, a protein which is able to transform endometrial cells into neoplastic tissue [58].

The microbiome could be involved in the initiation of inflammation (Figure 3), inducing the immunopathological changes which ultimately lead to the development of cancer [59]. The activation of immune receptors induces the cellular response, by activating the mitogen-activated protein kinase (MAPK), NF-κB, or PI3K/AKT signalling pathways. Activation of these signalling pathways induces the expression of pro-inflammatory cytokines (e.g., TNF-α, IL-6, and IL-8) and/or antimicrobial peptides, which are involved in the development of the inflammatory response [31].

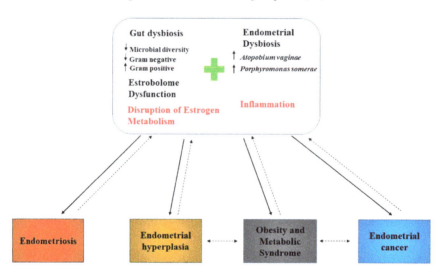

Figure 3. Endometrial and gut dysbiosis implication in endometrial cancer induction. The simultaneous presence of *Atopobium vaginae* and *Porphyromonas somerae* in the endometrium induce the production of pro-inflammatory cytokines, which are involved in endometrial carcinogenesis and other endometrial diseases.

As previously mentioned, the composition of the uterine microbiome is linked to several gynaecological pathologies, such as endometriosis, dysfunctional menstrual bleeding, and cancer [60] (Figure 3). Endometrial cancer is characterized by the simultaneous presence of two species, *Atopobium vaginae* and *Porphyromonas* [22]. In 2019, Caselli et al. performed an in-vitro analysis of the effect of *Atopobium vaginae* and *Porphyromonas somerae* on the expression of pro-inflammatory cytokines in endometrial cells using HEC-1A cells (human endometrial adenocarcinoma cells). The results of this study demonstrated that 24 h was sufficient to induce production of pro-inflammatory cytokines in endometrial cells cultured with *Atopobium vaginae* and *Porphyromonas somerae*. These cytokines produced in cells cultured with *Atopobium vaginae* and *Porphyromonas somerae* are not the same as those produced in cells cultured with *Lactobacillus vaginalis*. Thus, while *Lactobacillus vaginalis* induces the production of IL-8, *Atopobium vaginae* and *Porphyromonas somerae* induce the production of IL-1α, IL-1β, IL-17α, and TNFα, but not IL-8. This cytokine production was maintained over time without significant changes, suggesting a specific kinetic of cytokine induction, or a very gradual decrease in the ability of these bacteria to induce cytokine production. In the control group used with dead bacteria, it was observed that there was no production of cytokines, highlighting the need for the presence of *Atopobium vaginae* and *Porphyromonas somerae* to stimulate cytokine production in endometrial cells [61]. Several studies have demonstrated that IL1α and IL1β are overexpressed in various tumours including endometrial cancer, and promote cell proliferation, adhesion, invasion, and angiogenesis [62]. IL-17α, in turn, induces the production of other inflammatory proteins such as IL-8 and TNFα, stimulating the proliferation of endometrial cells, contributing to endometriosis and angiogenesis [63]. TNFα has been implicated in endometrial hyperplasia and, therefore, in endometrial cancer, evidencing an important role in metastasis and resistance to chemotherapy [64]. In addition to stimulating the production of the previously mentioned cytokines, Caselli et al. found that *Atopobium vaginae* and *Porphyromonas somerae* alter the transcription of other proteins, including CCL13, CCL8, CXCL2, IL22, and IL9. However, CCL13 production was also stimulated in the presence of *Lactobacillus vaginalis*. This implies the absence of a specific relationship between the production of CCL13 and the presence of *Atopobium vaginae* and *Porphyromonas somerae*. CCL8 and CXCL2 promote tumour invasion in various types of cancers, including endometrial cancer. Chemokine CXCL2 expression is induced by TNFα [61]. Interleukin IL-9 plays an important role in the immune response and cancer pathogenesis [65]. IL-22 induces breast cancer progression and endometrial cell proliferation through the production of CCL2 and IL-8 [61].

In another study, Lu et al. found that IL-6 and IL-17 mRNA levels are positively correlated with a relative abundance of *Micrococcus*, another Gram-positive bacterium belonging to the Phylum *Actinobacteria* related to endometrial cancer [31].

6. Modulation of Antitumoural Therapies Efficacy and Toxicity by Gut Microbiota

Endometrial cancer is mainly treated with surgery, to determine the stage of the tumour as an initial step to identify patients who could benefit from chemotherapy or radiation therapy. Immunotherapy is increasingly being investigated and seems to have favourable results in patients with microsatellite instability (MSI). In addition, recent studies have been conducted to establish whether the inhibition of immune checkpoints could be considered as a possible antitumour treatment method [66].

However, these treatments, particularly chemotherapy and radiotherapy, are very aggressive and can cause various side effects, especially at the intestinal level. Thus, up to 80% of patients exhibit intestinal symptoms such as abdominal pain and diarrhoea, among others, during treatment [67].

Consequently, recent studies have investigated the possibility of exploiting the microbiome to reduce the toxicity induced by antitumour therapies and improve the response to these therapies, incorporating, for example, probiotics as an adjuvant treatment, or designing microbial enzyme target molecules [68].

6.1. Immunotherapy

Recently, immunotherapy has emerged as an effective therapy with favourable results in killing tumour cells [69]. For some patients with recurrent or persistent metastatic gynaecological cancer, programmed cell death-1/programmed cell death-ligand 1 (PD-1/PD-L1) inhibitors are a possible option to enhance clinical outcomes [70].

The identification and elimination of tumour cells depends on cellular immunity mediated by T cells, which, through receptors (TCRs), bind with the specific antigen of the major histocompatibility complex (MHC) on the surface of tumour cells. The interaction of TCRs and MHC is regulated by a series of immune checkpoints, serving to activate or inhibit T cells. Cytotoxic T-lymphocyte-associated protein 4 (CTLA-4), PD-1, and PD-L1 are co-inhibitors which stop the immune response to prevent autoimmune diseases. In the tumour microenvironment, tumour and stromal cells overexpress co-inhibitory ligands and receptors. Thus, the binding of the PD-1 receptor with its PD-L1 ligand transmits inhibitory signals, blocking the immune activity of T cells, thus allowing tumour cells to escape the immune system [71]. Monoclonal antibodies against PD-1 (nivolumab), PD-L1 (pembrolizumab), and CTLA-4 (ipilimumab), reactivate the immune response of patients against cancer [72].

Recent studies have described the role of the microbiome in regulating tumour responses to immunotherapies targeting PD-L1 or cytotoxic T-lymphocyte-associated protein 4 (CTLA-4). Sivan et al. conducted studies on two groups of mice with subcutaneous melanomas and different intestinal microbiota, since the two groups were bred and raised in different laboratories. They obtained evidence that one of the two groups of mice included in the trial developed immune responses through induction and infiltration of antitumour CD8+ T cells, while the other group did not. After analysing the faecal microbiota of both groups, differences in composition were observed, where a greater amount of *Bifidobacterium* was found in the group that developed an antitumour immune response. This bacterium is capable of mediating dendritic cell reactivation by itself, which promotes the CD8+ T cells' response to eliminate tumour cells. The transfer of faecal *Bifidobacterium* in combination with the use of anti PD-L1 antibodies greatly improved the immune response, stimulating greater T cell production and helping to control the tumour [73].

In 2018, Routy et al., in a study comparing the faecal microbiota of a group of mice with non-small-cell lung cancer and renal carcinoma which responded positively to blocking immune checkpoints, and another group that did not respond, observed that in the group of mice that best responded to treatment with anti-PD-1, there was an enrichment in the groups of Firmicutes (*Clostridiales*), in addition to a significant increase in *Alistipes*, *Ruminococcus*, and *Eubacterium* species, and especially *Akkermansia muciniphila* species. In this last study, and unlike Sivan et al., Routy et al. found that the enrichment in the aforementioned species was accompanied by a relative decrease in other species, including *Bifidobacterium adolescentis*, *Bifidobacterium longum*, and *Parabacteroides distasonis*. Additionally, it was observed that the presence of *Enterococcus hirae* together with *Akkermansia muciniphila* enhanced the anti-PD-1 antitumour response in mice that best respond to anti-PD-1 antibodies. These two bacteria induce the production of IL-12, a Th1-type cytokine, in dendritic cells, stimulating the production of intestinal CD4+ T cells that express CCR9 receptors for chymosins in tumour beds, lymph nodes that drain the tumour, and in the mesenteric lymph nodes, exerting an adjuvant effect on the anti-PD-1 response. Conversely, it was observed that the group of mice that did not respond to anti-PD-1 had more *Corynebacterium aurimucosum* and *Staphylococcus haemolyticus* [74].

Gopalakrishnan et al. also investigated how gut microbiota can modulate the response to anti-PD-1. They saw that patients with metastatic melanoma, whose intestinal microbiome presented greater diversity and abundance in the Ruminococcaceae and *Faecalibacterium* families, developed a better systemic and antitumour immune response, showing greater antigen presentation, and an increase in the function of effector T cells in the periphery and the tumour microenvironment. Whereas the group of patients with metastatic melanoma, but whose intestinal microbiomes presented little diversity and a greater relative abundance in *Bacteroidales*, showed some alterations in the systemic and antitumour immune response due to limited intratumoural and myeloid lymphoid infiltration and low antigen presentation [75].

In summary, an abundance of *Clostridiales* in gut microbiome correlated to patients who respond positively to PD-1 blockade therapy, while the nonresponders' microbiomes were enriched with *Bacteroidale* [76]. In addition, the previously mentioned studies have demonstrated that there are three species (*Bifidobacterium*, *Akkermansia muciniphila*, and *Faecalibacterium*) that could be considered to be immune adjuvants in PD-1/PD-L1 immunotherapy. However, these species do not act by themselves, as they also influence the ecology and metabolism of the intestinal microbiota in response to immunotherapy. Furthermore, to support this hypothesis, the efficacy of inhibiting immune checkpoints has been shown to be reduced in patients who have received antibiotic treatment before or after immunotherapy [77].

In 2017, Chaput et al., analysing the gut microbiome of patients affected by metastatic melanoma treated with ipilimumab, revealed that enrichment with *Bacteroidetes* had a protective role against colitis, but also a poor tumour response, while enrichment with *Faecalibacterium* genus and other Firmicutes enhanced progression-free survival [78]. In another study, Cramer et al. reported that *Bacteroides fragilis* can be considered an immunogenic bacterium that acts as an anticancer probiotic, as its polysaccharide capsule induces IL-12-dependent TH1 immune responses. This bacterium enhances the effect of immunological treatment with anti-CTLA-4 [79]. In another study, Vétizou et al. also concluded that the composition of the microbiota, specifically the abundance of *Bacteroides fragilis* and/or *Bacteroides thetaiotaomicron* and *Burkholderiales*, modulates the response to a CTLA-4 blockade. The distribution of *Bacteroides fragilis* in the intestinal mucosa and its association with *Burkholderiales* stimulates pyrine-caspase1 inflammasome formation and activates the TLR2/TLR4 signalling pathway, which could explain the immunomodulatory effects that these bacteria have on CTLA-4. Although Ipilimumab, a monoclonal antibody to CTLA-4, is highly effective in immunotherapy, it can sometimes cause colitis. To counteract this, it has been observed that oral administration of *Bacteroides fragilis* and *Burkholderia cepacia* in mice can restore the response to anti-CTLA-4 and significantly reduce colitis. The efficacy of Ipilimumab is highly dependent on intestinal microbiota, so that enrichment with *Bacteroides fragilis* is necessary for the activation of CD4+ cells and obtaining favourable treatment results [80] (Table 3).

Table 3. Gut microbiota modulation of antitumoural therapies efficacy and toxicity.

Antitumoural Therapy		Author	Year	Sample Type Analized	Methods	Finding
Immunotherapy	anti-PD-L1	Sivan et al.	2015	Two groups of mice with subcutaneous melanomas and different intestinal microbiota, from different laboratories.	Transfer of faecal material within both group of mice before tumour implantation. 16S rRNA sequencing analysis	Gut microbiome of responder group: ↑*Bifidobacterium*
	anti-PD-1	Routy et al.	2018	Mice with non-small-cell lung cancer and renal carcinoma (responders to blocking immune checkpoints, and non-responders).	Faecal microbiota transplantation and 16S ribosomal rRNA of faecal samples	Gut microbiome of responder group: ↑Firmicutes (*Clostridiales*), ↑*Alistipes*, ↑*Ruminococcus*, ↑*Eubacterium* spp. ↑*Akkermansia muciniphila* ↑*Enterococcus hirae*, ↓*Bifidobacterium adolescentis*, ↓*Bifidobacterium longum* ↓*Parabacteroides distasonis* Gut microbiome of non-responder group: ↑*Corynebacterium aurimucosum*, ↑*Staphylococcus haemolyticus*
		Gopalakrishnan et al.	2018	Patients with metastatic melanoma (n = 112)	16S rRNA gene sequencing of oral, buccal and faecal samples, and tumour biopsies at treatment initiation and 6 months after treatment initiation.	Gut microbiome of responders group: ↑Diversity, ↑*Ruminococcaceae* ↑*Faecalibacterium* Non-responders group gut microbiome: ↓Diversity, ↑Bacteroidales
	anti-CTLA-4	Chaput et al.	2017	Patients with metastatic melanoma (n = 26)	16S rRNA gene sequencing at baseline and before each ipilimumab infusion in faecal samples.	Gut microbiome of responders group: ↑*Faecalibacterium*, ↑other Firmicutes Non-responders gut microbiome: ↑Bacteroidetes
		Cramer et al.	2017	Patients with metastatic melanoma and received ipilimumab (n = 34)	16S rRNA gene amplification and multiparallel sequencing of faecal samples.	*Bacteroides fragilis* enhances the effect of immunological treatment with anti-CTLA-4
		Vétizou et al.	2015	Mice with sarcomas	High-throughput pyrosequencing of 16S rRNA gene amplicons of faeces.	Gut microbiome of responders group: ↑*Bacteroides fragilis* ↑*Bacteroides* thetaiotaomicron ↑*Burkholderiales* ↑*Burkholderia cepacia*

Table 3. *Cont.*

Antitumoural Therapy		Author	Year	Sample Type Analized	Methods	Finding
Chemotherapy	cyclophosphamide	Ma et al.	2019	Mice treated with cyclophosphamide	High-throughput 454 pyrosequencing in faecal samples. Quantitative PCR targeting the domain bacteria and specific bacterial groups.	Gut microbiome involved in enhacing treatment response: *Enterococcus hirae* *Lactobacillus johnsonii* *Lactobacillus murinus* Segmented filamentous bacteria *Barnesiella intestinihominis*
	Gemcitabine	Chen et al.	2020	Transgenic mice with pancreatic cancer	Probiotic oral gavage of *Lactobacillus paracasei* and *Lactobacillus reuteri*. 16S rRNA Amplicon Sequencing.	↑*Lactobacillus paracasei*, *Lactobacillus reuteri* enhacing treatment response in transgenic mice.
	Irinotecan	Bhatt et al.	2020	Tumour xenograft model	16S rRNA Amplicon Sequencing	Changes in the composition of the intestinal microbiota induced by irinotecan: ↑Proteobacteria (*Enterobacteriaceae*), ↑Verrucomicrobia ↑*Akkermansia muciniphila*
	Doxorubicin	Hong et al.	2019	Patients with chemotherapeutic treatment for a solid tumour (*n* = 30) and non-cancer controls (*n* = 30)	Amplification and sequencing of 16S rRNA gene and ITS 1 DNA	Gut dysbiosis induced by doxorubicin: ↓*Streptococcus*, ↓*Actinomyces* ↓*Gemella*, ↓*Granulicatella* ↓*Veillonella*, ↑*Fusobacterium nucleatum* ↑*Prevotella oris*
		Yan et al.	2018	Healthy donors	16S rRNA Amplicon Sequencing of faecal samples	↑*Raoultella planticola*, *Klebsiella pneumoniae* and *Escherichia coli* involved in doxorubicin inactivation and degradation.
	Paclitaxel	Ramakrishna et al.	2019	Two groups of mice: sensitive and resistant to Paclitaxel-induced pain.	16S rRNA gene sequencing.	↓*Akkermansia muciniphila*

Table 3. *Cont.*

Antitumoural Therapy	Author	Year	Sample Type Analized	Methods	Finding
Toxicity induced by chemotherapy	Van Vliet et al.	2010	Mice colonic tissues	Elisa for measurement of intestinal permeability. PCR Mucosal cytokine measurements	Gut dysbosis associated to toxicity induced by chemotherapy: ↓*Bifidobacteria* ↓*Lactobacillus*, ↓*Faecalibacterium* ↓*Clostridium*
	Montassier et al.	2015	Patients with non-Hodgkin's lymphoma who received the same myeloablative conditioning regimen and no other concomitant therapy such as antibiotic (*n* = 28)	Amplification and sequencing of 16S rRNA genes in faecal samples	Gut dysbosis associated to toxicity induced by chemotherapy: ↑*Bacteroides*, ↑*Enterococcus* ↑Enterobacteriaceae ↓Firmicutes (*Ruminococcaceae*, Lachnospiraceae), ↓Actinobacteria (*Bifidobacterium*), ↑*Citrobacter*, ↓*Ruminococcus*, ↓*Coprococcus*, ↓*Dorea*, ↓*Lachnospira*, ↓*Roseburia*
Radiotherapy	Yan et al.	2007	Colon organ culture	Purification and analizing of proteins from *Lactobacillus*	*Lactobacillus rhamnosus*, *Lactobacillus casei* and *Lactobacillus acidophilus* have protective roles in minimizing the damage caused by radiation therapy
	Ciorba et al.	2012	Mice small intestine	Protein and nucleic acid analysis	Administration of *Lactobacillus rhamnosus* before radiotherapy decreases epithelial apoptosis and stimulates crypt survival in mice guts
	Delia et al.	2007	Patients who underwent surgery for sigmoid, rectal, or cervical cancer (*n* = 429)	Probiotic oral gavage of *Lactobacillus* spp. and *Bifidobacterium* spp.	Microbiome that can reduce gut toxicity induced by radiotherapy: *Lactobacillus* (*L. casei*, *L. plantarum*, *L. acidophilus*, and *L. delbrueckii subsp. bulgaricus*) Bifidobacteria (*B. longum*, *B. breve*, and *B. infantis*)

Table 3. *Cont.*

Antitumoural Therapy		Author	Year	Sample Type Analized	Methods	Finding
Targeted therapy	Trastuzumab	Di Modica et al.	2021	Female mice with breast cancer Patients with breast cancer (*n* = 24)	Faecal microbial transplantation in mice and faecal sample analysis of variable region V3 and V4 of the 16S rRNA gene for mice and human.	Gut microbiome of responders: ↑Clostridiales (Lachnospiraceae), ↑Bifidobacteriaceae, ↑Turicibacteracea, ↑Bacteroidales (Prevotellaceae) Gut microbiome of non-responders: ↑Bacteroidetes (Bacteroidia)
	Erlotinib and gefitinib	Flórez et al.	2016	Bacterial strains	Determination of minimum inhibitory concentrations	34 species of lactic acid bacteria, Bifidobacteria, and other intestinal bacteria are resistant to treatment with erlotinib and gefitinib
	Letrozole	Cao et al.	2020	Rats (8 normal controls and 30 with endometriosis)	Amplification and sequencing of 16S rRNA genes in faecal samples	↓Firmicutes/Bacteroidetes ratio, ↓inflammation, ↓Ruminococcaceae

However, whether endometrial microbiota can actually influence the efficacy of immunotherapy in endometrial cancers still needs to be investigated.

6.2. Chemotherapy

In patients with advanced cancers, cytotoxic drugs are used as the main therapy. However, these drugs often have strong adverse effects. Gut microbiota is considered a key element in enhancing the efficacy and reducing the toxicity of chemotherapy drugs, as well as improving the sensitivity to chemotherapy. Immunomodulation is one of the key mechanisms by which the microbiota intervenes in the response to different types of treatments.

The efficacy of cyclophosphamide, a cytotoxic alkylating agent used in chemotherapy, is modulated by the presence of Gram-positive bacteria such as *Enterococcus hirae*, *Lactobacillus johnsonii*, *Lactobacillus murinus*, and segmented filamentous bacteria. Furthermore, translocation of *Enterococcus hirae* improves the intratumoural CD8/Treg ratio. At the same time, *Barnesiella intestinihominis*, a Gram-negative bacterium, has been shown to enhance the infiltration of interferon-c-producing T cells into tumour tissue to enhance the effect of cyclophosphamide [77].

Gemcitabine is a chemotherapeutic agent belonging to the group of nucleoside (cytidine) analogues approved by the FDA to be used as a treatment for various solid tumours, including advanced endometrial cancer. This drug has the ability to kill cells in the S phase of DNA synthesis and blocks the progression of cells through the G1/S phase. Gemcitabine is metabolized into gemcitabine diphosphate and triphosphate, which, once incorporated into DNA, inhibits polymerase activity. Furthermore, apoptosis is induced through the recognition of incorporated gemcitabine by p53 and DNA-dependent kinases [81]. Chen et al. conducted a study on transgenic mice with pancreatic cancer treated with gemcitabine supplemented with *Lactobacillus*. In that study, *Lactobacillus paracasei*, a Gram-positive facultative heterofermentative lactic acid bacterium which is part of human and animal intestinal microbiota was used. *Lactobacillus paracasei* has been shown to inhibit Th2 cytokine production and modulate the Th1/Th2 balance by increasing IFN-γ levels. It was subsequently observed that the Th2 response produces tumourigenesis-promoting effects in patients with pancreatic cancer. Chen et al. used another probiotic, *Lactobacillus reuteri*, due to its antioxidant activity and ability to reduce levels of IL6 interleukin with tumorigenic activity. Gemcitabine treatment is known to cause increased levels of liver enzymes. After combining the treatment with probiotics, a decrease in the level of these enzymes was observed [82].

Irinotecan, another chemotherapeutic agent used for endometrial cancer, acts as a Topoisomerase I inhibitor [83]. Although its effectiveness as an anti-tumour treatment in various cancers is quite significant, this agent has several side effects at the gastrointestinal level, causing mucositis and diarrhoea on several occasions. Irinotecan is activated in-vivo on SN38, a potent inhibitor of Topoisomerase I, which delays the growth and proliferation of tumour and intestinal cells. SN38 is marked by glucuronic acid binding to form SN38-G, for subsequent elimination from the gastrointestinal tract. β-glucuronidase enzyme, produced by some intestinal bacteria, is capable of eliminating glucuronic acid from SN38-G, reactivating it to SN38, thus causing epithelial damage, shedding, diarrhoea, and weight loss in animal models. Bhatt et al., based on the relationship between SN38-G activation, β-glucuronidase activity, and intestinal toxicity produced by Irinotecan treatment, decided to investigate the effect of inhibiting this enzyme's activity to alleviate toxicity. In that study, it was observed that the use of amoxapine and pyrazolo 4-3-c quinoline, inhibitors of β-glucuronidase activity, protects the gastrointestinal epithelium by reducing the production of pro-inflammatory cytokines, and improves the response to treatment with Irinotecan. In addition, Irinotecan induces changes in the composition of the intestinal microbiota, increasing, above all, the levels of *Proteobacteria* (*Enterobacteriaceae*), in addition to *Verrucomicrobia* and *Akkermansia muciniphila*. The use of *GUS* gene (a gene that encodes the enzyme β-glucuronidase) inhibitors has been shown to reduce *Proteobacteria* levels [84].

Doxorubicin is a chemotherapeutic anticancer drug belonging to the anthracycline family, used to treat various types of cancers, including endometrial cancer. It is characterized by its ability to inhibit the growth of both cancer cells and bacteria through the generation of free radicals, DNA intercalation, alkylation and cross-linking of proteins, interference with DNA unwinding and Topoisimerase II, and direct membrane damage. However, the use of drugs belonging to the anthracycline family leads to the accumulation of toxic metabolites in healthy tissue [85]. In addition to the heart, the gut is also affected by the toxicity associated with the use of Doxorubicin. This drug causes damage to the intestinal epithelium by inducing apoptosis in the epithelial cells of the jejunum and damage to the mucosa, reducing the proliferation of crypts, so that fewer crypts are formed, and with smaller villi [86]. Oral mucositis, another reaction associated with doxorubicin-induced toxicity, produces an increase in salivary flow, gum inflammation, and sore formation. Oral mucositis produces dysbiosis, decreasing the levels of the *Streptococcus, Actinomyces, Gemella, Granulicatella,* and *Veillonella* genera, and increasing the levels of other Gram-negative bacteria such as *Fusobacterium nucleatum* and *Prevotella oris. Fusobacterium nucleatum* have pro-inflammatory and pro-apoptotic activity, contributing to the damage produced in the mucosa [87]. Conversely, bacteria of the intestinal microbiota have been implicated in the inactivation of some drugs, including doxorubicin. Yan et al. identified *Raoultella planticola* as a powerful inactivator of doxorubicin under anaerobic conditions, and demonstrated that this bacterium deglycosylates doxorubicin into the metabolites 7-deoxydoxorubicinol and 7-deoxydoxorubicinolone by the reductive deglycosylation mechanism. Subsequently, doxorubicin was anaerobically degraded by *Klebsiella pneumoniae* and *Escherichia coli* [85].

Paclitaxel, another chemotherapeutic agent used in the treatment of endometrial cancer, has neurological side effects, producing peripheral neuropathies. Ramakrishna et al. proposed that Paclitaxel lowers beneficial bacteria levels such as *Akkermansia muciniphila* which promotes barrier function. In addition, they observed that the *Porphyromonadaceae* family is involved in the dysbiosis produced by Paclitaxel, which, in turn, has been implicated in neurological damage produced in glial cells [88] (Table 3).

6.3. Radiotherapy

Radiation therapy is an effective method of antitumour treatment, based on the genotoxic effect on tumour cells, and through which cell death is induced by local irradiation, accompanied by systemic immunity and inflammation [89]. However, irradiation-mediated intestinal toxicity was observed in several cases, which involves an alteration in the composition of the microbiota, and leads to dysfunction of the intestinal barrier and apoptosis in intestinal crypts [90]. Yan et al. identified two soluble proteins produced by *Lactobacillus rhamnosus,* p75 and p40, which induce the activation of the AKT signalling pathway by stimulating cell proliferation, and inhibit the apoptosis induced by tumour necrosis factor, in epithelial cells. In addition to *Lactobacillus rhamnosus, Lactobacillus casei* and *Lactobacillus acidophilus* have also been shown to have protective roles in minimizing the damage caused by radiation therapy [91]. Ciorba et al. also found that administration of *Lactobacillus rhamnosus* before radiotherapy decreases epithelial apoptosis and stimulates crypt survival in mice guts. The cell wall of this bacterium, like all Gram-positive bacteria, is composed of peptidoglycan and lipoteichoic acids which act as Toll-like receptor-2 (TLR-2) ligands. The activation of TLR-2 leads to COX-2 expression and reactive oxygen species (ROS) production to activate the cytoprotective system NRF-2, a transcription factor that regulates the expression of detoxifying and antioxidant enzymes, thereby contributing to the protection of intestinal cells from damage caused by radiotherapy [92].

While Ciorba et al. did not find any radioprotective effect of *Bifidobacterium* [92], Delia et al., in a previous study, proved that VSL3, a mixture comprised of *Lactobacillus* (*Lactobacillus casei, Lactobacillus plantarum, Lactobacillus acidophilus,* and *Lactobacillus delbrueckii* subsp.

bulgaricus), Bifidobacteria (*Bifidobacterium longum, Bifidobacterium breve*, and *Bifidobacterium infantis*), and a species of *Streptococcus salivarius* subsp. *Thermophilus*, reduced the toxicity (diarrhoea) produced by radiotherapy [93] (Table 3).

6.4. Targeted Therapy

Recently, in addition to the previously mentioned traditional therapies, targeted molecular therapies have proven to be of essential importance in improving the long-term survival of cancer patients with specific biomarkers [94]. Trastuzumab, an FDA-approved drug which contains monoclonal antibodies targeting the *HER-2* receptor extracellular domain, is being tested for endometrial cancer, because in serous endometrial carcinoma the *HER-2* gene, which is responsible for the increase of cell proliferation, differentiation, and migration, is overexpressed [11]. Recently, Di Modica et al. analysed the gut microbiota composition of a group of breast cancer patients who responded favourably to adjuvant treatment with Trastuzumab. They found that in those patients with favourable results in response to treatment, *Clostridiales* (*Lachnospiraceae*), *Bifidobacteriaceae, Turicibacteraceae,* and *Bacteroidales* (*Prevotellaceae*) predominated, while in the other group of patients who did not respond to treatment, an enrichment in the phylum *Bacteroidetes* (*Bacteroidia*) was observed [95].

Erlotinib and gefitinib, two epidermal growth factor receptor (EGFR) and tyrosine kinase inhibitors, have also been tested in patients with endometrial cancer, as *EGFR* is overexpressed in 40–46% of Type I endometrial carcinoma cases, and in 34% of Type II endometrial carcinomas [11]. Flórez el al. demonstrated that 34 species of lactic acid bacteria, *Bifidobacteria*, and other intestinal bacteria are resistant to treatment with erlotinib and gefitinib, so that the abundance of these species was not altered after treatment [96].

Letrozole, an aromatase inhibitor that inhibits the production of local and circulating estrogens, has also been used in clinical trials as a treatment for endometrial cancer [97]. Cao et al., in a study with mice, found that Letrozole treatment produces a decrease in the Firmicutes/Bacteroidetes ratio, contributing to a decrease in inflammation. Furthermore, in the same study, it was observed that Letrozole altered the diversity of the intestinal microbiota in mice, significantly decreasing Ruminococcaceae levels [98] (Table 3).

6.5. Toxicity

It is evident that the intestinal microbiota can modulate the response to different antitumour treatments. However, in turn, the microbiota is itself altered in response to treatment [99]. Treatment of endometrial cancer can cause several symptoms in patients, one of which is vaginal atrophy, caused by cell damage as a result of radiation therapy. Patients with vaginal atrophy have less *Lactobacillus*, the first line of defense in the female urogenital tract. Damage to the vaginal epithelium caused by radiation therapy allows pathogens to penetrate the epithelium and causes inflammation that ultimately contributes to vaginal atrophy [100].

Chemotherapy, in turn, causes several side effects in patients, including gastrointestinal mucositis, which results in several symptoms in patients, such as nausea, diarrhoea, vomiting, and abdominal pain. Gastrointestinal mucositis is a lesion characterized by atrophy of the villi and the loss of enterocytes, which leads to epithelium deterioration and gut-barrier alteration [101]. Gut microbiota has been implicated in many of the pathological aspects of gastrointestinal mucositis caused by chemotherapy. After chemotherapy, the permeability of the intestinal mucosa increases due to the atrophy of the villi as a consequence of gastrointestinal mucositis. However, intestinal microbiota, especially *Bifidobacteria* and *Lactobacillus*, improves the functioning of the epithelial barrier, reducing its permeability by binding to TLR-2 receptors, which leads to protein kinase C phosphorylation and the production of proteins that form tight junctions. The levels of these bacteria and others involved in maintaining the normal permeability of the epithelial barrier (*Faecalibacterium, Ruminococcus, Coprococcus, Dorea, Lachnospira, Roseburia, Clostridium* and *Bifidobacterium*) decrease after chemotherapy, which explains the increased permeability of the intestinal mucosa as a result of mucositis [101,102]. Additionally, in another study, Montassier et al. noticed a decrease in both the number and diversity of intestinal microbiota after chemotherapy, which is associated with an increase in *Bacteroides, Enterococci,* and Enterobacteriaceae, and a decrease in Firmicutes (Ruminococcaceae, Lachnospiraceae) and Actinobacteria (*Bifidobacterium*). In the same study, they showed that bacteria that modulate the NF B signalling pathway to decrease the inflammatory response, such as *Faecalibacterium, Ruminococcus, Coprococcus, Dorea, Lachnospira, Roseburia* and *Clostridium*, decreased after chemotherapy, as did *Bifidobacterium*, whose function under normal conditions is to inhibit the inflammatory response. The decrease in these bacteria, which are also butyrate producers, implies a decrease in the production of short-chain fatty acids, and consequently the inflammatory response is not inhibited. Intestinal mucosa composition is also altered after chemotherapy. As a result of the reduction of butyrate-producing bacteria, butyrate is not produced, and therefore, mucin synthesis via MUC2 is not stimulated, which leads to tissue damage and translocation of bacteria due to alterations in the composition of the intestinal mucosa.

Conversely, an increase in *Citrobacter* was observed after chemotherapy. This bacterium stimulates NFB production and therefore stimulates the inflammatory response. In addition, it also participates in intestinal barrier degradation, using mucinases and glucosidases to digest mucin [101] (Table 3).

7. Modulation of Endometrial Microbiota

Commensal bacteria can protect their host from pathogen infections due to their ability to better adapt to the environment than pathogens, which allows them to compete successfully. In addition, they make better use of the available nutrients, leaving the pathogens without an energy source [103]. Consequently, there is a growing interest in modulating the endometrial microbiome composition and environment to break dysbiosis and prevent endometrial diseases.

Probiotics are live microorganisms that confer health benefits to their host. These bacteria can produce bioactive molecules that act on the body, promoting good health, with low toxicity and few side effects. Most of the studies carried out selected the *Lactobacillus rhamnosus* BPL005 strain as the best candidate to improve the female reproductive tract, due to its capacity in-vitro to reduce pH levels and produce organic acids such as lactate, which promotes the reduction of pathogenic bacteria [104]. Chenoll et al., with the aim of investigating whether strain *Lactobacillus rhamnosus* BPL005 could have beneficial effects against endometrial infections caused by pathogens, used human endometrial epithelial cells (HEEC) co-cultured with pathogenic bacteria (*Atopobium vaginae, Gardnerella vaginalis, Propionibacterium acnes,* and *Streptococcus agalactiae*) alone, and in combination with the strain *Lactobacillus rhamnosus* BPL005. The study showed that in the HEEC cells cultured with the strain *Lactobacillus rhamnosus* BPL005, there was a reduction of the pH, being less than 5. This low pH limits the growth of pathogens and inhibits their adhesion to endometrial cells. Another finding confirmed that *Lactobacillus rhamnosus* BPL005 decreased the levels of some metabolites like propionic acid produced by *Propionibacterium acnes* (linked to symptomatic bacterial vaginosis profiles) in endometrial cell cultures, leading to a drift towards a healthy organic acid profile. Furthermore, lactic acid produced by *Lactobacillus rhamnosus* BPL005 had a bactericidal effect against pathogen colonization in HEEC cells. These effects on pH and organic acid production were considered to be pathogen inhibition pathways to decrease pathogen colonization. Additionally, the *Lactobacillus rhamnosus* BPL005 strain produced bacteriocins, further protecting against vaginal pathogens [105].

Female genital microbiota modulation could also be used to protect against infection. Bacterial vaginosis is linked to endometrial microbial colonization, and a recent study found a polymicrobial *Gardnerella vaginalis* biofilm in the uterus of women with bacterial vaginosis [106]. The addition of the *Lactobacillus rhamnosus* BPL005 strain to HEEC cells colonized by pathogens increased proinflammatory cytokines such as IL-1RA and IL-

1β, and decreased the proinflammatory IL-6, IL-8, and MCP-1 cytokines, which were previously increased due to the pathogens' presence [105].

Recent studies have also shown that probiotic lactobacilli (*Lactobacillus reuteri RC-14* and *Lactobacillus rhamnosus GR-1*) can improve endometrial epithelial cells' barrier- function in response to the human immunodeficiency virus-1 (HIV-1). These bacterial strains are able to modulate the immune profile, indicating that female reproductive tract microbiota could be an important factor in the acquisition of resistance to viruses [107].

Prebiotics are compounds that serve as nutrients and promote the growth and activity of beneficial microorganisms with the aim of enhancing health. Lactoferrin is a prebiotic agent used to modify the endometrial microbiome. Lactoferrin, orally administrated during and after antibiotics treatment in women undergoing infertility treatment, can increase *Lactobacillus* levels in the endometria of non-*Lactobacillus* dominant patients after three months of use [108]. In addition, Lactoferrin administration showed effective results against bacterial vaginosis, preventing endometrial infections [104].

The use of prebiotics and probiotics can provide greater benefits than the use of antibiotics alone, which produces short-term results but which aggravates dysbiosis and promotes resistance over the long-term.

Finally, vaginal microbiota transplants (VMTs) (the transfer of cervicovaginal fluid from a healthy donor to a patient to restore their microenvironment) to patients suffering from symptomatic and recurrent vaginosis as a therapeutic alternative has shown positive treatment outcomes [109]. Currently, two Phase I/II clinical trials in the USA (NCT03769688 and NCT04046900) and one in Israel (NCT02236429) are recruiting participants to analyse the efficacy and safety of VMTs in women with bacterial vaginosis.

VMTs could be an effective tool for managing endometrial dysbiosis, as uterine colonization by microorganisms through vaginal-cervical ascension has been described previously [110,111].

VMTs could be used to modulate the vaginal microbiome by restoring the microenvironment for the prevention of endometrial cancer. Nevertheless, future studies with larger cohorts and randomized, placebo-controlled studies will be necessary to determine the efficacy and durability of VMTs for endometrial cancer prevention.

8. Conclusions

Due to the importance of the microbiome in many human physiological processes and recent advances in highly sensitive molecular techniques which facilitate the identification of microorganisms, several emergent studies have shown interest in investigating the relationship between gut and endometrial microbiome in endometrial cancer, one of the most common cancers in women worldwide, which occurs more frequently after menopause. There is evidence that the presence of both *Atopobium vaginae* and *Porphyromonas somerae* in the gynaecological tract is statistically related to endometrial cancer, particularly when vaginal pH is high. In endometrial cells, these two bacteria can also induce the production of IL-1α, IL-1β, IL-17α, and TNFα, pro-inflammatory cytokines which are involved in the carcinogenesis of various tumours. Because endometrial cancer is estrogen-dependent, an excess of estrogen in the body is considered to be an important risk factor for endometrial cancer. In this context, estrobolome (an aggregate of enteric bacterial genes whose products are capable of metabolizing estrogens) plays a fundamental role. These bacteria with β-glucuronidase activity can activate conjugated estrogens, transported from the liver to the intestine, though deconjugation. Consequently, estrobolome dysbiosis can lead to an estrogen increase, contributing to carcinogenesis. The microbiome is also involved in the body's response to treatment, so it can alleviate some of the side effects of various antitumour therapies and reduce their toxicity. However, the microbiome can also be altered in response to treatment. Due to the implication of the microbiome in various processes such as inflammation, estrogen metabolism, carcinogenesis, and antitumour treatments, we can conclude that modulating gut and endometrial microbiome in combination with traditional endometrial cancer treatments may provide an alternative method to achieve better antitumour therapy results and improve patient living conditions. Further research into metagenomic analysis in endometrial cancer is needed to improve our knowledge of this topic and to discover novel markers with therapeutic implications.

Author Contributions: Original idea for this article, conceptualization and provided overall supervision and coordination of the manuscript preparation, M.I.Q.-O., R.L.-V. and E.A.; generated the table and figures, which were revised by all authors; methodology, R.L.-V., S.B., A.G.-G., I.P.-A., A.L.-I., L.S.-A., J.P.-L., M.E.D.-R. and M.J.B.-P.; validation, R.L.-V., S.B., A.G.-G., I.P.-A., A.L.-I., L.S.-A., M.E.D.-R. and M.J.B.-P.; writing—original draft preparation, M.I.Q.-O., S.B., R.L.-V. and E.A.; writing—review and editing, all authors; funding acquisition, M.I.Q.-O. and E.A. All authors have read and agreed to the published version of the manuscript.

Funding: Maria Isabel Queipo-Ortuño is recipient of a "Miguel Servet Type II" program (CPI13/00003) from ISCIII, co-funded by the Fondo Europeo de Desarrollo Regional-FEDER, Madrid, Spain and also belongs to the regional "Nicolas Monardes" research program of the Consejería de Salud (C-0030-2018, Junta de Andalucía, Spain. Alicia González-González is recipient of a postdoctoral contract of ALIANZA MIXTA EN RED ANDALUCÍA-ROCHE EN ONCOLOGÍA MÉDICA DE PRECISIÓN (INVESTIGACIÓN BÁSICA/TRASLACIONAL). Aurora Laborda-Illanes was recipient of a predoctoral grant, PFIS-ISCIII (FI19-00112) co-funded by the Fondo Europeo de Desarrollo Regional-FEDER, Madrid, Spain. Lidia Sanchez-Alcoholado was recipient of a predoctoral grant (PE-0106-2019) from the Consejería de Salud y Familia (co-funded by the Fondo Europeo de Desarrollo Regional-FEDER, Andalucia, Spain).

Institutional Review Board Statement: Not applicable.

Informed Consent Statement: Not applicable.

Acknowledgments: We also thank Dwight Sangster for helping with the English language.

Conflicts of Interest: The authors declare no conflict of interest.

References

1. Yanaihara, A.; Otsuka, Y.; Iwasaki, S.; Aida, T.; Tachikawa, T.; Irie, T.; Okai, T. Differences in gene expression in the proliferative human endometrium. *Fertil. Steril.* **2005**, *83*, 1206–1215. [CrossRef] [PubMed]
2. Akhtar, M.; Al Hyassat, S.; Elaiwy, O.; Rashid, S.; Al-Nabet, A.D. Classification of Endometrial Carcinoma: New Perspectives Beyond Morphology. *Adv. Anat. Pathol.* **2019**, *26*, 421–427. [CrossRef] [PubMed]
3. Ferlay, J.; Soerjomataram, I.; Dikshit, R.; Eser, S.; Mathers, C.; Rebelo, M.; Parkin, D.M.; Forman, D.; Bray, F. Cancer Incidence and Mortality Worldwide: Sources, Methods and Major Patterns in GLOBOCAN 2012. *Int. J. Cancer* **2015**, *136*, E359–E386. [CrossRef]
4. Lortet-Tieulent, J.; Ferlay, J.; Bray, F.; Jemal, A. International Patterns and Trends in Endometrial Cancer Incidence, 1978–2013. *J. Natl. Cancer Inst.* **2017**, *110*, 354–361. [CrossRef]
5. Clarke, M.A.; Long, B.J.; Morillo, A.D.M.; Arbyn, M.; Bakkum-Gamez, J.N.; Wentzensen, N. Association of Endometrial Cancer Risk with Postmenopausal Bleeding in Women: A Systematic Review and Meta-Analysis. *JAMA Intern. Med.* **2018**, *178*, 1210–1222. [CrossRef]
6. Bray, F.; Loos, A.H.; Oostindier, M.; Weiderpass, E. Geographic and temporal variations in cancer of the corpus uteri: Incidence and mortality in pre- and postmenopausal women in Europe. *Int. J. Cancer* **2005**, *117*, 123–131. [CrossRef]
7. Bray, F.; Silva, I.D.S.; Moller, H.; Weiderpass, E. Endometrial Cancer Incidence Trends in Europe: Underlying Determinants and Prospects for Prevention. *Cancer Epidemiol. Biomark. Prev.* **2005**, *14*, 1132–1142. [CrossRef]
8. Ketabi, Z.; Mosgaard, B.J.; Gerdes, A.-M.; Ladelund, S.; Bernstein, I. Awareness of Endometrial Cancer Risk and Compliance with Screening in Hereditary Nonpolyposis Colorectal Cancer. *Obstet. Gynecol.* **2012**, *120*, 1005–1012. [CrossRef]
9. Tamura, K.; Kaneda, M.; Futagawa, M.; Takeshita, M.; Kim, S.; Nakama, M.; Kawashita, N.; Tatsumi-Miyajima, J. Genetic and genomic basis of the mismatch repair system involved in Lynch syndrome. *Int. J. Clin. Oncol.* **2019**, *24*, 999–1011. [CrossRef] [PubMed]
10. Pellat, A.; Netter, J.; Perkins, G.; Cohen, R.; Coulet, F.; Parc, Y.; Svrcek, M.; Duval, A.; André, T. Syndrome de Lynch: Quoi de neuf? *Bull. Cancer* **2019**, *106*, 647–655. [CrossRef] [PubMed]
11. Binder, P.S.; Mutch, D.G. Update on Prognostic Markers for Endometrial Cancer. *Women's Health* **2014**, *10*, 277–288. [CrossRef]
12. Corrado, G.; Laquintana, V.; Loria, R.; Carosi, M.; De Salvo, L.; Sperduti, I.; Zampa, A.; Cicchillitti, L.; Piaggio, G.; Cutillo, G.; et al. Endometrial cancer prognosis correlates with the expression of L1CAM and miR34a biomarkers. *J. Exp. Clin. Cancer Res.* **2018**, *37*, 139. [CrossRef]
13. Bokhman, J.V. Two pathogenetic types of endometrial carcinoma. *Gynecol. Oncol.* **1983**, *15*, 10–17. [CrossRef]

14. Levine, R.L.; Cargile, C.B.; Blazes, M.S.; Van Rees, B.; Kurman, R.J.; Ellenson, L.H. PTEN mutations and microsatellite instability in complex atypical hyperplasia, a precursor lesion to uterine endometrioid carcinoma. *Cancer Res.* **1998**, *58*, 6.
15. Sherman, M.E. Theories of Endometrial Carcinogenesis: A Multidisciplinary Approach. *Mod. Pathol.* **2000**, *13*, 295–308. [CrossRef] [PubMed]
16. Banno, K.; Yanokura, M.; Kisu, I.; Yamagami, W.; Susumu, N.; Aoki, D. MicroRNAs in endometrial cancer. *Int. J. Clin. Oncol.* **2013**, *18*, 186–192. [CrossRef] [PubMed]
17. Bansal, N.; Yendluri, V.; Wenham, R.M. The Molecular Biology of Endometrial Cancers and the Implications for Pathogenesis, Classification, and Targeted Therapies. *Cancer Control.* **2009**, *16*, 8–13. [CrossRef]
18. Liu, F.-S. Molecular Carcinogenesis of Endometrial Cancer. *Taiwan J. Obstet. Gynecol.* **2007**, *46*, 26–32. [CrossRef]
19. Buhtoiarova, T.N.; Brenner, C.A.; Singh, M. Endometrial Carcinoma: Role of Current and Emerging Biomarkers in Resolving Persistent Clinical Dilemmas. *Am. J. Clin. Pathol.* **2016**, *145*, 8–21. [CrossRef]
20. Van Nyen, T.; Moiola, C.P.; Colas, E.; Annibali, D.; Amant, F. Modeling Endometrial Cancer: Past, Present, and Future. *Int. J. Mol. Sci.* **2018**, *19*, 2348. [CrossRef] [PubMed]
21. Bulsa, M.; Urasińska, E. Triple negative endometrial cancer. *Ginekol. Polska* **2017**, *88*, 212–214. [CrossRef] [PubMed]
22. Walther-António, M.R.S.; Chen, J.; Multinu, F.; Hokenstad, A.; Distad, T.J.; Cheek, E.H.; Keeney, G.L.; Creedon, D.J.; Nelson, H.; Mariani, A.; et al. Potential contribution of the uterine microbiome in the development of endometrial cancer. *Genome Med.* **2016**, *8*, 1–15. [CrossRef] [PubMed]
23. Moreno, I.; Codoñer, F.M.; Vilella, F.; Valbuena, D.; Martinez-Blanch, J.F.; Jimenez-Almazán, J.; Alonso, R.; Alamá, P.; Remohí, J.; Pellicer, A.; et al. Evidence that the endometrial microbiota has an effect on implantation success or failure. *Am. J. Obstet. Gynecol.* **2016**, *215*, 684–703. [CrossRef] [PubMed]
24. Ravel, J.; Gajer, P.; Abdo, Z.; Schneider, G.M.; Koenig, S.S.K.; McCulle, S.L.; Karlebach, S.; Gorle, R.; Russell, J.; Tacket, C.O.; et al. Vaginal microbiome of reproductive-age women. *Proc. Natl. Acad. Sci. USA* **2011**, *108*, 4680–4687. [CrossRef]
25. Brotman, R.M.; Shardell, M.D.; Gajer, P.; Fadrosh, D.; Chang, K.; Silver, M.; Viscidi, R.P.; Burke, A.E.; Ravel, J.; Gravitt, P.E. Association between the vaginal microbiota, menopause status, and signs of vulvovaginal atrophy. *Menopause* **2014**, *21*, 450–458. [CrossRef]
26. Mitchell, C.M.; Haick, A.; Nkwopara, E.; Garcia, R.; Rendi, M.; Agnew, K.; Fredricks, D.; Eschenbach, D. Colonization of the upper genital tract by vaginal bacterial species in nonpregnant women. *Am. J. Obstet. Gynecol.* **2015**, *212*, 611.e1–611.e9. [CrossRef]
27. Fang, R.-L.; Chen, L.-X.; Shu, W.-S.; Yao, S.-Z.; Wang, S.-W.; Chen, Y.-Q. Barcoded sequencing reveals diverse intrauterine microbiomes in patients suffering with endometrial polyps. *Am. J. Transl. Res.* **2016**, *8*, 1581–1592.
28. Verstraelen, H.; Vilchez-Vargas, R.; Desimpel, F.; Jauregui, R.; Vankeirsbilck, N.; Weyers, S.; Verhelst, R.; De Sutter, P.; Pieper, D.H.; Van De Wiele, T. Characterisation of the human uterine microbiome in non-pregnant women through deep sequencing of the V1-2 region of the 16S rRNA gene. *PeerJ* **2016**, *4*, e1602. [CrossRef] [PubMed]
29. Chen, C.; Song, X.; Chunwei, Z.; Zhong, H.; Dai, J.; Lan, Z.; Li, F.; Yu, X.; Feng, Q.; Wang, Z.; et al. The microbiota continuum along the female reproductive tract and its relation to uterine-related diseases. *Nat. Commun.* **2017**, *8*, 1–11. [CrossRef]
30. Winters, A.D.; Romero, R.; Gervasi, M.T.; Gomez-Lopez, N.; Tran, M.R.; Garcia-Flores, V.; Pacora, P.; Jung, E.; Hassan, S.S.; Hsu, C.-D.; et al. Does the endometrial cavity have a molecular microbial signature? *Sci. Rep.* **2019**, *9*, 1–17. [CrossRef]
31. Lu, W.; He, F.; Lin, Z.; Liu, S.; Tang, L.; Huang, Y.; Hu, Z. Dysbiosis of the endometrial microbiota and its association with inflammatory cytokines in endometrial cancer. *Int. J. Cancer* **2021**, *148*, 1708–1716. [CrossRef] [PubMed]
32. Rajagopala, S.V.; Vashee, S.; Oldfield, L.M.; Suzuki, Y.; Venter, J.C.; Telenti, A.; Nelson, K.E. The Human Microbiome and Cancer. *Cancer Prev. Res.* **2017**, *10*, 226–234. [CrossRef]
33. Garrett, W.S. Cancer and the microbiota. *Science* **2015**, *348*, 80–86. [CrossRef]
34. Wang, F.; Meng, W.; Wang, B.; Qiao, L. Helicobacter pylori-induced gastric inflammation and gastric cancer. *Cancer Lett.* **2014**, *345*, 196–202. [CrossRef]
35. Mayrand, M.-H.; Duarte-Franco, E.; Rodrigues, I.; Walter, S.D.; Hanley, J.; Ferenczy, A.; Ratnam, S.; Coutlée, F.; Franco, E. Human Papillomavirus DNA versus Papanicolaou Screening Tests for Cervical Cancer. *N. Engl. J. Med.* **2007**, *357*, 1579–1588. [CrossRef] [PubMed]
36. Myšák, J.; Podzimek, S.; Sommerova, P.; Lyuya-Mi, Y.; Bartova, J.; Janatova, T.; Prochazkova, J.; Duškova, J. Porphyromonas gingivalis: Major Periodontopathic Pathogen Overview. *J. Immunol. Res.* **2014**, *2014*, 1–8. [CrossRef] [PubMed]
37. Hokenstad, A.; Mariani, A.; Walther-Antonio, M. Vaginal detection of Porphyromonas somerae is indicative of endometrial cancer diagnosis. *Gynecol. Oncol.* **2017**, *145*, 76. [CrossRef]
38. Gonzalez-Bosquet, J.; Pedra-Nobre, S.; Devor, E.; Thiel, K.; Goodheart, M.; Bender, D.; Leslie, K. Bacterial, Archaea, and Viral Transcripts (BAVT) Expression in Gynecological Cancers and Correlation with Regulatory Regions of the Genome. *Cancers* **2021**, *13*, 1109. [CrossRef] [PubMed]
39. Walsh, D.M.; Hokenstad, A.N.; Chen, J.; Sung, J.; Jenkins, G.D.; Chia, N.; Nelson, H.; Mariani, A.; Walther-Antonio, M.R.S. Postmenopause as a key factor in the composition of the Endometrial Cancer Microbiome (ECbiome). *Sci. Rep.* **2019**, *9*, 19213–19216. [CrossRef] [PubMed]
40. Amabebe, E.; Anumba, D.O.C. The Vaginal Microenvironment: The Physiologic Role of Lactobacilli. *Front. Med.* **2018**, *5*, 181. [CrossRef] [PubMed]

41. Mendling, W.; Palmeira-De-Oliveira, A.; Biber, S.; Prasauskas, V. An update on the role of Atopobium vaginae in bacterial vaginosis: What to consider when choosing a treatment? A mini review. *Arch. Gynecol. Obstet.* **2019**, *300*, 1–6. [CrossRef]
42. Groothuis, P.; Dassen, H.; Romano, A.; Punyadeera, C. Estrogen and the endometrium: Lessons learned from gene expression profiling in rodents and human. *Hum. Reprod. Updat.* **2007**, *13*, 405–417. [CrossRef]
43. Rodriguez, A.C.; Blanchard, Z.; Maurer, K.A.; Gertz, J. Estrogen Signaling in Endometrial Cancer: A Key Oncogenic Pathway with Several Open Questions. *Horm. Cancer* **2019**, *10*, 51–63. [CrossRef] [PubMed]
44. Van Weelden, W.J.; Massuger, L.F.A.G.; Pijnenborg, J.M.A.; Romano, A. Enitec Anti-estrogen Treatment in Endometrial Cancer: A Systematic Review. *Front. Oncol.* **2019**, *9*, 359. [CrossRef] [PubMed]
45. Zhu, B.T. Functional role of estrogen metabolism in target cells: Review and perspectives. *Carcinogenesis* **1998**, *19*, 1–27. [CrossRef]
46. Flores, R.; Shi, J.; Fuhrman, B.; Xu, X.; Veenstra, T.D.; Gail, M.H.; Gajer, P.; Ravel, J.; Goedert, J.J. Fecal microbial determinants of fecal and systemic estrogens and estrogen metabolites: A cross-sectional study. *J. Transl. Med.* **2012**, *10*, 253. [CrossRef] [PubMed]
47. Plottel, C.S.; Blaser, M.J. Microbiome and Malignancy. *Cell Host Microbe* **2011**, *10*, 324–335. [CrossRef] [PubMed]
48. Beaud, D.; Tailliez, P.; Anba-Mondoloni, J. Genetic characterization of the β-glucuronidase enzyme from a human intestinal bacterium, Ruminococcus gnavus. *Microbiology* **2005**, *151*, 2323–2330. [CrossRef] [PubMed]
49. Baker, J.M.; Al-Nakkash, L.; Herbst-Kralovetz, M.M. Estrogen–Gut microbiome axis: Physiological and clinical implications. *Maturitas* **2017**, *103*, 45–53. [CrossRef] [PubMed]
50. Pollet, R.M.; D'Agostino, E.H.; Walton, W.G.; Xu, Y.; Little, M.S.; Biernat, K.A.; Pellock, S.J.; Patterson, L.M.; Creekmore, B.; Isenberg, H.N.; et al. An Atlas of β-Glucuronidases in the Human Intestinal Microbiome. *Structure* **2017**, *25*, 967–977.e5. [CrossRef]
51. Parida, S.; Sharma, D. The Microbiome–Estrogen Connection and Breast Cancer Risk. *Cells* **2019**, *8*, 1642. [CrossRef]
52. Łaniewski, P.; Ilhan, Z.E.; Herbst-Kralovetz, M.M. The microbiome and gynaecological cancer development, prevention and therapy. *Nat. Rev. Urol.* **2020**, *17*, 232–250. [CrossRef]
53. Balkwill, F.; Mantovani, A. Inflammation and cancer: Back to Virchow? *Lancet* **2001**, *357*, 539–545. [CrossRef]
54. Modugno, F.; Ness, R.B.; Chen, C.; Weiss, N.S. Inflammation and Endometrial Cancer: A Hypothesis. *Cancer Epidemiol. Biomark. Prev.* **2005**, *14*, 2840–2847. [CrossRef] [PubMed]
55. Dossus, L.; Rinaldi, S.; Becker, S.; Lukanova, A.; Tjonneland, A.; Olsen, A.; Stegger, J.; Overvad, K.; Chabbert-Buffet, N.; Jimenez-Corona, A.; et al. Obesity, inflammatory markers, and endometrial cancer risk: A prospective case–control study. *Endocr. Relat. Cancer* **2010**, *17*, 1007–1019. [CrossRef]
56. Zhao, Y.; Nichols, J.E.; Bulun, S.E.; Mendelson, C.; Simpson, E.R. Aromatase P450 Gene Expression in Human Adipose Tissue. Role of a Jak/Stat Pathway in Regulation of the Adipose-Specific Promoter. *J. Biol. Chem.* **1995**, *270*, 16449–16457. [CrossRef] [PubMed]
57. Che, Q.; Liu, B.-Y.; Liao, Y.; Zhang, H.-J.; Yang, T.-T.; He, Y.-Y.; Xia, Y.-H.; Lu, W.; He, X.-Y.; Chen, Z.; et al. Activation of a positive feedback loop involving IL-6 and aromatase promotes intratumoral 17β-estradiol biosynthesis in endometrial carcinoma microenvironment. *Int. J. Cancer* **2014**, *135*, 282–294. [CrossRef]
58. St-Germain, M.-E.; Gagnon, V.; Parent, S.; Asselin, E. Regulation of COX-2 protein expression by Akt in endometrial cancer cells is mediated through NF-κB/IκB pathway. *Mol. Cancer* **2004**, *3*, 7. [CrossRef] [PubMed]
59. Francescone, R.; Hou, V.; Grivennikov, S.I. Microbiome, Inflammation, and Cancer. *Cancer J.* **2014**, *20*, 181–189. [CrossRef]
60. Pelzer, E.S.; Willner, D.; Buttini, M.; Huygens, F. A role for the endometrial microbiome in dysfunctional menstrual bleeding. *Antonie Van Leeuwenhoek* **2018**, *111*, 933–943. [CrossRef]
61. Caselli, E.; Soffritti, I.; D'Accolti, M.; Piva, I.; Greco, P.; Bonaccorsi, G. Atopobium Vaginae And Porphyromonas Somerae Induce Proinflammatory Cytokines Expression In Endometrial Cells: A Possible Implication For Endometrial Cancer? *Cancer Manag. Res.* **2019**, *11*, 8571–8575. [CrossRef]
62. Keita, M.; Bessette, P.; Pelmus, M.; AinMelk, Y.; Aris, A. Expression of interleukin-1 (IL-1) ligands system in the most common endometriosis-associated ovarian cancer subtypes. *J. Ovarian Res.* **2010**, *3*, 3. [CrossRef] [PubMed]
63. Hirata, T.; Osuga, Y.; Hamasaki, K.; Yoshino, O.; Ito, M.; Hasegawa, A.; Takemura, Y.; Hirota, Y.; Nose, E.; Morimoto, C.; et al. Interleukin (IL)-17A Stimulates IL-8 Secretion, Cyclooxygensase-2 Expression, and Cell Proliferation of Endometriotic Stromal Cells. *Endocrinology* **2008**, *149*, 1260–1267. [CrossRef] [PubMed]
64. Smith, H.O.; Stephens, N.D.; Qualls, C.R.; Fligelman, T.; Wang, T.; Lin, C.-Y.; Burton, E.H.; Griffith, J.K.; Pollard, J.W. The clinical significance of inflammatory cytokines in primary cell culture in endometrial carcinoma. *Mol. Oncol.* **2012**, *7*, 41–54. [CrossRef]
65. Tong, H.; Feng, H.; Hu, X.; Wang, M.-F.; Song, Y.-F.; Wen, X.-L.; Li, Y.-R.; Wan, X.-P. Identification of Interleukin-9 Producing Immune Cells in Endometrial Carcinoma and Establishment of a Prognostic Nomogram. *Front. Immunol.* **2020**, *11*, 11. [CrossRef] [PubMed]
66. Brooks, R.A.; Fleming, G.F.; Lastra, R.R.; Lee, N.K.; Moroney, J.W.; Son, C.H.; Tatebe, K.; Veneris, J.L. Current recommendations and recent progress in endometrial cancer. *CA Cancer J. Clin.* **2019**, *69*, 258–279. [CrossRef] [PubMed]
67. Andreyev, J. Gastrointestinal complications of pelvic radiotherapy: Are they of any importance? *Gut* **2005**, *54*, 1051–1054. [CrossRef]
68. Bhatt, A.P.; Redinbo, M.R.; Bultman, S.J. The role of the microbiome in cancer development and therapy. *CA Cancer J. Clin.* **2017**, *67*, 326–344. [CrossRef] [PubMed]
69. Steven, A.; Fisher, S.A.; Robinson, B.W.; Fong, K.M.; Van Zandwijk, N. Immunotherapy for lung cancer. *Respirology* **2016**, *21*, 821–833. [CrossRef]

70. Ventriglia, J.; Paciolla, I.; Pisano, C.; Cecere, S.C.; Di Napoli, M.; Tambaro, R.; Califano, D.; Losito, N.; Scognamiglio, G.; Setola, S.V.; et al. Immunotherapy in ovarian, endometrial and cervical cancer: State of the art and future perspectives. *Cancer Treat. Rev.* **2017**, *59*, 109–116. [CrossRef]
71. Yang, Y. Cancer immunotherapy: Harnessing the immune system to battle cancer. *J. Clin. Investig.* **2015**, *125*, 3335–3337. [CrossRef]
72. Kennedy, L.B.; Salama, A. A review of cancer immunotherapy toxicity. *CA Cancer J. Clin.* **2020**, *70*, 86–104. [CrossRef] [PubMed]
73. Sivan, A.; Corrales, L.; Hubert, N.; Williams, J.B.; Aquino-Michaels, K.; Earley, Z.M.; Benyamin, F.W.; Lei, Y.M.; Jabri, B.; Alegre, M.-L.; et al. Commensal Bifidobacterium promotes antitumor immunity and facilitates anti-pd-l1 efficacy. *Science* **2015**, *350*, 1084–1089. [CrossRef] [PubMed]
74. Routy, B.; Le Chatelier, E.; DeRosa, L.; Duong, C.P.M.; Alou, M.T.; Daillère, R.; Fluckiger, A.; Messaoudene, M.; Rauber, C.; Roberti, M.P.; et al. Gut microbiome influences efficacy of PD-1–based immunotherapy against epithelial tumors. *Science* **2018**, *359*, 91–97. [CrossRef] [PubMed]
75. Gopalakrishnan, V.; Spencer, C.N.; Nezi, L.; Reuben, A.; Andrews, M.C.; Karpinets, T.V.; Prieto, P.A.; Vicente, D.; Hoffman, K.; Wei, S.C.; et al. Gut microbiome modulates response to anti–PD-1 immunotherapy in melanoma patients. *Science* **2018**, *359*, 97–103. [CrossRef] [PubMed]
76. Borella, F.; Carosso, A.R.; Cosma, S.; Preti, M.; Collemi, G.; Cassoni, P.; Bertero, L.; Benedetto, C. Gut Microbiota and Gynecological Cancers: A Summary of Pathogenetic Mechanisms and Future Directions. *ACS Infect. Dis.* **2021**, *7*, 987–1009. [CrossRef] [PubMed]
77. Ma, W.; Mao, Q.; Xia, W.; Dong, G.; Yu, C.; Jiang, F. Gut Microbiota Shapes the Efficiency of Cancer Therapy. *Front. Microbiol.* **2019**, *10*, 1050. [CrossRef]
78. Chaput, N.; Lepage, P.; Coutzac, C.; Soularue, E.; Le Roux, K.; Monot, C.; Boselli, L.; Routier, E.; Cassard, L.; Collins, M.; et al. Baseline gut microbiota predicts clinical response and colitis in metastatic melanoma patients treated with ipilimumab. *Ann. Oncol.* **2017**, *28*, 1368–1379. [CrossRef]
79. Cramer, P.; Bresalier, R.S. Gastrointestinal and Hepatic Complications of Immune Checkpoint Inhibitors. *Curr. Gastroenterol. Rep.* **2017**, *19*, 3. [CrossRef]
80. Vétizou, M.; Pitt, J.M.; Daillère, R.; Lepage, P.; Waldschmitt, N.; Flament, C.; Rusakiewicz, S.; Routy, B.; Roberti, M.P.; Duong, C.P.M.; et al. Anticancer immunotherapy by CTLA-4 blockade relies on the gut microbiota. *Science* **2015**, *350*, 1079–1084. [CrossRef]
81. Grisham, R.N.; Adaniel, C.; Hyman, D.M.; Ma, W.; Iasonos, A.; Aghajanian, C.; Konner, J. Gemcitabine for Advanced Endometrial Cancer: A Review of the MSKCC Experience. *Int. J. Gynecol. Cancer* **2012**, *22*, 807–811. [CrossRef]
82. Chen, S.-M.; Chieng, W.-W.; Huang, S.-W.; Hsu, L.-J.; Jan, M.-S. The synergistic tumor growth-inhibitory effect of probiotic Lactobacillus on transgenic mouse model of pancreatic cancer treated with gemcitabine. *Sci. Rep.* **2020**, *10*, 1–12. [CrossRef]
83. Nishio, S.; Shimokawa, M.; Tasaki, K.; Nasu, H.; Yoshimitsu, T.; Matsukuma, K.; Terada, A.; Tsuda, N.; Kawano, K.; Ushijima, K. A phase II trial of irinotecan in patients with advanced or recurrent endometrial cancer and correlation with biomarker analysis. *Gynecol. Oncol.* **2018**, *150*, 432–437. [CrossRef] [PubMed]
84. Bhatt, A.P.; Pellock, S.J.; Biernat, K.A.; Walton, W.G.; Wallace, B.D.; Creekmore, B.C.; Letertre, M.M.; Swann, J.; Wilson, I.D.; Roques, J.R.; et al. Targeted inhibition of gut bacterial β-glucuronidase activity enhances anticancer drug efficacy. *Proc. Natl. Acad. Sci. USA* **2020**, *117*, 7374–7381. [CrossRef]
85. Yan, A.; Culp, E.; Perry, J.; Lau, J.T.; MacNeil, L.T.; Surette, M.G.; Wright, G.D. Transformation of the Anticancer Drug Doxorubicin in the Human Gut Microbiome. *ACS Infect. Dis.* **2018**, *4*, 68–76. [CrossRef]
86. Rigby, R.; Carr, J.; Orgel, K.; King, S.L.; Lund, P.K.; Dekaney, C.M. Intestinal bacteria are necessary for doxorubicin-induced intestinal damage but not for doxorubicin-induced apoptosis. *Gut Microbes* **2016**, *7*, 414–423. [CrossRef]
87. Hong, B.-Y.; Sobue, T.; Choquette, L.; Dupuy, A.K.; Thompson, A.; Burleson, J.A.; Salner, A.L.; Schauer, P.K.; Joshi, P.; Fox, E.; et al. Chemotherapy-induced oral mucositis is associated with detrimental bacterial dysbiosis. *Microbiome* **2019**, *7*, 1–18. [CrossRef] [PubMed]
88. Ramakrishna, C.; Corleto, J.; Ruegger, P.M.; Logan, G.D.; Peacock, B.B.; Mendonca, S.; Yamaki, S.; Adamson, T.; Ermel, R.; McKemy, D.; et al. Dominant Role of the Gut Microbiota in Chemotherapy Induced Neuropathic Pain. *Sci. Rep.* **2019**, *9*, 1–16. [CrossRef]
89. DeMaria, S.; Formenti, S.C. Radiation as an immunological adjuvant: Current evidence on dose and fractionation. *Front. Oncol.* **2012**, *2*, 153. [CrossRef]
90. Barker, H.E.; Paget, J.T.E.; Khan, A.; Harrington, K. The tumour microenvironment after radiotherapy: Mechanisms of resistance and recurrence. *Nat. Rev. Cancer* **2015**, *15*, 409–425. [CrossRef] [PubMed]
91. Yan, F.; Cao, H.; Cover, T.; Whitehead, R.; Washington, M.K.; Polk, D.B. Soluble Proteins Produced by Probiotic Bacteria Regulate Intestinal Epithelial Cell Survival and Growth. *Gastroenterology* **2007**, *132*, 562–575. [CrossRef]
92. Ciorba, M.A.; Riehl, T.E.; Rao, M.S.; Moon, C.; Ee, X.; Nava, G.; Walker, M.R.; Marinshaw, J.M.; Stappenbeck, T.S.; Stenson, W.F. Lactobacillus probiotic protects intestinal epithelium from radiation injury in a TLR-2/cyclo-oxygenase-2-dependent manner. *Gut* **2011**, *61*, 829–838. [CrossRef] [PubMed]
93. Delia, P. Use of probiotics for prevention of radiation-induced diarrhea. *World J. Gastroenterol.* **2007**, *13*, 912. [CrossRef] [PubMed]
94. Mitamura, T.; Dong, P.; Ihira, K.; Kudo, M.; Watari, H. Molecular-targeted therapies and precision medicine for endometrial cancer. *Jpn. J. Clin. Oncol.* **2019**, *49*, 108–120. [CrossRef]

95. Di Modica, M.; Gargari, G.; Regondi, V.; Bonizzi, A.; Arioli, S.; Belmonte, B.; De Cecco, L.; Fasano, E.; Bianchi, F.; Bertolotti, A.; et al. Gut Microbiota Condition the Therapeutic Efficacy of Trastuzumab in HER2-Positive Breast Cancer. *Cancer Res.* **2021**, *81*, 2195–2206. [CrossRef] [PubMed]
96. Flórez, A.B.; Sierra, M.; Ruas-Madiedo, P.; Mayo, B. Susceptibility of lactic acid bacteria, bifidobacteria and other bacteria of intestinal origin to chemotherapeutic agents. *Int. J. Antimicrob. Agents* **2016**, *48*, 547–550. [CrossRef]
97. Berstein, L.; Maximov, S.; Gershfeld, E.; Meshkova, I.; Gamajunova, V.; Tsyrlina, E.; Larionov, A.; Kovalevskij, A.; Vasilyev, D. Neoadjuvant therapy of endometrial cancer with the aromatase inhibitor letrozole: Endocrine and clinical effects. *Eur. J. Obstet. Gynecol. Reprod. Biol.* **2002**, *105*, 161–165. [CrossRef]
98. Cao, Y.; Jiang, C.; Jia, Y.; Xu, D.; Yu, Y. Letrozole and the Traditional Chinese Medicine, Shaofu Zhuyu Decoction, Reduce Endometriotic Disease Progression in Rats: A Potential Role for Gut Microbiota. *Evid. Based Complement. Altern. Med.* **2020**, *2020*, 1–14. [CrossRef]
99. Helmink, B.A.; Khan, M.A.W.; Hermann, A.; Gopalakrishnan, V.; Wargo, J.A. The microbiome, cancer, and cancer therapy. *Nat. Med.* **2019**, *25*, 377–388. [CrossRef]
100. Chase, D.; Goulder, A.; Zenhausern, F.; Monk, B.; Herbst-Kralovetz, M. The vaginal and gastrointestinal microbiomes in gynecologic cancers: A review of applications in etiology, symptoms and treatment. *Gynecol. Oncol.* **2015**, *138*, 190–200. [CrossRef]
101. Montassier, E.; Gastinne, T.; Vangay, P.; Al-Ghalith, G.A.; Des Varannes, S.B.; Massart, S.; Moreau, P.; Potel, G.; De La Cochetière, M.F.; Batard, E.; et al. Chemotherapy-driven dysbiosis in the intestinal microbiome. *Aliment. Pharmacol. Ther.* **2015**, *42*, 515–528. [CrossRef] [PubMed]
102. van Vliet, M.J.; Harmsen, H.J.M.; de Bont, E.S.J.M.; Tissing, W.J.E. The Role of Intestinal Microbiota in the Development and Severity of Chemotherapy-Induced Mucositis. *PLoS Pathog.* **2010**, *6*, e1000879. [CrossRef] [PubMed]
103. Benner, M.; Ferwerda, G.; Joosten, I.; Van Der Molen, R.G. How uterine microbiota might be responsible for a receptive, fertile endometrium. *Hum. Reprod. Updat.* **2018**, *24*, 393–415. [CrossRef] [PubMed]
104. Molina, N.M.; Sola-Leyva, A.; Saez-Lara, M.J.; Plaza-Diaz, J.; Tubić-Pavlović, A.; Romero, B.; Clavero, A.; Mozas-Moreno, J.; Fontes, J.; Altmäe, S. New Opportunities for Endometrial Health by Modifying Uterine Microbial Composition: Present or Future? *Biomolecules* **2020**, *10*, 593. [CrossRef] [PubMed]
105. Chenoll, E.; Moreno, I.; Sánchez, M.; Garcia-Grau, I.; Silva, Á.; González-Monfort, M.; Genovés, S.; Vilella, F.; Seco-Durban, C.; Simón, C.; et al. Selection of New Probiotics for Endometrial Health. *Front. Cell. Infect. Microbiol.* **2019**, *9*, 114. [CrossRef] [PubMed]
106. Swidsinski, A.; Verstraelen, H.; Loening-Baucke, V.; Swidsinski, S.; Mendling, W.; Halwani, Z. Presence of a Polymicrobial Endometrial Biofilm in Patients with Bacterial Vaginosis. *PLoS ONE* **2013**, *8*, e53997. [CrossRef]
107. Dizzell, S.; Nazli, A.; Reid, G.; Kaushic, C. Protective Effect of Probiotic Bacteria and Estrogen in Preventing HIV-1-Mediated Impairment of Epithelial Barrier Integrity in Female Genital Tract. *Cells* **2019**, *8*, 1120. [CrossRef]
108. Kyono, K.; Hashimoto, T.; Kikuchi, S.; Nagai, Y.; Sakuraba, Y. A pilot study and case reports on endometrial microbiota and pregnancy outcome: An analysis using 16S rRNA gene sequencing among IVF patients, and trial therapeutic intervention for dysbiotic endometrium. *Reprod. Med. Biol.* **2019**, *18*, 72–82. [CrossRef]
109. Lev-Sagie, A.; Goldman-Wohl, D.; Cohen, Y.; Dori-Bachash, M.; Leshem, A.; Mor, U.; Strahilevitz, J.; Moses, A.E.; Shapiro, H.; Yagel, S.; et al. Vaginal microbiome transplantation in women with intractable bacterial vaginosis. *Nat. Med.* **2019**, *25*, 1500–1504. [CrossRef]
110. Romero, R.; Gomez-Lopez, N.; Winters, A.D.; Jung, E.; Shaman, M.; Bieda, J.; Panaitescu, B.; Pacora, P.; Erez, O.; Greenberg, J.M.; et al. Evidence that intra-amniotic infections are often the result of an ascending invasion—A molecular microbiological study. *J. Périnat. Med.* **2019**, *47*, 915–931. [CrossRef]
111. Vornhagen, J.; Armistead, B.; Santana-Ufret, V.; Gendrin, C.; Merillat, S.; Coleman, M.; Quach, P.; Boldenow, E.; Alishetti, V.; Leonhard-Melief, C.; et al. Group B streptococcus exploits vaginal epithelial exfoliation for ascending infection. *J. Clin. Investig.* **2018**, *128*, 1985–1999. [CrossRef] [PubMed]

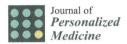

Journal of
Personalized
Medicine

Review

Exploring the Oral Microbiome in Rheumatic Diseases, State of Art and Future Prospective in Personalized Medicine with an AI Approach

Silvia Bellando-Randone [1,†], Edda Russo [1,†], Vincenzo Venerito [2], Marco Matucci-Cerinic [1,3], Florenzo Iannone [2], Sabina Tangaro [4] and Amedeo Amedei [1,*]

1. Department of Clinical and Experimental Medicine, University of Florence, Largo Brambilla 3, 50134 Florence, Italy; silvia.bellandorandone@unifi.it (S.B.-R.); edda.russo@unifi.it (E.R.); marco.matuccicerinic@unifi.it (M.M.-C.)
2. Rheumatology Unit, Department of Emergency and Organ Transplantations, University of Bari "Aldo Moro", 70121 Bari, Italy; vincenzo.venerito@uniba.it (V.V.); florenzo.iannone@uniba.it (F.I.)
3. Unit of Immunology, Rheumatology, Allergy and Rare Diseases (UnIRAR), IRCCS San Raffaele Hospital, 20132 Milan, Italy
4. Dipartimento Interateneo di Fisica "M. Merlin", Istituto Nazionale di Fisica Nucleare, Sezione di Bari, 70121 Bari, Italy; sabina.tangaro@uniba.it
* Correspondence: amedeo.amedei@unifi.it; Tel.: +39-(0)5-5275-8330
† Equal contribution.

Abstract: The oral microbiome is receiving growing interest from the scientific community, as the mouth is the gateway for numerous potential etiopathogenetic factors in different diseases. In addition, the progression of niches from the mouth to the gut, defined as "oral–gut microbiome axis", affects several pathologies, as rheumatic diseases. Notably, rheumatic disorders (RDs) are conditions causing chronic, often intermittent pain affecting the joints or connective tissue. In this review, we examine evidence which supports a role for the oral microbiome in the etiology and progression of various RDs, including rheumatoid arthritis (RA), Sjogren's syndrome (SS), and systemic lupus erythematosus (SLE). In addition, we address the most recent studies endorsing the oral microbiome as promising diagnostic biomarkers for RDs. Lastly, we introduce the concepts of artificial intelligence (AI), in particular, machine learning (ML) and their general application for understanding the link between oral microbiota and rheumatic diseases, speculating the application of a possible AI approach-based that can be applied to personalized medicine in the future.

Keywords: oral microbiota; microbiome; rheumatology diseases; biomarkers; artificial intelligence; machine learning; rheumatoid arthritis; Sjogren's syndrome; systemic lupus erythematosus

Citation: Bellando-Randone, S.; Russo, E.; Venerito, V.; Matucci-Cerinic, M.; Iannone, F.; Tangaro, S.; Amedei, A. Exploring the Oral Microbiome in Rheumatic Diseases, State of Art and Future Prospective in Personalized Medicine with an AI Approach. *J. Pers. Med.* 2021, 11, 625. https://doi.org/10.3390/jpm11070625

Academic Editor: J. Luis Espinoza

Received: 12 May 2021
Accepted: 28 June 2021
Published: 30 June 2021

Publisher's Note: MDPI stays neutral with regard to jurisdictional claims in published maps and institutional affiliations.

Copyright: © 2021 by the authors. Licensee MDPI, Basel, Switzerland. This article is an open access article distributed under the terms and conditions of the Creative Commons Attribution (CC BY) license (https://creativecommons.org/licenses/by/4.0/).

1. Introduction

The human body is a symbiotic ecosystem containing trillions of microorganisms classified into the domains of the *Eukarya* (and their viruses), *Bacteria*, *Archaea*. These communities have been named as microbiota, while the term microbiome describes either the collective genome of the microorganisms that reside in an environmental niche. The microbiota is on all surfaces of our body exposed to the external environment, from the respiratory to the gastrointestinal and urogenital tract.

A balanced composition of the microbiome is of paramount significance, influencing healthy and pathological states through many biological activities as regulation of metabolic processes, energy extraction, defense from pathogenic microorganisms, production of vitamins, and modulation of the immune system [1–4]. A healthy microbiome is described by high diversity, while the loss of variety may lead to "dysbiosis", a crucial condition of disequilibrium between pathogenic and commensal bacteria. Human microbiota has been studied in several tissue sites as skin, oral, subgingival, nasal, lung, and vessels.

Currently, the oral microbiome is receiving growing interest from the scientific community, as the mouth is the gateway for different potential etiopathogenetic factors in numerous diseases. Thus, also the commensal oral microbiome has an important role in the maintenance of oral and systemic health. Due to the abundance of nutrients, the human oral cavity represents an ideal habitat for the most varied and distinctive communities of microorganism in the human body, however, to date, these communities remain relatively understudied as compared to the gut ones [3,5]. The ecological oral niche consists of five distinct areas: saliva, teeth, tongue, gingival sulcus and periodontal pocket, and the remaining oral mucosa. Concerning the microbiota composition of the oral niches, it has been observed that the mouth bacterial microflora is organized as a highly interconnected chain of microbiomes across the human body, creating a kind of micro-biosphere, composed of small multiple ecological niches with different groups of microorganisms [6]. The progression of niches from the mouth to the intestine is defined as "oral–gut microbiome axis", rather that the oral microbiome alone, it is the complexity of the interrelationships between the different microbiomes through this axis that affects the healthy status. However, transfer of oral bacteria to the gut is therefore common. Members of the oral and oropharyngeal microbiota reach the gut through swallowed saliva, nutrients, and drinks.

Multiple reports on the composition of the microflora within the oral niches show higher levels of the genus *Corynebacterium* in gingival plaques [7] and higher levels of the phylum *Firmicutes* in buccal mucosa and saliva [8]. In addition, fungi have also been detected as members of the healthy oral microbiota (belonging to the oral Mycobiota) [9].

It has been observed that several factors are the main causes for oral microflora dysbiosis, including poor oral hygiene, dietary habits, gingival inflammation, dysfunction of the salivary glands, smoking, genetic difference [10,11]. In addition, changes in the salivary concentration of nutrients, oxygen, and pH can induce the selection of different microorganisms involved in the formation of their own niche via biofilm development or nutrient metabolism [12]. However, a dysbiotic oral microbiome is involved in a number of oral infectious diseases, such as periodontitis, dental caries, alveolar bone loss, endodontic infection, and tonsillitis [13], and finally seem to be involved in pathogenesis of more systemic diseases [14–16]. It has been speculated that the dysbiosis in the oral cavity is guided by "keystone pathogens", which can regulate community microbiome variations. Due to the high vascularity of the mouth and the manipulation of a host response, the dysbiotic oral microflora can influence the activities at other body districts. As previously cited, this condition suggests potential implications of the oral microbiome not only in oral diseases but also in a number of systemic pathologies [17–19] and notably, several cancer types [20]. Recently, many scientists have focused on the potential role of the commensal bacteria in the pathogenesis of systemic autoimmune diseases as rheumatic diseases (RDs).

2. The Oral Microbiome in Rheumatic Diseases

The etiopathogenesis of systemic autoimmune diseases is still almost unknown, but a complex interplay of environmental and genetic factors associated at stochastic events lead to loss of immunological tolerance and autoimmunity [21]. Numerous advances in understanding RDs pathogenesis have provided a mechanistic framework for studying host–microbiota interactions and candidate pathobionts. The gut microbiome is the most deeply evaluated also in RDs but several studies of the human skin, oral, subgingival, nasal, lung, and vascular microbiota suggest that dysbiosis is a common feature across rheumatic diseases, in particular, rheumatoid arthritis (RA), connective tissue diseases, and primary vasculitides and it might impact their symptoms and disease course [22] (Figure 1).

The introduction of high-throughput methods in microbiome analysis like sequencing of 16S rRNA, NGS (Next Generation Sequencing), and metabolomics gave the possibilities for large cohort studies which showed that microbiota may have a protective, neutral, or provocative role in the context of autoimmunity as Yurkovetskiy et al. pointed out [23].

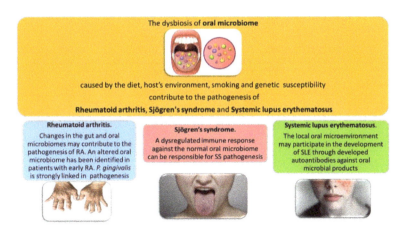

Figure 1. The dysbiosis of oral microbiome in rheumatic diseases.

For example, commensals may have direct effects as the well established molecular mimicry that may be a potential ligand to autoimmunity through the existence of nonselective T cell receptors with cross-reactivity to self-antigens [23–25].

Moreover, in recent years, saliva analysis has also played a central role in the definitions of biomarkers for the diagnosis, prognosis, and treatment of oral and systemic disease. Recent advances in salivary biomarker diagnostics have broadened the discovery of microbial pathogens associated with systemic and oral diseases [26]. While host biomarkers are subjected to individual biological variation, oral microbiome is relatively conserved among unrelated individuals. Indeed, the analysis of the oral microbial changes could be considered in the future as a screening biomarker also for rheumatic diseases, leading to a personalized medicine approach. In this review, we will focus on the oral–gut microbiota axis and we will evaluate the most recent studies endorsing it as a promising diagnostic biomarker for RDs; in addition, we will explore new perspectives in microbiome research trough a machine learning approach.

3. Oral Microbiome and Rheumatoid Arthritis

Rheumatoid arthritis (RA) is a systemic chronic autoimmune inflammatory disease characterized by destruction of bone in multiple joints and auto-antibody production such as rheumatoid factor and in particular, anticitrullinated protein antibodies (ACPAs), the most powerful and earlier diagnostic biomarkers [27–29]. Periodontal disease (PD) and tobacco use seem to be related to ACPA production, RA etiopathogenesis still remains unclear. The idea that oral microbiota is involved in inducing or driving of RA progression is supported by the high frequency of periodontal inflammatory disorders in RA patients and its association with anti-CCP antibody levels [30] (Figure 2).

In addition, animal models have reported that RA alters, qualitatively and quantitatively, the oral microbiome, highlighting the bidirectional link between host and microbiota [31]. The discovery that post-translational protein citrullination primarily determines autoantibody reactivity in RA has clarified microbial contributions to its pathogenesis [32].

Periodontitis is characterized by a chronic inflammation caused by oral bacteria and leucocyte infiltration with progressive destruction of the alveolar bone and it seems to share the same pathogenetic mechanisms with RA: accumulation of leucocyte infiltration, release of inflammatory cytokines, and mediators such as prostaglandin E2 (PGE2), tumour necrosis factor (TNF)-α, and several other citokines, such as interleukin (IL)-1b, IL-6, IL-17, IL-33, IL-12, IL-18r [33]. In a recent study, salivary cytokine analysis showed that IL-17 was markedly increased in RA patients with periodontitis, but not periodontitis without RA [34].

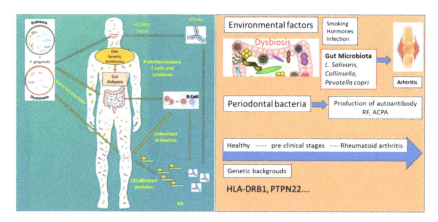

Figure 2. Genetic and environmental factors involved in the pathogenesis of rheumatoid arthritis.

P. gingivalis is considered the keystone pathogen in periodontitis and the most extensively studied in RA and it was found to deregulate local immune responses and to promote dysbiosis. The clinical association of *P. gingivalis* and RA has been investigated by many studies, most commonly by molecular detection of bacterial DNA from plaque or gingival crevicular fluid, or by bacterial culture, by measuring serum antibody reactivity and its role in the development of experimental arthritis, has been explored in animal models [35,36]. *P. gingivalis* was first proposed as a crucial agent in RA onset, expressing a bacterial protein arginine deiminase (PPAD) that can citrullinate free L-arginine and C-terminal arginine residues in cleaved peptides [37]. C-terminal citrullination of both bacterial and host protein has been hypothesized to break immunological tolerance and initiate the ACPA response in RA [38]. Sato et al. [39] also showed that *P. gingivalis* exacerbate arthritis by modulating the gut microbiota and increasing the proportion of Th17 (T helper 17) cells in mesenteric lymph nodes. Another proof of the link between RA and oral inflammation is the evidence that the treatment of periodontal disease may improve RA symptoms [40].

Furthermore, microbiome of periodontally healthy individuals with and without RA has been evaluated. The subgingival microbiota differed significantly between RA and healthy individuals. In the absence of periodontitis, *Porphyromonas gingivalis* and *A. actinomycetemcomitans* did not differ significantly between groups [41]. In contrast, *Cryptobacterium curtum* was increased in RA patients [35]. *Aggregatibacter actinomycetemcomitans*, a periodontal bacterium, was recently proposed to connect periodontitis to RA for its ability to induce citrullinated autoantigens through the bacterial pore-forming toxin leukotoxin A (LtxA), which is its primary virulence factor [42]. LtxA induces the citrullination of a wide range of RA autoantigens which are subsequently released by the dying neutrophil in a process that is reminiscent of NETosis but is biologically distinct. Exposure to *A. actinomycetemcomitans* by anti-LtxA antibody reactivity was observed in a large RA subset [42], a finding that has been replicated in an independent Dutch cohort [43,44]. HLA-DRB1 shared epitope risk alleles associated with ACPAs only in RA patients with evidence of *A. actinomycetemcomitans* exposure, suggesting that LtxA-induced protein citrullination may play a role in ACPA production in genetically susceptible subjects [42].

Several other bacteria have been implicated in RA pathogenesis. Recently, Brusca et al. [45] found that there were more organisms besides *P. gingivalis* which cause periodontal disease (i.e., *Anaerglobus geminatus* and *Prevotella/Leptotrichia*) and were linked to the ACPA presence.

In the oral flora, bacteria such as *P. intermedia/Tannerella forsythia* were found and high titers of antibodies against these microorganisms have been detected in the serum and synovial fluids of RA patients [46]. Otherwise, IgG antibodies to *P. intermedia* and

C. ochracea were found to be associated with a lower RF prevalence [47,48]. Oral microbiota seems to have a crucial role not only in RA pathogenesis but also in exacerbation of joint involvement and in treatment response. In fact, it has been shown that dysbiosis may exacerbate arthritis through the oral inoculation of *P. gingvalis* using animal models, even if the mechanism underlying the exacerbation is not entirely elucidated [49]. In a collagen-type II experimental arthritis in mice, periodontitis caused by *P. gingivalis* and *Provotellanigrescens* exacerbated arthritis through TLR2-dependent antigen-specific Th17 immune response [49].

Regarding oral microbiota in early RA patients compared to those with advanced phases, Wolff et al. showed that patients with early RA showed a high PD prevalence at disease onset [50] and that microbiota of their subgingival biofilm was similar to that of patients with chronic RA. Scher JU et al. reported that the subgingival microbiota in patients with new-onset RA was distinct from healthy controls [51].

Prevotella and *Leptotrichia* were found in subgingival microbiota from new-onset RA patients but not from healthy controls and this was unrelated to periodontal disease. The abundance of *P. gingivalis* was directly associated with periodontitis severity but it did not correlate with ACPAs, while *Anaeroglobus geminatus* correlated with ACPAs and the rheumatoid factor [52]. Zhang et al., in a large Chinese study, demonstrated that changes in the dental, saliva, or gut microbiome identified RA patients from healthy controls. In particular, treatment-naive RA patients had an increased abundance of *Lactobacillus salivarius* in the microbiota of all three sites, in particular those with high disease activity [53], while *Haemophilus* species were depleted in RA patients and negatively correlated with serum levels of autoantibodies.

Mikules et al. showed that dysbiosis was partially resolved following treatment with disease modifying anti-rheumatic drugs [54], further stressing the bidirectional crosstalk between the microbiota and their hosts. Interestingly, Ceccarelli et al. demonstrated a significant association between the percentage of *P. gingivalis* on the total tongue biofilm and RA disease activity (DAS28) [55].

Furthermore, studies have shown that RA patients have altered gut and mouth microbiomes that are partly normalized after disease modifying antirheumatic drugs (DMARDs) and could predict response to treatment [56]. Zhang, X. et al. showed that patients that responded well to treatment were characterized by a greater number of virulence factors before treatment and also by the reduction in *Holdemania filiformis* and *Bacteroides* sp. after treatment. They also reported that the effect on the gut microbiome was moderate compared to the oral microbiome [53].

4. Link between Oral Microbiome and Sjogren's Syndrome

Sjogren's syndrome (SS) is an autoimmune disease characterized by autoantibody production (frequently directed against ribonucleoproteins TRIM21/Ro52/SS-A, Ro60, and La/SS-B), destruction of exocrine glands (in particular, salivary and lacrimal) by lymphocytes, and of extraglandular epithelial tissues [57]. SS can co-exist or pre-exist with other RD and then, it is known as secondary Sjogren's syndrome. Exocrine glands infiltration causes a reduction of production of saliva and tear film, leading to an alteration of mucosal barrier function and favoring dysbiosis and colonization with pathobionts [58]. From a clinical point of view, the most frequent symptoms are dryness of mouth and eyes while extraglandular manifestations include arthritis, peripheral neuropathy, cutaneous vasculitis, respiratory dysfunction, and tubulointerstitial nephritis [59]. The condition of dry mouth imposes a very significant burden on many oral functions, such as speaking and eating, reducing greatly the life quality of patients but also making patients at a considerable risk for severe oral and dental diseases. However, SS is considered benign, even patients have an increased risk of developing lymphoma. Genetic predisposition and environmental factors are the most important etiopathogenetic SS factors [60], but, as recently suggested, also the dysbiosis may play a significant role in SS pathogenesis. Oral and gut microbiome in SS have been explored to evaluate a possible interplay between human microbiome and SS clinical manifestations and disease severity. In fact, SS alters the saliva composition, which in turn induces alterations in the oral microbiome, certain organisms e.g., *Capnocytophaga, Dialister, Fusobacterium, Helicobacter, Streptococcus*, and *Veilonella* were found in abundance in SS, while *Porphyromona sgingivalis* and *Actinobacillus actinomycetemcomitans* were not detected in any SS patient [61]. On the other hand, it has been hypothesized that dysbiosis and bacterial translocation propagate local and systemic inflammation, modulating SS severity (Figure 3).

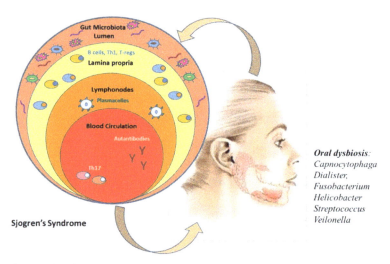

Figure 3. Oral dysbiosis in Sjogren's syndrome.

In recent years, there have been five studies focused on SS microbiome and exploring different oral niches: one each from saliva [62], tongue [63], and oral washings [64] and two from buccal mucosa [65]. Interesting results have been reported on oral microbiota composition in primary SS (pSS). Van der Meulen et al. [14] examined the bacterial composition by 16S rRNA sequencing of the oral microbiome in 37 pSS patients, 86 non-SS sicca patients, and 24 healthy controls. They found that buccal mucosa microbiome of pSS and non-SS sicca patients differed from healthy controls, with a higher *Firmicutes/Proteobacteria* ratio observed in both SS and non-SS sicca patients. These data highlight how oral dryness may favor dysbiosis. In a similar study, evaluating chewing-stimulated whole saliva *Porphyromonas endodontalis, Prevotella intermedia, Fusobacterium nucleatum vincentii, Streptococcus intermedius, Tannerella* spp., and *Treponema* spp. were only detected in the context of oral dryness (SS and non-SS sicca patients), while *Porphyromonas pasteri* showed increased abundance in healthy controls [66]. De Pavia et al. found that patients with primary SS had increased levels of *Lactobacillus* spp., *S. mutans*, and *Candida albicans* within their supragingival plaque samples. Samples from the oral mucosa and tongue also showed increased prevalence of *Staphylococcus* aureus and *Candida albicans*. The greatest shift in microbial differences was observed in patients who had a saliva reduction [63]. Furthermore, increasing evidence suggests a role for cross-reactivity of commensal oral and gut bacteria with SSA/Ro60 in the SS etiopathogenesis [67]. The key role of activated B cells has been established in the pathogenesis of Sjogren's syndrome. Their activation leads to the production of autoantibodies and hypergammaglobulinemia seen in some SS patients [68]. Moreover, it has been demonstrated that the von Willebrand factor type A, a microbial protein shared by different commensal oral/gut bacteria, could activate Ro60 reactive T cells, promoting autoantibody responses against Ro60. In fact, *Corynebacterium amycolatum* has been shown to colonize the lacrimal duct, making C. amycolatum Ro60 a candidate ortholog for the development of anti-Ro60 antibodies in SS [69].

It is possible that a dysregulated immune response against the normal microbiome can be one of the potential pathways starting the autoimmune responses in SS. Considering that oral infections are a common problem in SS patients, this pathway might also be involved in amplification of autoimmune responses in this disease [70]. However, whether oral dysbiosis is merely a consequence of oral dryness and decreased antimicrobial properties of saliva or an active driver of systemic and target tissue inflammation in patients with SS is still unknown. The microbiome of the buccal mucosa is not specific enough for pSS and therefore not useful for characterizing SS patients in clinical practice. It is unlikely that one specific bacterial taxon in the buccal mucosa microbiome is involved in SS etiology. Regarding the gut microbiota, Moon J et al. showed that gut dysbiosis was partly correlated to dry eye severity [71]. Furthermore, SS showed significant gut dysbiosis compared to controls and environmental dry eye syndrome, while dry eye patients showed compositional changes of gut microbiome somewhere in between Sjögren's syndrome and controls. Cano Ortiz et al. demonstrated that the SS patients had gut dysbiosis associated with increased serum levels of proinflammatory cytokines including IL-6, IL-12, IL-17, and TNF-alpha (systemic inflammation) and zonulin (intestinal permeability) that resulted in increased systemic microbial exposure [72].

5. Oral Microbiome on Systemic Lupus Erythematosus

Systemic lupus erythematosus (SLE) is a prototypic autoimmune disease affecting multiple organs, particularly in females of childbearing age. SLE is characterized by loss of tolerance to various self-antigens with autoantibody production to nuclear and cytoplasmic antigens and immune complex deposition, reflecting dysregulation of both the innate and adaptive immune systems [73]. Among clinical features, oral manifestations are common (in 5–40% of cases) and often are the first SLE manifestation [74]. A recent study suggested that the local oral microenvironment is involved in the development of oral SLE lesions and/or systemic lesions [70]. Among environmental factors implicated in SLE pathogenesis, the role of the microbiome has gained increasing interest in the last years. Gut microbiota has been shown to be associated with an imbalance in the proportions of Th17 and Treg cells [75] in SLE patients while the potential participation of oral microbiome remains elusive.

Moreover, intestinal dysbiosis has been demonstrated, consisting of an imbalance of specific gut flora in SLE patients compared with healthy controls (with a significantly lower *Firmicutes/Bacteroidetes* ratio and an associated over representation of oxidative phosphorylation and glycan utilization pathways) [76].

Furthermore, it has been recently shown that a mechanism through which the bacteria may drive autoimmunity in SLE is by the production of amyloid–DNA complexes, which can trigger an immune cascade involving TLR9 stimulation, IFNs type 1 transcription, and antinuclear antibody production [77].

Nonetheless, the frequent and early involvement of the oral mucosa in SLE suggests that the local oral microenvironment may participate in the development of oral SLE lesions and/or may contribute to systemic involvement through the generation of circulating autoantibodies against oral microbial products. In addition, the viral infections (i.e., EBV and CMV) that have been implicated in SLE pathogenesis may also arise in the oral cavity. Li et al. found that in SLE patients, the oral microbiota was inbalanced and diversity was reduced but no difference was found between new-onset and treated SLE patients. The abundances of *Lactobacillaceae*, *Veillonellaceae*, and *Moraxellaceae* were increased in patients with systemic lupus erythematosus, whereas those of families were decreased, such as *Corynebacteriaceae*, *Micrococcaceae*, *Sphingomonadaceae*, *Halomonadaceae*, *Xanthomonadaceae* [78].

Finally, the genus *Veillonella* was found to be increased in SLE patients with oral ulcers. A recent study showed that the genera *Haemophilus* and *Veillonella* were among the main members of the oral microbiota in healthy adults [79]. Additionally, *Haemophilus parainfluenzae* was abundant in patients with Behçet's disease [80]. The expression of oral ulcers in these autoimmune diseases may be related to overabundance of the genera *Veillonella* and *Haemophilus* in the oral environment.

SLE is also associated with alterations of gut microbiota. Fecal microbiome from SLE mice can induce the production of anti-dsDNA antibodies in germ free mice and stimulate the inflammatory response, and alter the expression of SLE susceptibility genes in these mice. The *Firmicutes*-to-*Bacteroidetes* ratio has been demonstrated to be consistently reduced in SLE patients, regardless of ethnicity. The relative abundance of Lactobacillus differs from the animal model used (MRL/lpr mice or NZB/W F1 mice). This may indicate that interactions between gut microbes and the host, rather than the enrichment of some gut microbes, are especially relevant for the SLE development. *Enterococcus gallinarum* and *Lactobacillus reuteri*, both of which are possible gut pathobionts, become translocated into systemic tissue if the gut epithelial barrier is impaired. The microbes then interact with the host immune systems, activating the type I IFN pathway and inducing autoantibody production. In addition, molecular mimicry may critically link the gut microbiome to systemic lupus erythematosus. Gut commensals of SLE patients share protein epitopes with the Ro60 autoantigen. *Ruminococcus gnavus* strain cross-reacted with native DNA, triggering an anti-double-stranded DNA antibody response [81]. Expansion of *R. gnavus* in SLE patients is paralleled to an increase in disease activity and lupus nephritis. Such insights into the link between the gut microbiota and SLE enhance our understanding of SLE pathogenesis and will identify biomarkers predicting active disease.

6. Oral Microbiota as Promising Diagnostic Biomarkers for Rheumatology Diseases

With the improvement in NGS tools available to investigators, we have a greater understanding of the dysbiotic oral microbiome diversity and its effect on a number of systemic pathologies, indicating the potential of oral microbiota as a non-invasive diagnostic tool. In general, the oral cavity would be an ideal site for analyzing biomarkers because samples are comparatively easy to obtain. Indeed, saliva is a non-invasive collection method that does not cause discomfort and pain to patients. To analyze the oral microbiome, each oral micro-habitat has to be sampled with an adequate methodology. For oral mucosa, the use of nylon sterile microbrushes [20,82] and sterile brushes [83] have been reported. Sterile Gracey curettes are used for teeth hard tissues [84] or plaque sampling on endodontics paper cones [85], sterile toothpicks [86], sterile microbrushes, and floss [86]. For saliva sampling, non-stimulated saliva [87] has been used, but other studies rather used oral rinse (saliva after rinsing), to obtain a higher fraction of microbes possibly adhered to oral surfaces [88].

Previous studies reported the possibility of clinical use of oral bacteria in various kinds of tumors such as pancreatic cancer, lung cancer, esophageal [89], and oral cancers [90,91]. Regarding rheumatology diseases, [53] as previously reported, recent studies suggest that RA has a correlation with oral microbiome and may be affected by its dynamic variations. A new research study of 2018 may provide the impetus for a RA diagnostic testing via biomarkers identified in the oral microbiome [92]. The investigators compared the oral microbiota profiles of RA patients, osteoarthritis (OA) patients, and healthy subjects, which showed significant differences between RA patients, OA patients, and the healthy controls. Using the information on the structural changes in the oral microbiota, eight oral bacterial biomarkers were identified to differentiate RA from osteoarthritis, notably *Actinomyces, Neisseria, Neisseria subflava, Haemophilus parainfluenzae, Haemophilus, Veillonella dispar, Prevotella,* and *Veillonella*. This report provides proof of oral microbiota as an informative source for discovering non-invasive biomarkers for arthritis screening.

In a very recent study, saliva samples were collected from RA high-risk individuals, who were positive for ACPA and have no clinical arthritis, from RA patients and healthy controls [93]. In the "pre-clinical" stages, salivary microbial diversity was significantly reduced compared to RA patients and healthy controls. Individuals at high-risk for RA showed a reduction in the abundance of genus *Defluviitaleaceae*_UCG-011 and the species *Neisseria oralis*, but an expansion of *Prevotella*_6. Interestingly, the authors observed a characteristic compositional change of salivary microbes in individuals at high-risk for RA, suggesting that oral microbiota dysbiosis occurs in the "pre-clinical" stage of RA and are correlated with systemic autoimmune features. These findings support the hypothesis that microbiome changes occurring in mucosal sites such as the oral cavity might contribute to disease pathogenesis in the initial RA stages. For this reason, manipulating the microbes by traditional dietary modifications, probiotics, and antibiotics and by currently employed disease-modifying agents seems to modulate the disease process and its "progression" [94].

Future studies should explore the use of oral microbiota dysbiosis as a biomarker of disease and the manipulation of oral microbiota therapeutically to change RA disease progression.

7. Future Direction: Artificial Intelligence (AI) and Its Application in the Prediction of the Link between Oral Microbiome and Rheumatic Diseases

Despite current failures in analysis and research design, advances in high-throughput sequencing techniques have created a significant quantity of sequencing data, bringing fresh insights into the oral microbiota and rheumatic diseases relationship. The next step would be to use AI techniques like machine learning (ML) and deep learning (DL) to predict rheumatic disease states from the oral microbiota. Consistent collection of host information across research is required to employ AI-based techniques for predicting oral microbiome–rheumatic diseases connections.

ML is a subset of AI that relies on mathematical models to discern trends and patterns from data without the use of explicit instructions [95]. ML-based methods that integrate multiple omics (for instance genomics, metabolomics, imaging, microbiome, etc.) and clinical data enable the definition of robust and sensitive multidimensional biomarkers related to complex diseases. In microbiome research, ML algorithms find important features from the given feature set (phylogeny, relative abundance, or functional profiles from the microbiome data) for more accurate prediction of the phenotype of interest, e.g., disease state.

In rheumatology, ML can represent a step towards precision medicine, leading to the improvement of patient profiling and treatment personalization [96,97]. Notably, ML can be split into two parts: supervised and unsupervised learning [95]. Supervised learning leads algorithms to solve a pre-defined problem. To provide a forecast, the ML software must be trained per acceptably large amount of data that had been previously labeled by humans [95]. It is also possible to identify the most relevant features for classification. On the other hand, supervised methods include decision tree algorithm, logistic regression, as well as more complex algorithms like random forest and artificial neural networks.

In recent years, both supervised and unsupervised methods were incrementally used in microbiome research. A glimpse of how precision microbiome medicine can become a reality was provided by Zeevi et al. who used a decision-tree with a gradient boosting model integrating 800 people's blood parameters, dietary habits, anthropometrics, physical activity, and microbiome profile to predict postprandial glycemic response [98]. Similarly, in the oncology setting, supervised ML methods on microbiota data were used to predict chemotherapy effectiveness and tolerability [99]. ML had also been used to analyze how bacteria contribute to drug metabolism [100]. In oral microbiome research, ML has proven useful to predict atherosclerotic cardiovascular disease (ACVD). In a study including 43 patients with ACVD and 86 age- and sex-matched non-ACVD individuals, a random forest algorithm based on 43 unique operational taxonomic units (OTUs) was able to predict ACVD with area under the curve (AUC) of 0.93 [101]

In rheumatology, the use of ML in microbiome research remains largely unexplored. In this regard, although promising, the results seem less consistent than in other areas as of few studies with a limited sample size have been carried out only on fecal samples. In particular, in a cohort of 39 patients with juvenile idiopathic arthritis, a random forest algorithm was used to discriminate patients from healthy controls (AUC 0.80) by integrating information of 12 genera including *Anaerostipes*, *Dialister*, *Lachnospira*, and *Roseburia* from fecal samples [102]. Size and quality of datasets are of utmost importance in ML.

The future of oral microbiome-systemic link studies relies on the development of larger datasets, meaning more consistent validation and testing performance. This is to say, in deploying any ML approach to microbiome in rheumatology, researchers actually face issues consisting in the scarcity of data sharing of rheumatic patient datasets. In contrast with other research areas such as oncology and dermatology [103,104], there is a lack of dedicated open repositories integrating either labeled clinical features, histopathologic visual contents, and/or microbiome data from patients with rheumatic diseases [97]. In the absence of large annotated datasets, the potential of ML methods involving oral microbiome data in predicting therapy response remains largely unexploited. For being finally adopted in real-life clinical settings and making microbiome-led precision medicine comes true in rheumatology, data and code sharing must be strongly advocated. The use of proper study designs and the gathering of detailed host personal data in future oral microbiome analysis could help to improve AI-based oral healthcare research, which could have significant clinical benefits such as the ability to predict systemic disease condition from the oral microbiota.

8. Conclusions

Microbiome research in rheumatic diseases is expanding significantly, offering unique opportunities to better understand aspects of pathogenesis, the potential for patient stratification, and its application towards personalized therapeutic strategies. Oral microbiota seems to be a promising diagnostic and prognostic biomarker and a useful tool that may help to guide the disease comprehension. Today, new perspectives in microbiome biomarkers research are represented by artificial intelligence approaches such as machine learning (ML). In rheumatology, AI can represent a step towards precision medicine, leading to the improvement of patient profiling and treatment personalization (Tables 1 and 2).

Table 1. Literature data linking the oral microbiota with the pathogenesis of progression of rheumatic diseases.

Authors	Journal	Finding
Gomez-Banuelos, E.; et al. [35]	*J. Clin. Med.* **2019**	The subgingival microbiota differes significantly between RA and healthy individuals
Rosenstein, E.D.; et al. [37]	*Inflammation* **2004**	*P. gingivalis* expresses a bacterial protein arginine deiminase (PPAD) that can citrullinate free L-arginine and C-terminal arginine residues in cleaved peptides
Sato; et al. [39]	*Sci. Rep.* **2017**	*P. gingivalis* exacerbate arthritis by modulating the gut microbiota and increasing the proportion of Th17 (T helper 17) cells in mesenteric lymph nodes
Brusca, S.B.; et al. [45]	*Curr. Opin. Rheumatol.* **2014**	Several organisms, besides P. Gingivalis, cause periodontal disease (i.e., *Anaerglobus geminatus* and *Prevotella/Leptotrichia*) and are linked to the ACPA presence
Scher, J.U.; et al. [51]	*Arthritis Res. Ther.* **2013**	An alteration in the bacterial taxa of several mucosal sites (including oral, lung, and intestinal microbiomes) is required for the transition from a pre-clinical, autoimmune phase of RA into clinically classifiable disease
Ceccarelli, F.; et al. [55]	*Clin. Exp. Immunol.* **2018**	A significant association between the percentage of *P. Gingivalis* on the total tongue biofilm and RA disease activity (DAS28) was found
Szymula, A.; et al. [67]	*Clin. Immunol.* **2014**	A role for cross-reactivity of commensal oral and gut bacteria with SSA/Ro60 in the Sjogren Syndrome aetiopathogenesis

Table 1. *Cont.*

Authors	Journal	Finding
Horta-Baas, G.; et al. [86]	*J. Immunol. Res.* **2017**	Both gut and oral microbiota differ in early stages of RA from healthy controls, with a reduction of *Bifidobacterium* and *Bacteroides* and an increase in *Prevotella*
van der Meulen, T.A.; et al. [14]	*Rheumatology (Oxford)* **2018**	Buccal mucosa microbiome of primary Sjogren Syndrome (pSS) and non-SS sicca patients differ from healthy controls, with a higher *Firmicutes/Proteobacteria* ratio observed in both SS and non-SS sicca patients.
Greiling, T.M.; et al. [69]	*Sci. Transl. Med.* **2018**	*Corynebacterium amycolatum* has been shown to colonize the lacrimal duct, making *C. amycolatum* Ro60, a candidate ortholog for the development of anti-Ro60 antibodies in SS
Li, B.Z. et al. [78]	*Arch. Oral Biol.* **2020**	In SLE patients, the oral microbiota was imbalanced and diversity was reduced but no difference was found between new-onset and treated SLE patients

Table 2. Literature data in which AI tools is used to study the oral-gut microbiota axis of rheumatic diseases.

Authors	Disease	Number of Patients	Algorithm	Outcome
Qian, X.; et al. [102]	Juvenile Idiopathic Arthritis	39	Random Forest	Discrimination between patients and healthy controls

Author Contributions: S.B.-R., E.R., M.M.-C. and A.A. conceptualized the review; S.B.-R., E.R. and V.V. wrote the paper; S.B.-R., E.R., V.V. and S.T. performed the collected the data; E.R. drawed the figures; M.M.-C., S.T., F.I. and A.A. corrected the final version; S.B.-R., E.R., A.A., M.M.-C. Funding Acquisition; all authors did critical revision of the manuscript. All authors have read and agreed to the published version of the manuscript.

Funding: The research has been founded with a grant from the Foundation 'Ente Cassa di Risparmio di Firenze' FCR 2019.

Informed Consent Statement: Not applicable.

Data Availability Statement: Not applicable.

Acknowledgments: The authors thank Elisangela Miceli for English revisions.

Conflicts of Interest: Authors declare no conflict of interest.

References

1. Human Microbiome Project Consortium. A framework for human microbiome research. *Nature* **2012**, *486*, 215–221. [CrossRef] [PubMed]
2. Ackerman, J. The ultimate social network. *Sci. Am.* **2012**, *306*, 36–43. [CrossRef] [PubMed]
3. Human Microbiome Project Consortium. Structure, function and diversity of the healthy human microbiome. *Nature* **2012**, *486*, 207–214. [CrossRef]
4. Russo, E.; Taddei, A.; Ringressi, M.N.; Ricci, F.; Amedei, A. The interplay between the microbiome and the adaptive immune response in cancer development. *Therap. Adv. Gastroenterol.* **2016**, *9*, 594–605. [CrossRef] [PubMed]
5. Li, K.; Bihan, M.; Yooseph, S.; Methe, B.A. Analyses of the microbial diversity across the human microbiome. *PLoS ONE* **2012**, *7*, e32118. [CrossRef] [PubMed]
6. Avila, M.; Ojcius, D.M.; Yilmaz, O. The oral microbiota: Living with a permanent guest. *DNA Cell Biol.* **2009**, *28*, 405–411. [CrossRef] [PubMed]
7. Segata, N.; Haake, S.K.; Mannon, P.; Lemon, K.P.; Waldron, L.; Gevers, D.; Huttenhower, C.; Izard, J. Composition of the adult digestive tract bacterial microbiome based on seven mouth surfaces, tonsils, throat and stool samples. *Genome Biol.* **2012**, *13*, R42. [CrossRef]
8. Xu, X.; He, J.; Xue, J.; Wang, Y.; Li, K.; Zhang, K.; Guo, Q.; Liu, X.; Zhou, Y.; Cheng, L.; et al. Oral cavity contains distinct niches with dynamic microbial communities. *Environ. Microbiol.* **2015**, *17*, 699–710. [CrossRef]
9. Krom, B.P.; Kidwai, S.; Ten Cate, J.M. Candida and other fungal species: Forgotten players of healthy oral microbiota. *J. Dent. Res.* **2014**, *93*, 445–451. [CrossRef]

10. Kilian, M.; Chapple, I.L.; Hannig, M.; Marsh, P.D.; Meuric, V.; Pedersen, A.M.; Tonetti, M.S.; Wade, W.G.; Zaura, E. The oral microbiome—An update for oral healthcare professionals. *Br. Dent. J.* **2016**, *221*, 657–666. [CrossRef]
11. Marsh, P.D.; Head, D.A.; Devine, D.A. Prospects of oral disease control in the future—An opinion. *J. Oral Microbiol.* **2014**, *6*, 26176. [CrossRef]
12. Laubichler, M.D.; Renn, J. Extended evolution: A conceptual framework for integrating regulatory networks and niche construction. *J. Exp. Zool. B Mol. Dev. Evol.* **2015**, *324*, 565–577. [CrossRef]
13. Dewhirst, F.E.; Chen, T.; Izard, J.; Paster, B.J.; Tanner, A.C.; Yu, W.H.; Lakshmanan, A.; Wade, W.G. The human oral microbiome. *J. Bacteriol.* **2010**, *192*, 5002–5017. [CrossRef]
14. van der Meulen, T.A.; Harmsen, H.J.M.; Bootsma, H.; Liefers, S.C.; Vich Vila, A.; Zhernakova, A.; Fu, J.; Wijmenga, C.; Spijkervet, F.K.L.; Kroese, F.G.M.; et al. Dysbiosis of the buccal mucosa microbiome in primary Sjogren's syndrome patients. *Rheumatology (Oxford)* **2018**, *57*, 2225–2234. [CrossRef]
15. Moutsopoulos, N.M.; Konkel, J.E. Tissue-Specific Immunity at the Oral Mucosal Barrier. *Trends Immunol.* **2018**, *39*, 276–287. [CrossRef]
16. Wei, Y.; Shi, M.; Zhen, M.; Wang, C.; Hu, W.; Nie, Y.; Wu, X. Comparison of Subgingival and Buccal Mucosa Microbiome in Chronic and Aggressive Periodontitis: A Pilot Study. *Front. Cell. Infect. Microbiol.* **2019**, *9*, 53. [CrossRef]
17. Genco, R.J.; Grossi, S.G.; Ho, A.; Nishimura, F.; Murayama, Y. A Proposed Model Linking Inflammation to Obesity, Diabetes, and Periodontal Infections. *J. Periodontol.* **2005**, *76* (Suppl. 11S), 2075–2084. [CrossRef]
18. Beck, J.D.; Offenbacher, S. Systemic effects of periodontitis: Epidemiology of periodontal disease and cardiovascular disease. *J. Periodontol.* **2005**, *76*, 2089–2100. [CrossRef]
19. Sudhakara, P.; Gupta, A.; Bhardwaj, A.; Wilson, A. Oral Dysbiotic Communities and Their Implications in Systemic Diseases. *Dent. J.* **2018**, *6*, 10. [CrossRef]
20. Michaud, D.S.; Fu, Z.; Shi, J.; Chung, M. Periodontal Disease, Tooth Loss, and Cancer Risk. *Epidemiol. Rev.* **2017**, *39*, 49–58. [CrossRef]
21. Goris, A.; Liston, A. The immunogenetic architecture of autoimmune disease. *Cold Spring Harb. Perspect. Biol.* **2012**, *4*. [CrossRef] [PubMed]
22. Konig, M.F. The microbiome in autoimmune rheumatic disease. *Best Pract. Res. Clin. Rheumatol.* **2020**, *34*, 101473. [CrossRef] [PubMed]
23. Yurkovetskiy, L.A.; Pickard, J.M.; Chervonsky, A.V. Microbiota and autoimmunity: Exploring new avenues. *Cell Host Microbe* **2015**, *17*, 548–552. [CrossRef] [PubMed]
24. Benagiano, M.; D'Elios, M.M.; Amedei, A.; Azzurri, A.; van der Zee, R.; Ciervo, A.; Rombola, G.; Romagnani, S.; Cassone, A.; Del Prete, G. Human 60-kDa heat shock protein is a target autoantigen of T cells derived from atherosclerotic plaques. *J. Immunol.* **2005**, *174*, 6509–6517. [CrossRef]
25. Amedei, A.; Bergman, M.P.; Appelmelk, B.J.; Azzurri, A.; Benagiano, M.; Tamburini, C.; van der Zee, R.; Telford, J.L.; Vandenbroucke-Grauls, C.M.; D'Elios, M.M.; et al. Molecular mimicry between Helicobacter pylori antigens and H+, K+ –adenosine triphosphatase in human gastric autoimmunity. *J. Exp. Med.* **2003**, *198*, 1147–1156. [CrossRef]
26. Malamud, D. Saliva as a diagnostic fluid. *Dent. Clin. N. Am.* **2011**, *55*, 159–178. [CrossRef]
27. Schellekens, G.A.; de Jong, B.A.; van den Hoogen, F.H.; van de Putte, L.B.; van Venrooij, W.J. Citrulline is an Essential Constituent of Antigenic Determinants Recognized by Rheumatoid Arthritis-specific Autoantibodies. 1998. *J. Immunol.* **2015**, *195*, 8–16.
28. Puszczewicz, M.; Iwaszkiewicz, C. Role of anti-citrullinated protein antibodies in diagnosis and prognosis of rheumatoid arthritis. *Arch. Med. Sci.* **2011**, *7*, 189–194. [CrossRef]
29. Sakkas, L.I.; Chen, P.F.; Platsoucas, C.D. T-cell antigen receptors in rheumatoid arthritis. *Immunol. Res.* **1994**, *13*, 117–138. [CrossRef]
30. Dissick, A.; Redman, R.S.; Jones, M.; Rangan, B.V.; Reimold, A.; Griffiths, G.R.; Mikuls, T.R.; Amdur, R.L.; Richards, J.S.; Kerr, G.S. Association of periodontitis with rheumatoid arthritis: A pilot study. *J. Periodontol.* **2010**, *81*, 223–230. [CrossRef]
31. Correa, J.D.; Saraiva, A.M.; Queiroz-Junior, C.M.; Madeira, M.F.; Duarte, P.M.; Teixeira, M.M.; Souza, D.G.; da Silva, T.A. Arthritis-induced alveolar bone loss is associated with changes in the composition of oral microbiota. *Anaerobe* **2016**, *39*, 91–96. [CrossRef]
32. Firestein, G.S.; McInnes, I.B. Immunopathogenesis of Rheumatoid Arthritis. *Immunity* **2017**, *46*, 183–196. [CrossRef]
33. Araujo, V.M.; Melo, I.M.; Lima, V. Relationship between Periodontitis and Rheumatoid Arthritis: Review of the Literature. *Mediat. Inflamm.* **2015**, *2015*, 259074. [CrossRef]
34. Correa, J.D.; Fernandes, G.R.; Calderaro, D.C.; Mendonca, S.M.S.; Silva, J.M.; Albiero, M.L.; Cunha, F.Q.; Xiao, E.; Ferreira, G.A.; Teixeira, A.L.; et al. Oral microbial dysbiosis linked to worsened periodontal condition in rheumatoid arthritis patients. *Sci. Rep.* **2019**, *9*, 8379. [CrossRef]
35. Gomez-Banuelos, E.; Mukherjee, A.; Darrah, E.; Andrade, F. Rheumatoid Arthritis-Associated Mechanisms of Porphyromonas gingivalis and Aggregatibacter actinomycetemcomitans. *J. Clin. Med.* **2019**, *8*, 1309. [CrossRef]
36. Potempa, J.; Mydel, P.; Koziel, J. The case for periodontitis in the pathogenesis of rheumatoid arthritis. *Nat. Rev. Rheumatol.* **2017**, *13*, 606–620. [CrossRef]
37. Rosenstein, E.D.; Greenwald, R.A.; Kushner, L.J.; Weissmann, G. Hypothesis: The humoral immune response to oral bacteria provides a stimulus for the development of rheumatoid arthritis. *Inflammation* **2004**, *28*, 311–318. [CrossRef]

38. Wegner, N.; Wait, R.; Sroka, A.; Eick, S.; Nguyen, K.A.; Lundberg, K.; Kinloch, A.; Culshaw, S.; Potempa, J.; Venables, P.J. Peptidylarginine deiminase from Porphyromonas gingivalis citrullinates human fibrinogen and alpha-enolase: Implications for autoimmunity in rheumatoid arthritis. *Arthritis Rheum.* **2010**, *62*, 2662–2672. [CrossRef]
39. Sato, K.; Takahashi, N.; Kato, T.; Matsuda, Y.; Yokoji, M.; Yamada, M.; Nakajima, T.; Kondo, N.; Endo, N.; Yamamoto, R.; et al. Aggravation of collagen-induced arthritis by orally administered Porphyromonas gingivalis through modulation of the gut microbiota and gut immune system. *Sci. Rep.* **2017**, *7*, 6955. [CrossRef]
40. Bialowas, K.; Radwan-Oczko, M.; Dus-Ilnicka, I.; Korman, L.; Swierkot, J. Periodontal disease and influence of periodontal treatment on disease activity in patients with rheumatoid arthritis and spondyloarthritis. *Rheumatol. Int.* **2020**, *40*, 455–463. [CrossRef]
41. Eriksson, K.; Fei, G.; Lundmark, A.; Benchimol, D.; Lee, L.; Hu, Y.O.O.; Kats, A.; Saevarsdottir, S.; Catrina, A.I.; Klinge, B.; et al. Periodontal Health and Oral Microbiota in Patients with Rheumatoid Arthritis. *J. Clin. Med.* **2019**, *8*, 630. [CrossRef]
42. Konig, M.F.; Abusleme, L.; Reinholdt, J.; Palmer, R.J.; Teles, R.P.; Sampson, K.; Rosen, A.; Nigrovic, P.A.; Sokolove, J.; Giles, J.T.; et al. Aggregatibacter actinomycetemcomitans-induced hypercitrullination links periodontal infection to autoimmunity in rheumatoid arthritis. *Sci. Transl. Med.* **2016**, *8*, 369ra176. [CrossRef]
43. Konig, M.F.; Andrade, F. A Critical Reappraisal of Neutrophil Extracellular Traps and NETosis Mimics Based on Differential Requirements for Protein Citrullination. *Front. Immunol.* **2016**, *7*, 461. [CrossRef]
44. Volkov, M.; Dekkers, J.; Loos, B.G.; Bizzarro, S.; Huizinga, T.W.J.; Praetorius, H.A.; Toes, R.E.M.; van der Woude, D. Comment on "Aggregatibacter actinomycetemcomitans-induced hypercitrullination links periodontal infection to autoimmunity in rheumatoid arthritis". *Sci. Transl. Med.* **2018**, *10*. [CrossRef]
45. Brusca, S.B.; Abramson, S.B.; Scher, J.U. Microbiome and mucosal inflammation as extra-articular triggers for rheumatoid arthritis and autoimmunity. *Curr. Opin. Rheumatol.* **2014**, *26*, 101–107. [CrossRef]
46. Caminer, A.C.; Haberman, R.; Scher, J.U. Human microbiome, infections, and rheumatic disease. *Clin. Rheumatol.* **2017**, *36*, 2645–2653. [CrossRef]
47. Goh, C.E.; Kopp, J.; Papapanou, P.N.; Molitor, J.A.; Demmer, R.T. Association Between Serum Antibodies to Periodontal Bacteria and Rheumatoid Factor in the Third National Health and Nutrition Examination Survey. *Arthritis Rheumatol.* **2016**, *68*, 2384–2393. [CrossRef]
48. Roszyk, E.; Puszczewicz, M. Role of human microbiome and selected bacterial infections in the pathogenesis of rheumatoid arthritis. *Reumatologia* **2017**, *55*, 242–250. [CrossRef]
49. Hamamoto, Y.; Ouhara, K.; Munenaga, S.; Shoji, M.; Ozawa, T.; Hisatsune, J.; Kado, I.; Kajiya, M.; Matsuda, S.; Kawai, T.; et al. Effect of Porphyromonas gingivalis infection on gut dysbiosis and resultant arthritis exacerbation in mouse model. *Arthritis Res. Ther.* **2020**, *22*, 249. [CrossRef]
50. Wolff, B.; Berger, T.; Frese, C.; Max, R.; Blank, N.; Lorenz, H.M.; Wolff, D. Oral status in patients with early rheumatoid arthritis: A prospective, case-control study. *Rheumatology (Oxford)* **2014**, *53*, 526–531. [CrossRef]
51. Scher, J.U.; Abramson, S.B. Periodontal disease, Porphyromonas gingivalis, and rheumatoid arthritis: What triggers autoimmunity and clinical disease? *Arthritis Res. Ther.* **2013**, *15*, 122. [CrossRef] [PubMed]
52. Scher, J.U.; Ubeda, C.; Equinda, M.; Khanin, R.; Buischi, Y.; Viale, A.; Lipuma, L.; Attur, M.; Pillinger, M.H.; Weissmann, G.; et al. Periodontal disease and the oral microbiota in new-onset rheumatoid arthritis. *Arthritis Rheum.* **2012**, *64*, 3083–3094. [CrossRef] [PubMed]
53. Zhang, X.; Zhang, D.; Jia, H.; Feng, Q.; Wang, D.; Liang, D.; Wu, X.; Li, J.; Tang, L.; Li, Y.; et al. The oral and gut microbiomes are perturbed in rheumatoid arthritis and partly normalized after treatment. *Nat. Med.* **2015**, *21*, 895–905. [CrossRef] [PubMed]
54. Mikuls, T.R.; Payne, J.B.; Yu, F.; Thiele, G.M.; Reynolds, R.J.; Cannon, G.W.; Markt, J.; McGowan, D.; Kerr, G.S.; Redman, R.S.; et al. Periodontitis and Porphyromonas gingivalis in patients with rheumatoid arthritis. *Arthritis Rheumatol.* **2014**, *66*, 1090–1100. [CrossRef]
55. Ceccarelli, F.; Orru, G.; Pilloni, A.; Bartosiewicz, I.; Perricone, C.; Martino, E.; Lucchetti, R.; Fais, S.; Vomero, M.; Olivieri, M.; et al. Porphyromonas gingivalis in the tongue biofilm is associated with clinical outcome in rheumatoid arthritis patients. *Clin. Exp. Immunol.* **2018**, *194*, 244–252. [CrossRef]
56. Phillips, R. Rheumatoid arthritis: Microbiome reflects status of RA and response to therapy. *Nat. Rev. Rheumatol.* **2015**, *11*, 502. [CrossRef]
57. Brito-Zeron, P.; Baldini, C.; Bootsma, H.; Bowman, S.J.; Jonsson, R.; Mariette, X.; Sivils, K.; Theander, E.; Tzioufas, A.; Ramos-Casals, M. Sjogren syndrome. *Nat. Rev. Dis. Primers* **2016**, *2*, 16047. [CrossRef]
58. Lynge Pedersen, A.M.; Belstrom, D. The role of natural salivary defences in maintaining a healthy oral microbiota. *J. Dent.* **2019**, *80* (Suppl. 1), S3–S12. [CrossRef]
59. Mariette, X.; Criswell, L.A. Primary Sjogren's Syndrome. *N. Engl. J. Med.* **2018**, *378*, 931–939. [CrossRef]
60. Lessard, C.J.; Li, H.; Adrianto, I.; Ice, J.A.; Rasmussen, A.; Grundahl, K.M.; Kelly, J.A.; Dozmorov, M.G.; Miceli-Richard, C.; Bowman, S.; et al. Variants at multiple loci implicated in both innate and adaptive immune responses are associated with Sjogren's syndrome. *Nat. Genet.* **2013**, *45*, 1284–1292. [CrossRef]
61. Sharma, D.; Sandhya, P.; Vellarikkal, S.K.; Surin, A.K.; Jayarajan, R.; Verma, A.; Kumar, A.; Ravi, R.; Danda, D.; Sivasubbu, S.; et al. Saliva microbiome in primary Sjogren's syndrome reveals distinct set of disease-associated microbes. *Oral Dis.* **2020**, *26*, 295–301. [CrossRef]

62. Siddiqui, H.; Chen, T.; Aliko, A.; Mydel, P.M.; Jonsson, R.; Olsen, I. Microbiological and bioinformatics analysis of primary Sjogren's syndrome patients with normal salivation. *J. Oral Microbiol.* **2016**, *8*, 31119. [CrossRef]
63. de Paiva, C.S.; Jones, D.B.; Stern, M.E.; Bian, F.; Moore, Q.L.; Corbiere, S.; Streckfus, C.F.; Hutchinson, D.S.; Ajami, N.J.; Petrosino, J.F.; et al. Altered Mucosal Microbiome Diversity and Disease Severity in Sjogren Syndrome. *Sci. Rep.* **2016**, *6*, 23561. [CrossRef]
64. Zhou, Z.; Ling, G.; Ding, N.; Xun, Z.; Zhu, C.; Hua, H.; Chen, X. Molecular analysis of oral microflora in patients with primary Sjogren's syndrome by using high-throughput sequencing. *PeerJ* **2018**, *6*, e5649. [CrossRef]
65. Leung, K.C.; Leung, W.K.; McMillan, A.S. Supra-gingival microbiota in Sjogren's syndrome. *Clin. Oral Investig.* **2007**, *11*, 415–423. [CrossRef]
66. Rusthen, S.; Kristoffersen, A.K.; Young, A.; Galtung, H.K.; Petrovski, B.E.; Palm, O.; Enersen, M.; Jensen, J.L. Dysbiotic salivary microbiota in dry mouth and primary Sjogren's syndrome patients. *PLoS ONE* **2019**, *14*, e0218319. [CrossRef]
67. Szymula, A.; Rosenthal, J.; Szczerba, B.M.; Bagavant, H.; Fu, S.M.; Deshmukh, U.S. T cell epitope mimicry between Sjogren's syndrome Antigen A (SSA)/Ro60 and oral, gut, skin and vaginal bacteria. *Clin. Immunol.* **2014**, *152*, 1–9. [CrossRef]
68. Komai, K.; Shiozawa, K.; Tanaka, Y.; Yoshihara, R.; Tanaka, C.; Sakai, H.; Yamane, T.; Murata, M.; Tsumiyama, K.; Hashiramoto, A.; et al. Sjogren's syndrome patients presenting with hypergammaglobulinemia are relatively unresponsive to cevimeline treatment. *Mod. Rheumatol.* **2009**, *19*, 416–419. [CrossRef]
69. Greiling, T.M.; Dehner, C.; Chen, X.; Hughes, K.; Iniguez, A.J.; Boccitto, M.; Ruiz, D.Z.; Renfroe, S.C.; Vieira, S.M.; Ruff, W.E.; et al. Commensal orthologs of the human autoantigen Ro60 as triggers of autoimmunity in lupus. *Sci. Transl. Med.* **2018**, *10*. [CrossRef]
70. Nikitakis, N.G.; Papaioannou, W.; Sakkas, L.I.; Kousvelari, E. The autoimmunity-oral microbiome connection. *Oral Dis.* **2017**, *23*, 828–839. [CrossRef]
71. Moon, J.; Choi, S.H.; Yoon, C.H.; Kim, M.K. Gut dysbiosis is prevailing in Sjogren's syndrome and is related to dry eye severity. *PLoS ONE* **2020**, *15*, e0229029. [CrossRef]
72. Cano-Ortiz, A.; Laborda-Illanes, A.; Plaza-Andrades, I.; Membrillo Del Pozo, A.; Villarrubia Cuadrado, A.; Rodriguez Calvo de Mora, M.; Leiva-Gea, I.; Sanchez-Alcoholado, L.; Queipo-Ortuno, M.I. Connection between the Gut Microbiome, Systemic Inflammation, Gut Permeability and FOXP3 Expression in Patients with Primary Sjogren's Syndrome. *Int. J. Mol. Sci.* **2020**, *21*, 8733. [CrossRef]
73. Lisnevskaia, L.; Murphy, G.; Isenberg, D. Systemic lupus erythematosus. *Lancet* **2014**, *384*, 1878–1888. [CrossRef]
74. Brennan, M.T.; Valerin, M.A.; Napenas, J.J.; Lockhart, P.B. Oral manifestations of patients with lupus erythematosus. *Dent. Clin. N. Am.* **2005**, *49*, 127–141. [CrossRef]
75. Lopez, P.; de Paz, B.; Rodriguez-Carrio, J.; Hevia, A.; Sanchez, B.; Margolles, A.; Suarez, A. Th17 responses and natural IgM antibodies are related to gut microbiota composition in systemic lupus erythematosus patients. *Sci. Rep.* **2016**, *6*, 24072. [CrossRef]
76. Hevia, A.; Milani, C.; Lopez, P.; Cuervo, A.; Arboleya, S.; Duranti, S.; Turroni, F.; Gonzalez, S.; Suarez, A.; Gueimonde, M.; et al. Intestinal dysbiosis associated with systemic lupus erythematosus. *mBio* **2014**, *5*, e01548-14. [CrossRef]
77. Spaulding, C.N.; Dodson, K.W.; Chapman, M.R.; Hultgren, S.J. Fueling the Fire with Fibers: Bacterial Amyloids Promote Inflammatory Disorders. *Cell Host Microbe* **2015**, *18*, 1–2. [CrossRef]
78. Li, B.Z.; Zhou, H.Y.; Guo, B.; Chen, W.J.; Tao, J.H.; Cao, N.W.; Chu, X.J.; Meng, X. Dysbiosis of oral microbiota is associated with systemic lupus erythematosus. *Arch. Oral Biol.* **2020**, *113*, 104708. [CrossRef]
79. Bik, E.M.; Long, C.D.; Armitage, G.C.; Loomer, P.; Emerson, J.; Mongodin, E.F.; Nelson, K.E.; Gill, S.R.; Fraser-Liggett, C.M.; Relman, D.A. Bacterial diversity in the oral cavity of 10 healthy individuals. *ISME J.* **2010**, *4*, 962–974. [CrossRef]
80. Coit, P.; Mumcu, G.; Ture-Ozdemir, F.; Unal, A.U.; Alpar, U.; Bostanci, N.; Ergun, T.; Direskeneli, H.; Sawalha, A.H. Sequencing of 16S rRNA reveals a distinct salivary microbiome signature in Behcet's disease. *Clin. Immunol.* **2016**, *169*, 28–35. [CrossRef]
81. Ma, Y.; Xu, X.; Li, M.; Cai, J.; Wei, Q.; Niu, H. Gut microbiota promote the inflammatory response in the pathogenesis of systemic lupus erythematosus. *Mol. Med.* **2019**, *25*, 35. [CrossRef] [PubMed]
82. Zaura, E.; Keijser, B.J.; Huse, S.M.; Crielaard, W. Defining the healthy "core microbiome" of oral microbial communities. *BMC Microbiol.* **2009**, *9*, 259. [CrossRef] [PubMed]
83. Mager, D.L.; Ximenez-Fyvie, L.A.; Haffajee, A.D.; Socransky, S.S. Distribution of selected bacterial species on intraoral surfaces. *J. Clin. Periodontol.* **2003**, *30*, 644–654. [CrossRef] [PubMed]
84. Eren, A.M.; Borisy, G.G.; Huse, S.M.; Mark Welch, J.L. Oligotyping analysis of the human oral microbiome. *Proc. Natl. Acad. Sci. USA* **2014**, *111*, E2875–E2884. [CrossRef]
85. Hall, M.W.; Singh, N.; Ng, K.F.; Lam, D.K.; Goldberg, M.B.; Tenenbaum, H.C.; Neufeld, J.D.; Beiko, R.G.; Senadheera, D.B. Inter-personal diversity and temporal dynamics of dental, tongue, and salivary microbiota in the healthy oral cavity. *NPJ Biofilms Microbiomes* **2017**, *3*, 2. [CrossRef]
86. Mark Welch, J.L.; Rossetti, B.J.; Rieken, C.W.; Dewhirst, F.E.; Borisy, G.G. Biogeography of a human oral microbiome at the micron scale. *Proc. Natl. Acad. Sci. USA* **2016**, *113*, E791–E800. [CrossRef]
87. Lim, Y.; Totsika, M.; Morrison, M.; Punyadeera, C. The saliva microbiome profiles are minimally affected by collection method or DNA extraction protocols. *Sci. Rep.* **2017**, *7*, 8523. [CrossRef]
88. Ghannoum, M.A.; Jurevic, R.J.; Mukherjee, P.K.; Cui, F.; Sikaroodi, M.; Naqvi, A.; Gillevet, P.M. Characterization of the oral fungal microbiome (mycobiome) in healthy individuals. *PLoS Pathog.* **2010**, *6*, e1000713. [CrossRef]
89. Chen, X.; Winckler, B.; Lu, M.; Cheng, H.; Yuan, Z.; Yang, Y.; Jin, L.; Ye, W. Oral Microbiota and Risk for Esophageal Squamous Cell Carcinoma in a High-Risk Area of China. *PLoS ONE* **2015**, *10*, e0143603. [CrossRef]

90. Schmidt, B.L.; Kuczynski, J.; Bhattacharya, A.; Huey, B.; Corby, P.M.; Queiroz, E.L.; Nightingale, K.; Kerr, A.R.; DeLacure, M.D.; Veeramachaneni, R.; et al. Changes in abundance of oral microbiota associated with oral cancer. *PLoS ONE* **2014**, *9*, e98741. [CrossRef]
91. Farrell, J.J.; Zhang, L.; Zhou, H.; Chia, D.; Elashoff, D.; Akin, D.; Paster, B.J.; Joshipura, K.; Wong, D.T. Variations of oral microbiota are associated with pancreatic diseases including pancreatic cancer. *Gut* **2012**, *61*, 582–588. [CrossRef]
92. Chen, B.; Zhao, Y.; Li, S.; Yang, L.; Wang, H.; Wang, T.; Bin, S.; Gai, Z.; Heng, X.; Zhang, C.; et al. Variations in oral microbiome profiles in rheumatoid arthritis and osteoarthritis with potential biomarkers for arthritis screening. *Sci. Rep.* **2018**, *8*, 17126. [CrossRef]
93. Tong, Y.; Zheng, L.; Qing, P.; Zhao, H.; Li, Y.; Su, L.; Zhang, Q.; Zhao, Y.; Luo, Y.; Liu, Y. Oral Microbiota Perturbations Are Linked to High Risk for Rheumatoid Arthritis. *Front. Cell Infect. Microbiol.* **2019**, *9*, 475. [CrossRef]
94. Sandhya, P.; Danda, D.; Sharma, D.; Scaria, V. Does the buck stop with the bugs?: An overview of microbial dysbiosis in rheumatoid arthritis. *Int. J. Rheum. Dis.* **2016**, *19*, 8–20. [CrossRef]
95. LeCun, Y.; Bengio, Y.; Hinton, G. Deep learning. *Nature* **2015**, *521*, 436–444. [CrossRef]
96. Venerito, V.; Angelini, O.; Fornaro, M.; Cacciapaglia, F.; Lopalco, G.; Iannone, F. A Machine Learning Approach for Predicting Sustained Remission in Rheumatoid Arthritis Patients on Biologic Agents. *J. Clin. Rheumatol.* **2021**. [CrossRef]
97. Venerito, V.; Angelini, O.; Cazzato, G.; Lopalco, G.; Maiorano, E.; Cimmino, A.; Iannone, F. A convolutional neural network with transfer learning for automatic discrimination between low and high-grade synovitis: A pilot study. *Intern. Emerg. Med.* **2021**. [CrossRef]
98. Zeevi, D.; Korem, T.; Zmora, N.; Israeli, D.; Rothschild, D.; Weinberger, A.; Ben-Yacov, O.; Lador, D.; Avnit-Sagi, T.; Lotan-Pompan, M.; et al. Personalized Nutrition by Prediction of Glycemic Responses. *Cell* **2015**, *163*, 1079–1094. [CrossRef]
99. Cammarota, G.; Ianiro, G.; Ahern, A.; Carbone, C.; Temko, A.; Claesson, M.J.; Gasbarrini, A.; Tortora, G. Gut microbiome, big data and machine learning to promote precision medicine for cancer. *Nat. Rev. Gastroenterol. Hepatol.* **2020**, *17*, 635–648. [CrossRef]
100. Dasgupta, Y.; Golovine, K.; Nieborowska-Skorska, M.; Luo, L.; Matlawska-Wasowska, K.; Mullighan, C.G.; Skorski, T. Drugging DNA repair to target T-ALL cells. *Leuk. Lymphoma* **2018**, *59*, 1746–1749. [CrossRef]
101. Kato-Kogoe, N.; Sakaguchi, S.; Kamiya, K.; Omori, M.; Gu, Y.H.; Ito, Y.; Nakamura, S.; Nakano, T.; Tamaki, J.; Ueno, T.; et al. Characterization of Salivary Microbiota in Patients with Atherosclerotic Cardiovascular Disease: A Case-Control Study. *J. Atheroscler. Thromb.* **2021**. [CrossRef] [PubMed]
102. Qian, X.; Liu, Y.X.; Ye, X.; Zheng, W.; Lv, S.; Mo, M.; Lin, J.; Wang, W.; Wang, W.; Zhang, X.; et al. Gut microbiota in children with juvenile idiopathic arthritis: Characteristics, biomarker identification, and usefulness in clinical prediction. *BMC Genom.* **2020**, *21*, 286. [CrossRef] [PubMed]
103. Tangaro, S.; Bellotti, R.; De Carlo, F.; Gargano, G.; Lattanzio, E.; Monno, P.; Massafra, R.; Delogu, P.; Fantacci, M.E.; Retico, A.; et al. MAGIC-5: An Italian mammographic database of digitised images for research. *Radiol. Med.* **2008**, *113*, 477–485. [CrossRef] [PubMed]
104. Esteva, A.; Kuprel, B.; Novoa, R.A.; Ko, J.; Swetter, S.M.; Blau, H.M.; Thrun, S. Dermatologist-level classification of skin cancer with deep neural networks. *Nature* **2017**, *542*, 115–118. [CrossRef]

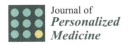

Article

Different Associations between Tonsil Microbiome, Chronic Tonsillitis, and Intermittent Hypoxemia among Obstructive Sleep Apnea Children of Different Weight Status: A Pilot Case-Control Study

Hai-Hua Chuang [1,2,3,4], Jen-Fu Hsu [2,5], Li-Pang Chuang [2,6], Cheng-Hsun Chiu [2,5], Yen-Lin Huang [2,7], Hsueh-Yu Li [2,8], Ning-Hung Chen [2,6], Yu-Shu Huang [2,9], Chun-Wei Chuang [10], Chung-Guei Huang [10,11], Hsin-Chih Lai [10,11] and Li-Ang Lee [2,8,*]

[1] Department of Family Medicine, Chang Gung Memorial Hospital, Taipei Branch and Linkou Main Branch, Taoyuan 33305, Taiwan; chhaihua@cgmh.org.tw
[2] College of Medicine, Chang Gung University, Taoyuan 33302, Taiwan; jeff0724@gmail.com (J.-F.H.); r5243@cgmh.org.tw (L.-P.C.); chchiu@cgmh.org.tw (C.-H.C.); dochempath@cgmh.org.tw (Y.-L.H.); hyli38@cgmh.org.tw (H.-Y.L.); nhchen@cgmh.org.tw (N.-H.C.); yushuhuang1212@gmail.com (Y.-S.H.)
[3] Department of Industrial Engineering and Management, National Taipei University of Technology, Taipei 10608, Taiwan
[4] Obesity Institute, Genomic Medicine Institute, Geisinger, Danville, PA 17822, USA
[5] Department of Pediatrics, Chang Gung Memorial Hospital, Linkou Main Branch, Taoyuan 33305, Taiwan
[6] Department of Pulmonary and Critical Care Medicine, Chang Gung Memorial Hospital, Linkou Main Branch, Taoyuan 33305, Taiwan
[7] Department of Pathology, Chang Gung Memorial Hospital, Linkou Main Branch, Taoyuan 33305, Taiwan
[8] Department of Otorhinolaryngology-Head and Neck Surgery, Chang Gung Memorial Hospital, Linkou Main Branch, Taoyuan 33305, Taiwan
[9] Department of Child Psychiatry, Chang Gung Memorial Hospital, Linkou Main Branch, Taoyuan 33305, Taiwan
[10] Department of Laboratory Medicine, Chang Gung Memorial Hospital, Linkou Main Branch, Taoyuan 33305, Taiwan; whitereverie5336@gmail.com (C.-W.C.); joyce@cgmh.org.tw (C.-G.H.); hclai@mail.cgu.edu.tw (H.-C.L.)
[11] Department of Medical Biotechnology and Laboratory Science, Graduate Institute of Biomedical Sciences, Chang Gung University, Taoyuan 33302, Taiwan
* Correspondence: 5738@cgmh.org.tw; Tel.: +886-3328-1200 (ext. 3968)

Citation: Chuang, H.-H.; Hsu, J.-F.; Chuang, L.-P.; Chiu, C.-H.; Huang, Y.-L.; Li, H.-Y.; Chen, N.-H.; Huang, Y.-S.; Chuang, C.-W.; Huang, C.-G.; et al. Different Associations between Tonsil Microbiome, Chronic Tonsillitis, and Intermittent Hypoxemia among Obstructive Sleep Apnea Children of Different Weight Status: A Pilot Case-Control Study. J. Pers. Med. **2021**, 11, 486. https://doi.org/10.3390/jpm11060486

Academic Editor: Lucrezia Laterza

Received: 4 May 2021
Accepted: 26 May 2021
Published: 28 May 2021

Publisher's Note: MDPI stays neutral with regard to jurisdictional claims in published maps and institutional affiliations.

Copyright: © 2021 by the authors. Licensee MDPI, Basel, Switzerland. This article is an open access article distributed under the terms and conditions of the Creative Commons Attribution (CC BY) license (https://creativecommons.org/licenses/by/4.0/).

Abstract: The tonsil microbiome is associated with chronic tonsillitis and obstructive sleep apnea (OSA) in children, and the gut microbiome is associated with host weight status. In this study, we hypothesized that weight status may be associated with clinical profiles and the tonsil microbiome in children with OSA. We prospectively enrolled 33 non-healthy-weight (cases) and 33 healthy-weight (controls) pediatric OSA patients matched by the proportion of chronic tonsillitis. Differences in the tonsil microbiome between the non-healthy-weight and healthy-weight subgroups and relationships between the tonsil microbiome and clinical variables were investigated. Non-healthy weight was associated with significant intermittent hypoxemia (oxygen desaturation index, mean blood saturation (SpO_2), and minimal SpO_2) and higher systolic blood pressure percentile, but was not related to the tonsil microbiome. However, chronic tonsillitis was related to Acidobacteria in the non-healthy-weight subgroup, and oxygen desaturation index was associated with Bacteroidetes in the healthy-weight subgroup. In post hoc analysis, the children with mean $SpO_2 \leq 97\%$ had reduced α and β diversities and a higher abundance of Bacteroidetes than those with mean $SpO_2 > 97\%$. These preliminary findings are novel and provide insights into future research to understand the pathogenesis of the disease and develop personalized treatments for pediatric OSA.

Keywords: children; intermittent hypoxemia; microbiome; obstructive sleep apnea; tonsil; weight status

1. Introduction

Obstructive sleep apnea (OSA) is a chronic disorder characterized by intermittent partial or complete upper airway obstruction during sleep. The prevalence of pediatric OSA is estimated to be 1–4%, with adenotonsillar hypertrophy and overweight/obesity being the two most important risk factors [1–3]. Pediatric OSA is of great clinical significance since evidence has shown a wide range of detrimental long-term effects associated with the condition [1]. For example, children with OSA show higher risks of neurobehavioral impairment [4], metabolic alterations [5], and cardiovascular dysfunction [6].

The role of microbiota in the development and aggravation of OSA has gained increasing attention. Previous studies have reported that the gut microbiota is involved in the pathogenesis of OSA [7,8], obesity [9,10], and hypertension [11,12]. For example, the transplant of fecal microbiota has been shown to elicit sleep disturbance [8], obesity [13], and hypertension [12] in animal models. The gut microbiota has also been associated with intermittent hypoxia and systemic inflammation [7,10], which are both well-documented manifestations of OSA [14–16]. More recent studies have suggested that, in addition to the gut microbiota, OSA is linked to alterations in various other microbiomes in the human body such as the nasal cavity [17], adenoids [18], tonsils [19], oropharynx [20], oral cavity [21], lungs [22], and urine [21]. In children who snore, the adenotonsillar microbiome has been shown to interact with the regional mucosal immune system such as interleukin-8 and heat shock protein 27 [23].

Tonsil size is one of the most important predictors for apnea-hypopnea index (AHI) in preschoolers and school-age children [24]. Therefore, the influence of the tonsil microbiome may be significant on OSA in young children. Two main methods are used to detect bacterial communities on tonsils: swab cultures and culture-free molecular tests based on 16S ribosomal RNA or ribosomal DNA sequencing [25]. Notably, molecular tests enable metagenomic studies to better detect slow-growing, uncultivable, and rare bacteria [26]. The advent of metagenomics has led to an increase in investigations on human microbiota. However, studies on the tonsil microbiomes in pediatric OSA patients and their relationships with patient characteristics, disease severity, and hypertension are still lacking. To the best of our knowledge, the clinical significance of tonsil microbiota in children with OSA has not been comprehensively elucidated.

We hypothesized that the tonsil microbiome may be associated with the weight status and anthropometrics of pediatric OSA patients. Furthermore, the relationships between the tonsil microbiome, OSA severity, intermittent hypoxemia, and hypertension may differ across patients with various demographic and clinical parameters. Therefore, among a cohort of children with OSA, the first aim of this study was to investigate differences in the tonsil microbiome between non-healthy-weight and healthy-weight subgroups. The second aim was to perform post hoc analysis to understand the correlations between the tonsil microbiome and other variables of interest, including OSA severity, intermittent hypoxemia, and hypertension.

2. Materials and Methods

2.1. Ethical Considerations

This was a prospective case-control study. Consecutive pediatric patients referred to the Department of Otolaryngology at Chang Gung Memorial Hospital (Linkou Main Branch, Taoyuan, Taiwan) for adenotonsillectomy between 1 March 2017 and 31 January 2019 were recruited. The Institutional Review Board of Chang Gung Medical Foundation approved this study (201507279A3), and all procedures were conducted in compliance with the Declaration of Helsinki 1975. Written informed consent was obtained from all parents and participants ≥6 years of age.

2.2. Patient Selection and Grouping

All of the participants underwent comprehensive history-taking, physical examinations, and standard in-lab polysomnography (PSG). The protocol was previously published [15]. The inclusion criteria were: (1) age 5–12 years, and (2) AHI $\geq$ 5.0 events/h or AHI $\geq$ 2.0 events/h plus at least one morbidity (such as elevated blood pressure (BP), daytime sleepiness, learning problems, growth failure, or enuresis) [14,27,28]. Patients with craniofacial, neuromuscular, or chronic inflammatory disorders (such as atopic dermatitis, asthma, or autoimmune disease) were excluded [14,15]. The subjects were further divided into two subgroups according to body mass index (BMI) z-score: "non-healthy-weight" ($\leq$ −2.0 kg/m^2 and $\geq$ 1.0 kg/m^2) group, and "healthy-weight" (> −2.0 kg/m^2 and <1.0 kg/m^2) group [29]. Both groups were matched by the proportion of chronic tonsillitis. Chronic tonsillitis was defined as symptoms of tonsillitis that persisted for a period longer than three months [30]. Patients with acute inflammation, such as rhinosinusitis, tonsillitis, gastrointestinal infection, or other conditions that needed antibiotic treatment did not undergo surgery after the diseases diminished for at least 2 weeks [15]. Subjective OSA symptoms (evaluated using the Chinese version of the OSA-18 questionnaire [31,32]), tonsil size (rated using the Brodsky grading scale [33]), the adenoidal-nasopharyngeal ratio (ANR) (measured using lateral radiography of the nasopharynx [34]), and allergic rhinitis were recorded. Figure 1 shows the flow diagram of the study.

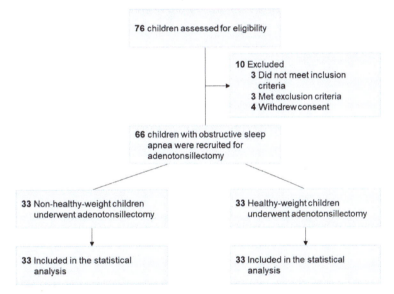

Figure 1. Flow diagram of the study. Seventy-six children with obstructive sleep apnea were assessed for eligibility. However, three did not meet the inclusion criteria, three met the exclusion criteria, and four withdrew consent. Therefore, a total of 66 children were recruited. The non-healthy-weight group included 33 children, and the healthy-weight group included 33 children. Both groups were matched by the proportion of chronic tonsillitis. All participants underwent adenotonsillectomy. Therefore, 66 participants were included in the primary analysis.

2.3. Polysomnography Variables

We assessed OSA severity variables (AHI, respiratory disturbance index (RDI), oxygen desaturation index (ODI), mean pulse oxygen saturation (SpO$_2$), and minimal SpO$_2$) by standard full-night, in-lab PSG, according to the 2012 American Academy of Sleep Medicine Manual [35]. Briefly, the AHI was defined as the sum of all apneas ($\geq$ 90% decrease in airflow for a duration of $\geq$ 2 breaths) plus hypopneas ($\geq$ 50% decrease in airflow and either $\geq$ 3% desaturation or electroencephalographic arousal, for a duration of $\geq$ 2 breaths) divided by the number of hours of total sleep time. The patients were then categorized as having either severe (obstructive AHI $\geq$ 10.0 events/h) or non-severe (obstructive AHI $\geq$ 2.0 events/h to < 10.0 events/h) OSA [36]. The RDI was defined as the average number of respiratory disturbances (obstructive apneas, hypopneas, and respiratory-event-related arousals) per hour. The ODI was calculated as the average number of respiratory events with a 3% drop in SpO_2 per hour. Furthermore, sleep stages were scored from electroencephalography records according to conventional criteria. PSG scoring was performed by a technician blinded to the clinical status of the children. Details of the PSG protocol were described previously [15,37].

2.4. Nocturnal Blood Pressure

Before the PSG exam, nocturnal BP was measured three times with a standard sphyg-momanometer between 10:00 and 11:00 PM. The detailed procedure of measuring BP is described elsewhere [38]. Age, sex, and height-corrected percentiles of systolic BP (SBP) and diastolic BP (DBP) were recorded for each child [39]. Pediatric hypertension was defined as an average clinic SBP and/or DBP $\geq$ 95th percentile [39].

2.5. Tonsil Microbiota

The current study chose tonsil as the primary site for investigation since previous research suggested that the adenoidal microbiome was compatible with the tonsillar microbiome at the phylum level [23]. Also, since bacterial colonies were mainly observed in the tonsil crypts rather than in the tonsil follicles, the superficial tonsils with crypts were used for molecular examinations.

Tonsils with crypts were excised using sterile scissors during adenotonsillectomy. The specimens were rinsed with normal saline to remove superficial debris several times after harvesting. Genomic DNA was immediately extracted from the superficially biopsied specimens (3 mm × 3 mm × 3 mm) using an EasyPrep Genomic DNA Extraction Kit (Biotools Co., Ltd., New Taipei, Taiwan). Tonsil tissue was treated with 4 μL of RNase A (100 mg/mL) for 5 min at room temperature followed by 20 μL of Proteinase K at 56 °C until completely lysed, and then 200 μL ethanol (96–100%) for 15 s [40]. The quality and quantity of genomic DNA were measured using a NanoPhotometer P360 system (Implen, Westlake Village, CA, USA). Polymerase chain reaction (PCR) was used to amplify the V3–V4 regions of the gene encoding for 16S rRNA in bacteria using composite primers, including the forward primer 5'-TCGTCGGCAGCGTCAGATGTGTATAAGAGACAGCCTAYGGGRBGCASCAG-3' and the reverse primer 5'-GTCTCGTGGGCTCGGAGATGTGTATAAGAGACAGGGACTACNNGGG TATCTAAT-3' [41]. Amplicons were purified using a QiaQuick PCR Purification Kit (Qiagen, Hilden, Germany). PCR amplicons were sequenced using the Illumina HiSeq 2500 platform (Illumina, Inc., San Diego, CA, USA) following the manufacturer's instructions to generate 250 bp paired-end reads.

All of the paired-end reads were assembled using FLASH software (version 1.2.7; http://ccb.jhu.edu/software/FLASH/ (accessed on 5 February 2019)) [42], and reads with a quality score < 20 were removed using QIIME software (version 1.7; http://qiime.org/ (accessed on 5 February 2019)) [43]. Sequences were chimera-checked using UCHIME software (http://drive5.com/uchime/ (accessed on 5 February 2019)) [44] and filtered from the dataset before the operational taxonomic unit (OTU) picking of 97% sequence identity using USEARCH (version 7) [45]. Taxonomy classification was annotated according to the Greengenes database (version 13.8; http://greengenes.secondgenome.com/ (accessed on 5 February 2019)) [46]. Multiple sequences were aligned using PyNAST software (version 1.2; https://pypi.org/project/pynast/ (accessed on 5 February 2019)) against the Greengenes core set database to identify the relationships between different OTUs [47]. We used Graphical Phylogenetic Analysis to visualize microbial genomes and metagenomes [48]. Detailed protocols of bioinformatics were described previously [41,49]. During data collection and analysis, the investigators were blinded to group allocation.

2.6. Sample Size Estimation

The sample size was estimated using primary outcome effects (BMI z-score) based on a priori study criteria [15] (healthy-weight group = 0.52 ± 1.12 and non-healthy-weight group = 1.53 ± 1.05). We used a two-tailed Wilcoxon–Mann–Whitney test to calculate the sample size (effect size = 0.93; type I error = 0.05; power = 0.95), which generated a sample size of 33 in each group.

2.7. Statistical Analysis

The D'Agostino and Pearson normality test showed that most variables had non-normal distribution. Therefore, descriptive statistics were expressed as the median, interquartile range (IQR), or frequency. Differences in variables of interest between specific (weight, OSA severity, BP) subgroups were determined using the Mann–Whitney U test, Kruskal–Wallis test, or chi-square test as appropriate. Analysis of similarity was performed to compare bacterial communities [50]. The α diversity (the diversity within each sample) of the tonsil sample was calculated using the observed richness based on the frequency of OTUs and genera in the sequence collections [51]. The β diversity (the number of species shared between two groups) was calculated using the weighted UniFrac measure [52]. Spearman's correlation test was used to determine associations among major (>0.1% abundance and present in >90% of samples [49]) or minor phyla with the patient characteristics. Overall taxonomic or phylum-level abundances were included when determining the most discriminatory taxa between the two groups. Statistical significance was established at $p < 0.05$. p-values were corrected for multiple comparisons using the Benjamini–Hochberg method at 0.1 and reported as q-values when appropriate [53]. All statistical analyses were conducted using R software (versions 2.15.3 and 3.6.1, R Foundation for Statistical Computing, Vienna, Austria; http://www.r-project.org/ (accessed on 26 February 2021)) and Graph Pad Prism software (version 9.00; Graph Pad Software Inc., San Diego, CA, USA).

3. Results

3.1. Participants' Characteristics

Figure 1 demonstrates the study flow diagram. Seventy-six Taiwanese children of Han ancestry with OSA were assessed for eligibility, 10 of whom were excluded from this study. Therefore, a total of 66 children with OSA (16 girls and 50 boys; median age, 6.5 years (IQR, 6.0–9.0); median BMI, 17.1 kg/m^2 (IQR, 15.2–22.7); median AHI, 8.5 events/hour (IQR, 4.1–19.5); median SBP, 103 mmHg (IQR, 95–114); median DBP, 64 mmHg (IQR, 58–71)) were enrolled.

The children were further divided into two subgroups according to BMI z-score: non-healthy-weight subgroup (cases; $n = 33$), and healthy-weight subgroup (controls; $n = 33$). In the non-healthy-weight subgroup, 30 (91%) children had a BMI z-score $\geq$ 1.0 kg/m^2 and three (9%) had a BMI z-score ≤ -2.0 kg/m^2. All participants underwent adenotonsillectomy and were included for primary statistical analysis. The median time interval between PSG and adenotonsillectomy was 1 week (IQR: 6–19 weeks).

3.2. Differences in Participants' Characteristics, PSG Variables, BP, and Tonsil Microbiome between the Different Weight Status Subgroups

3.2.1. Differences in Participants' Characteristics, PSG Variables, and BP between the Different Weight Status Subgroups

As expected, there was no significant difference in the proportion of chronic tonsillitis between the two subgroups (Table 1). Furthermore, there were no statistically significant differences in the proportions of male sex, allergic rhinitis, tonsil size, ANR, OSA-18 score, AHI, RDI, N1 stage, N2 stage, N3 stage, rapid eye movement (REM) stage, and DBP percentile. Notably, the non-healthy-weight group had significantly higher age, BMI z-score, ODI, SBP, DBP, and SBP percentile, and lower mean SpO$_2$ and minimal SpO$_2$ than the healthy-weight group. The difference in the tonsil size between children with chronic tonsillitis (3 (IQR, 3–3)) and children without chronic tonsillitis (3 (IQR, 3–4)) did not reach a statistical significance ($p = 0.13$).

Table 1. Patient characteristics, polysomnography variables, and blood pressures of the different weight status subgroups.

Variables	Non-Healthy-Weight Subgroup	Healthy-Weight Subgroup	p-Value [1]
	Patient Characteristics		
Age (years)	7.0 (6.0–8.0)	6.0 (5.0–7.5)	0.015 *
Male sex, n (%)	28 (85)	22 (67)	0.150
Chronic tonsillitis	6 (18)	10 (30)	0.389
Allergic rhinitis, n (%)	22 (67%)	25 (76%)	0.587
BMI (kg/m^2) z-score	2.01 (1.46–2.38)	−0.36 (−1.16–0.18)	<0.001 *
Tonsil size	3 (3–4)	2 (3–4)	0.461
ANR	0.73 (0.62–0.83)	0.81 (0.72–0.87)	0.053
OSA-18 score	80 (69–92)	81 (70–91)	0.928
	Polysomnography variables		
AHI (events/h)	9.6 (5.0–25.2)	5.4 (3.9–16.5)	0.074
RDI (events/h)	12.1 (5.3–27.6)	6.1 (4.9–17.9)	0.158
ODI (events/h)	7.3 (3.6–22.3)	3.2 (1.6–9.3)	0.006 *
Mean SpO$_2$ (%)	97 (96–98)	98 (97–98)	0.030 *
Minimal SpO$_2$ (%)	89 (83–91)	91 (88–93)	0.022 *
N1 stage	13 (6–21)	9 (6–13)	0.142
N2 stage	38 (33–46)	41 (36–44)	0.807
N3 stage	28 (23–30)	28 (22–36)	0.663
REM stage	18 (13–22)	21 (16–25)	0.221
	Blood pressure variables		
Systolic BP, mmHg	111 (100–121)	98 (87–107)	0.001 *
Diastolic BP, mmHg	67 (61–76)	60 (58–68)	0.011 *
Systolic BP percentile (%)	84 (55–91)	48 (25–89)	0.018 *
Diastolic BP percentile (%)	75 (55–87)	68 (50–77)	0.174

Note: Data are summarized as median (interquartile range) or n (%) as appropriate. Abbreviations: AHI, apnea–hypopnea index; ANR, adenoid–nasopharyngeal ratio; BMI, body mass index; BP, blood pressure; ODI, oxygen desaturation index; OSA, obstructive sleep apnea; RDI, respiratory disturbance index; REM, rapid eye movement; SpO$_2$, pulse oxygen saturation. [1] Data were compared using the Mann–Whitney U test for continuous variables, and the chi-square test for categorical variables. * Significant differences $p < 0.05$.

Furthermore, the differences in participants' characteristics, PSG variables, and BP between the overweight and underweight subgroups were not statistically significant (Supplementary Table S1). These variables were also comparable across the overweight, underweight, and healthy-weight subgroups (all $p > 0.05$).

3.2.2. Differences in Tonsil Microbiome between the Different Weight Status Subgroups

After quality assessment, a total of 4,207,400 16S rRNA paired-end reads with an average of 105,185 ± 19,957 paired-end reads per sample passed the filters. Figure 2A,B show OTU trees of the non-healthy-weight subgroup (OTU = 9318) and healthy-weight subgroup (OTU = 9886). Figure 2C shows that both subgroups shared 6539 OTUs; otherwise, there were 2779 and 3347 deferential OTUs in the non-healthy-weight and healthy-weight subgroups, respectively. However, there were no significant differences in α diversity, β diversity, and relative abundances of the top 10 tonsil families between the non-healthy-weight and healthy-weight subgroups (Figure 2D–F; all $p > 0.05$). Furthermore, the α diversity, β diversity, and relative abundance of the top 10 tonsil families of the over-weight were comparable with those of the underweight subgroups ($p = 0.064$, 0.106, 0.492, respectively). Moreover, the differences in α diversity, β diversity, and relative abundances of the top 10 tonsil families across the overweight, underweight, and healthy-weight subgroups ($p = 0.088$, 0.119, 0.700, respectively).

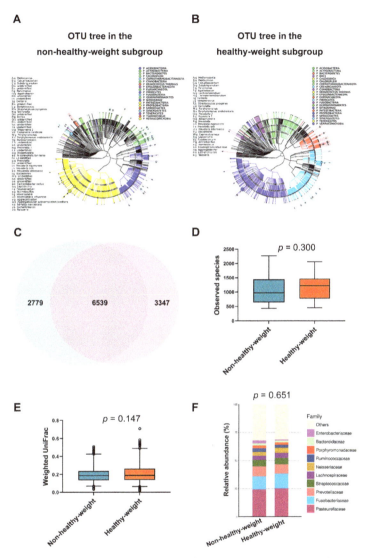

Figure 2. Tonsil microbiome in children with obstructive sleep apnea. (**A**) The operational taxonomic unit (OTU) tree of the non-healthy-weight subgroup (n = 33) included 9318 OTUs, assessed by Graphical Phylogenetic Analysis. (**B**) The OTU tree of the healthy-weight subgroup (n = 33) included 9886 OTUs. (**C**) A Venn diagram demonstrated that both subgroups shared 6539 OTUs; otherwise, the non-healthy-weight subgroup had 2779 deferential OTUs and the healthy-weight subgroup had 3347 deferential OTUs. (**D**) The α diversities of both subgroups were equal (p = 0.300; Mann–Whitney U test). (**E**) Furthermore, the β diversity of the non-healthy-weight subgroup was comparable to that of the healthy-weight group (p = 0.147; Mann–Whitney U test). (**F**) The relative abundances of the top 10 tonsil families in the non-healthy-weight subgroup were similar to those in the healthy-weight subgroup (p = 0.651; analysis of similarity test).

Fifty-five phyla were identified from the tonsil samples. There were six major phyla (>0.1% abundance and present in >90% of the samples [49]), including *Proteobacteria*, *Firmicutes*, *Bacteroidetes*, *Fusobacteria*, *Actinobacteria*, and *Epsilonbacteraeota*, and 49 minor phyla. In descending order of median relative abundance, the 10 most common phyla were *Proteobacteria*, *Firmicutes*, *Bacteroidetes*, *Fusobacteria*, *Actinobacteria*, *Epsilonbacteraeota*, *Patescibacteria*, *Cyanobacteria*, *Tenericutes*, and *Acidobacteria*.

Figure 3A,B demonstrate the similar distributions of the relative abundances of these phyla in the non-healthy-weight and healthy-weight subgroups ($p > 0.05$). Furthermore, the relative abundances of these phyla in the overweight and underweight subgroups were comparable ($p = 0.536$). Additionally, the differences in the 10 most common phyla across the overweight, underweight, and healthy-weight subgroups were not statistically significant ($p = 0.814$).

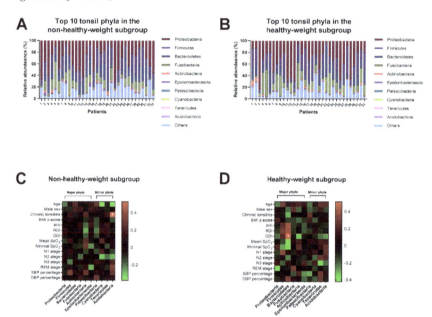

Figure 3. The top 10 tonsil phyla in both weight status subgroups. The relative abundances of the top 10 tonsil phyla in the non-healthy-weight subgroup (**A**) and the healthy-weight subgroup (**B**) ($p = 0.651$; analysis of similarity test). Chronic tonsillitis was significantly associated with a relative abundance of Acidobacteria in the non-healthy-weight subgroup ($r = 0.53$, $q = 0.015$) (**C**), whereas the oxygen desaturation index (ODI) was significantly associated with Bacteroidetes in the healthy-weight subgroup ($r = 0.52$, $q = 0.020$) (**D**). Abbreviations: AHI, apnea–hypopnea index; BMI, body mass index; RDI, respiratory disturbance index; REM, rapid eye movement; SpO$_2$, pulse oxygen saturation.

3.2.3. Associations of Tonsil Phyla, Participants' Characteristics, PSG Variables, and BPs in the Different Weight Status Subgroups

In the non-healthy-weight group, age was related to Cyanobacteria and Acidobacteria, chronic tonsillitis was correlated with Acidobacteria, and SBP percentile was associated with Firmicutes (Figure 3C). The positive relationship between chronic tonsillitis and Acidobacteria remained significant after applying the Benjamini–Hochberg method ($r = 0.53$, $q = 0.015$).

Although there were several weak associations between the PSG variables (AHI, RDI, ODI, mean SpO$_2$, minimal SpO$_2$), DBP percentile, and Bacteroidetes, ODI and Actinobacteria, stage 1 sleep and Firmicutes, stage 3 sleep and Tenericutes, and REM stage and Proteobacteria, only the significant positive association between ODI and Bacteroidetes persisted after applying the Benjamini–Hochberg method ($r = 0.52$, $q = 0.020$) (Figure 3D).

3.3. Post Hoc Analysis

After studying the differences between the two weight subgroups, we wondered whether other classifications may be associated with the tonsil microbiome. We performed median splits of the participants' characteristics, PSG variables, and BPs. The α diversities of the tonsil microbiome were not associated with age ≥ 6 years, male sex, chronic tonsillitis, BMI z-score ≥ 1.00, AHI ≥ 9.0 events/h, RDI ≥ 9.0 events/h, ODI ≥ 5.0 events/h, minimal SpO$_2$ ≤ 90%, N1 stage ≥ 10%, N2 stage ≥ 40%, N3 stage ≤ 26%, REM stage ≥ 19%, SBP percentile ≥ 70%, and DSBP percentile ≥ 70%. In addition, differences in the tonsil microbiome between various (moderate-to-severe OSA and mild OSA; severe OSA, and non-severe OSA; hypertension and non-hypertension) subgroups did not reach statistical significance.

Interestingly, both α (Figure 4A) and β (Figure 4B) diversity indices of the mean SpO$_2$ ≤ 97% subgroup were significantly lower than those of the mean SpO$_2$ > 97% subgroup (p = 0.030 and 0.0005, respectively). The relative abundances of the top 10 tonsil phyla in the mean SpO$_2$ ≤ 97% subgroup were significantly different from those in the mean SpO$_2$ > 97% subgroup (p = 0.014; analysis of similarity test) (Figure 4C). Notably, the relative abundance of Bacteroidetes in the mean SpO$_2$ ≤ 97% subgroup was significantly higher than that in the mean SpO$_2$ > 97% subgroup (q = 0.026) (Figure 4D).

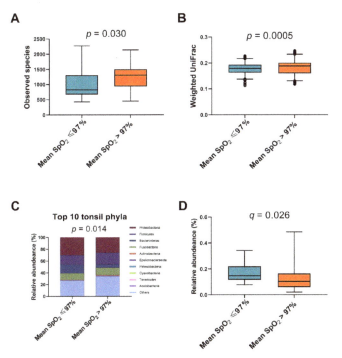

Figure 4. Comparison of the tonsil microbiome between the mean oxygen saturation (SpO$_2$) ≤ 97% and > 97% subgroups. (**A**) The α diversity of the mean SpO$_2$ ≤ 97% subgroup was significantly lower than that of the mean SpO$_2$ > 97% subgroup (p = 0.030; Mann–Whitney U test). (**B**) The β diversity of the mean SpO$_2$ ≤ 97% subgroup was significantly lower than that of the SpO$_2$ > 97% subgroup (p = 0.0005; Mann–Whitney U test). (**C**) The relative abundances of the top 10 tonsil phyla in the mean SpO$_2$ ≤ 97% subgroup were significantly different from those in the mean SpO$_2$ > 97% subgroup (p = 0.014; analysis of similarity test). (**D**) Furthermore, the relative abundance of Bacteroidetes in the mean SpO$_2$ ≤ 97% subgroup was significantly higher than that in the mean SpO$_2$ > 97% subgroup (q = 0.026; Mann–Whitney U test).

4. Discussion

In the following paragraphs, we address several novel and interesting findings of this study regarding the relationships of the tonsil microbiome with weight status, OSA severity, and hypoxemia among a sample of pediatric OSA patients.

Some clinical parameters were significantly different between the non-healthy-weight and healthy-weight subgroups. The non-healthy-weight subgroup had more profound intermittent hypoxemia (ODI, mean SpO_2, and minimal SpO_2) and a higher SBP percentile, which is consistent with the well-known connections between obesity and manifestations of OSA. However, no significant association was observed between the tonsil microbiome and weight status. The data did not support our primary hypothesis. Notably, although weight status was not directly associated with the tonsil microbiome in the overall cohort, relationships between the tonsil microbiome and other clinical parameters differed between the patients with different weight statuses. Chronic tonsillitis was related to Acidobacteria in the non-healthy-weight subgroup, while ODI was associated with Bacteroidetes in the healthy-weight subgroup. In post hoc analysis, we found that the children with or without a mean $SpO_2 \leq 97\%$ had significantly different microbial profiles, especially with regards to Bacteroidetes. It seemed that, instead of weight status, hypoxemia status was the key differentiating factor for the tonsil microbiota among pediatric OSA patients.

Previous studies have suggested that the presence and severity of OSA are associated with microbial profiles [19,20,23]. Yang et al. used 16S ribosomal DNA sequencing to investigate the oropharyngeal microbiome and demonstrated that adults with OSA had less oropharyngeal species diversity and altered abundance compared with non-OSA controls, and that the relative abundance of *Neisseria* (a genus of Proteobacteria) increased with higher OSA severity [20]. In our results, neither Proteobacteria nor *Neisseria* was related to AHI ($p = 0.905$ and 0.246, respectively). However, the children with a mean $SpO_2 \leq 97\%$ had less tonsillar species diversity and altered abundance compared to those with a mean $SpO_2 > 97\%$. Again, this suggested that the degree of intermittent hypoxemia may be more influential on the tonsil microbiome than OSA severity.

Johnston et al. investigated the tonsillar crypt microbiota in children with recurrent tonsillitis [54] and OSA [19], and found that Fusobacteria, Proteobacteria, Bacteroidetes, and Firmicutes were major phyla of the tonsil specimens in both groups (α diversity: $p = 0.66$; β diversity: $p = 0.52$) [19]. In another study on the adenotonsillar microbiome of children who snored [23], Kim and colleagues also reported similar major phyla, namely Proteobacteria, Actinobacteria, Firmicutes, Fusobacteria, Bacteroidetes, and Tenericutes. They further demonstrated that α diversity indices were related to some patient characteristics such as sex, emotional stress, and interleukin-8, and that β diversity indices were related to heat shock protein 70. These findings suggest possible connections between demographic characteristics, clinical symptoms, regional mucosal immune environment, and tonsil microbiome.

Our data are compatible with the results of the previous studies concerning the general picture of the tonsil microbiome. Moreover, we found a positive correlation between chronic tonsillitis and Acidobacteria in the non-healthy-weight subgroup. To the best of our knowledge, this is the first study to suggest that Acidobacteria may be implicated in tonsillar infections among pediatric OSA patients. Acidobacteria are Gram-negative rod-shaped bacteria. The majority of Acidobacteria strains have been described as aerobes, and they are ubiquitous in soil [55]. An increasing number of studies have investigated Acidobacteria in humans. For example, Acidobacteria are reported to be the fifth most dominant phyla in the bronchoalveolar lavage of adults with OSA [22]. In addition, both Acidobacteria and obesity are associated with an increase in the fecal levels of valeric acid [56,57]. Furthermore, Acidobacteria are shown to be significantly enriched in patients with chronic endodontic infection [58]. These observations provide indirect evidence for possible connections between tonsillar Acidobacteria infection, OSA, and obesity, and future investigations are warranted to confirm the causality.

The other novel finding of our study is the significant association between intermittent hypoxemia and Bacteroidetes in the healthy-weight subgroup. Members of the phylum Bacteroidetes are Gram-negative, rod-shaped, anaerobic or aerobic bacteria, and they are commonly found in the oral cavity and gastrointestinal tract. The abundance of Bacteroidetes and the Bacteroidetes–Firmicutes ratio are reported to be decreased in obese individuals compared to lean individuals [59]. However, our data suggested that it was the healthy-weight pediatric OSA patients in whom ODI significantly interacted with Bacteroidetes. Bacteroidetes of the tonsils may thus be implicated in the pathophysiology of OSA.

Previous studies have suggested associations between OSA and alterations in the composition and diversity of fecal microbiota. In a murine model, intermittent hypoxia exposure led to a lower abundance of Bacteroidetes in the feces [60], and reintroduction of a normoxic environment did not reverse the negative alterations of the gut microbiota [61]. In a sample of adults with OSA, Ko et al. found that fecal *Bacteroides* (a major genus of Bacteroidetes) were not associated with AHI or intermittent hypoxemia [62]. However, the results were very different for the oral microbiome. Xu et al. reported a higher abundance of oral Bacteroidetes in children with OSA [21]. Consistent with this finding, we also found a higher abundance of Bacteroidetes in pediatric OSA patients with a lower mean SpO_2. The discrepancy between fecal and oral microbiota as well as the differences between patients with and without profound hypoxia are very interesting and may be explained by the oxygen concentration level at different sites and the aerotolerant abilities of different bacteria.

The environments of sites in the human body impact which microorganisms can inhabit these sites. Unlike the environment of the intestine, which is extremely low in oxygen concentration [63], to survive in the oral cavity, bacteria need to overcome the challenge of atmospheric oxygen exposure. Moreover, mouth breathing is very common in children with OSA [64] and positively associated with AHI [65]. OSA-related mouth breathing further increases exposure of the tonsil microbiome to atmospheric oxygen. *Bacteroides* species are among the most aerotolerant anaerobes and are able to tolerate oxygen in room air for up to 3 days [66]. On the other hand, *Fusobacterium* species (a genus of Fusobacteria) and *Clostridium* species (a genus of Firmicutes) are less aerotolerant anaerobes. Intermittent hypoxemia (in terms of mean $SpO_2 \leq 97\%$) further enhances the survival advantage of Bacteroidetes relative to other aerobes of the tonsils. Mouse models of chronic intermittent hypoxia would be helpful to further validate these inferences [60].

Several limitations should be addressed in this study. First, the patient number of the underweight subgroup was too small and insufficient to make a conclusion. Future studies with a larger sample size of each weight status subgroup are warranted to further understand how obesity or underweight may impact the tonsil microbiome and its interaction with OSA. Second, the study cohort was predominantly male and mostly Han in ethnicity, which may limit the generalizability of the results. Third, some of the children may have had co-existing chronic tonsillitis, which would interfere with the analysis of the tonsil microbiome. However, the proportions of sex and chronic tonsillitis were comparable in both weight subgroups to minimize confounding effects from baseline characteristics. Forth, the study was cross-sectional and thus unable to conclude the direction of associations or causal effects. The relationships between the microbiota and OSA need to be further explored. Also, future prospective investigations on the effects of OSA treatment on the tonsil microbiome with a larger sample size will be of interest.

5. Conclusions

The advent of metagenomics has led to an increase in investigations on human microbiota. The tonsil microbiome plays a role in pediatric OSA, and it seems to have different effects depending on weight status. We preliminarily found that chronic tonsillitis was related to Acidobacteria in children with OSA and non-healthy weight, and that ODI was associated with Bacteroidetes in the children with OSA and healthy weight. In addition, children with OSA with or without mean $SpO_2 \leq 97\%$ had significantly different microbial profiles, particularly with regards to Bacteroidetes. Future studies to investigate associations among alterations of the tonsil microbiome and exacerbations or reductions of OSA severity are warranted. Furthermore, this study also suggests the possibility of personalized treatment of pediatric OSA based on the tonsil microbiome.

Supplementary Materials: The following are available online at https://www.mdpi.com/article/10.3390/jpm11060486/s1, Table S1: Patient characteristics, polysomnography variables, and blood pressures of the over-weight and under-weight subgroups.

Author Contributions: Conceptualization, H.-H.C., J.-F.H., C.-G.H., H.-C.L., and L.-A.L.; methodology, L.-P.C., Y.-L.H., H.-Y.L., Y.-S.H., C.-W.C., C.-G.H., H.-C.L., and L.-A.L.; software, J.-F.H., N.-H.C., C.-W.C., C.-G.H., and H.-C.L.; validation, H.-H.C., C.-H.C., Y.-L.H., H.-Y.L., N.-H.C., Y.-S.H., C.-G.H., H.-C.L., and L.-A.L.; formal analysis, H.-H.C. and L.-A.L.; investigation, H.-H.C., L.-P.C., C.-H.C., Y.-L.H., H.-Y.L., Y.-S.H., C.-G.H., and L.-A.L.; resources, L.-P.C., C.-H.C., Y.-L.H., Y.-S.H., C.-G.H., H.-C.L., and L.-A.L.; data curation, J.-F.H., C.-H.C., H.-Y.L., N.-H.C., Y.-S.H., C.-G.H., and H.-C.L.; writing—original draft, H.-H.C., J.-F.H., L.-P.C., C.-W.C., and L.-A.L.; writing—review and editing, C.-H.C., Y.-L.H., H.-Y.L., N.-H.C., Y.-S.H., C.-G.H., and H.-C.L.; visualization, H.-H.C. and L.-A.L.; supervision, C.-H.C., H.-Y.L., N.-H.C., Y.-S.H., and H.-C.L.; project administration, L.-A.L.; funding acquisition, H.-H.C. and L.-A.L. All authors have read and agreed to the published version of the manuscript.

Funding: This research was funded by the Chang Gung Medical Foundation, Taiwan, grant numbers CMRPG1J0041, EMRPD1I0411, and 1K0391 (H.-H.C.), and CMRPG3F1091, 3F1092, 3F1093, and 3J1701 (L.-A.L.). The APC was funded by the Chang Gung Medical Foundation, Taiwan.

Institutional Review Board Statement: The study was conducted according to the guidelines of the Declaration of Helsinki and approved by the Institutional Review Board of the Chang Gung Medical Foundation, Taoyuan, Taiwan (protocol code 201507279A3 and date of approval 15 April 2016).

Informed Consent Statement: Informed consent was obtained from all subjects involved in the study.

Data Availability Statement: The data presented in this study are available upon request from the corresponding author. The data are not publicly available due to ethical restrictions.

Acknowledgments: The authors would like to thank Ruo-Chi Wang and Chung-Fang Hsiao (Department of Otorhinolaryngology, Head and Neck Surgery, Linkou Chang Gung Memorial Hospital, Taoyuan City, Taiwan) for their technical assistance.

Conflicts of Interest: The authors declare no conflict of interest. The funders had no role in the design of the study; in the collection, analyses, or interpretation of data; in the writing of the manuscript, or in the decision to publish the results.

References

1. Marcus, C.L.; Brooks, L.J.; Draper, K.A.; Gozal, D.; Halbower, A.C.; Jones, J.; Schechter, M.S.; Sheldon, S.H.; Spruyt, K.; Ward, S.D.; et al. Diagnosis and management of childhood obstructive sleep apnea syndrome. *Pediatrics* **2012**, *130*, 576–584. [CrossRef] [PubMed]
2. Andersen, I.G.; Holm, J.C.; Homoe, P. Obstructive sleep apnea in children and adolescents with and without obesity. *Eur. Arch. Otorhinolaryngol.* **2019**, *276*, 871–878. [CrossRef] [PubMed]
3. Wang, J.; Zhao, Y.; Yang, W.; Shen, T.; Xue, P.; Yan, X.; Chen, D.; Qiao, Y.; Chen, M.; Ren, R.; et al. Correlations between obstructive sleep apnea and adenotonsillar hypertrophy in children of different weight status. *Sci. Rep.* **2019**, *9*, 11455. [CrossRef] [PubMed]
4. Madaeva, I.; Berdina, O.; Polyakov, V.; Kolesnikov, S. Obstructive Sleep Apnea and Hypertension in Adolescents: Effect on Neurobehavioral and Cognitive Functioning. *Can. Respir. J.* **2016**, *2016*, 3950914. [CrossRef]
5. Shalitin, S.; Deutsch, V.; Tauman, R. Hepcidin, soluble transferrin receptor and IL-6 levels in obese children and adolescents with and without type 2 diabetes mellitus/impaired glucose tolerance and their association with obstructive sleep apnea. *J. Endocrinol. Investig.* **2018**, *41*, 969–975. [CrossRef]
6. Smith, D.F.; Hossain, M.M.; Hura, A.; Huang, G.; McConnell, K.; Ishman, S.L.; Amin, R.S. Inflammatory Milieu and Cardiovascular Homeostasis in Children With Obstructive Sleep Apnea. *Sleep* **2017**, *40*. [CrossRef]
7. Tripathi, A.; Melnik, A.V.; Xue, J.; Poulsen, O.; Meehan, M.J.; Humphrey, G.; Jiang, L.; Ackermann, G.; McDonald, D.; Zhou, D.; et al. Intermittent Hypoxia and Hypercapnia, a Hallmark of Obstructive Sleep Apnea, Alters the Gut Microbiome and Metabolome. *mSystems* **2018**, *3*. [CrossRef] [PubMed]

8. Badran, M.; Khalyfa, A.; Ericsson, A.; Gozal, D. Fecal microbiota transplantation from mice exposed to chronic intermittent hypoxia elicits sleep disturbances in naive mice. *Exp. Neurol.* **2020**, *334*, 113439. [CrossRef]
9. Turnbaugh, P.J.; Ley, R.E.; Mahowald, M.A.; Magrini, V.; Mardis, E.R.; Gordon, J.I. An obesity-associated gut microbiome with increased capacity for energy harvest. *Nature* **2006**, *444*, 1027–1031. [CrossRef]
10. Cox, A.J.; West, N.P.; Cripps, A.W. Obesity, inflammation, and the gut microbiota. *Lancet Diabetes Endocrinol.* **2015**, *3*, 207–215. [CrossRef]
11. Pevsner-Fischer, M.; Blacher, E.; Tatirovsky, E.; Ben-Dov, I.Z.; Elinav, E. The gut microbiome and hypertension. *Curr. Opin. Nephrol. Hypertens.* **2017**, *26*, 1–8. [CrossRef] [PubMed]
12. Durgan, D.J.; Ganesh, B.P.; Cope, J.L.; Ajami, N.J.; Phillips, S.C.; Petrosino, J.F.; Hollister, E.B.; Bryan, R.M., Jr. Role of the Gut Microbiome in Obstructive Sleep Apnea-Induced Hypertension. *Hypertension* **2016**, *67*, 469–474. [CrossRef]
13. Ridaura, V.K.; Faith, J.J.; Rey, F.E.; Cheng, J.; Duncan, A.E.; Kau, A.L.; Griffin, N.W.; Lombard, V.; Henrissat, B.; Bain, J.R.; et al. Gut microbiota from twins discordant for obesity modulate metabolism in mice. *Science* **2013**, *341*, 1241214. [CrossRef] [PubMed]
14. Huang, Y.S.; Guilleminault, C.; Hwang, F.M.; Cheng, C.; Lin, C.H.; Li, H.Y.; Lee, L.A. Inflammatory cytokines in pediatric obstructive sleep apnea. *Medicine (Baltimore)* **2016**, *95*, e4944. [CrossRef]
15. Chuang, H.H.; Huang, C.G.; Chuang, L.P.; Huang, Y.S.; Chen, N.H.; Li, H.Y.; Fang, T.J.; Hsu, J.F.; Lai, H.C.; Chen, J.Y.; et al. Relationships Among and Predictive Values of Obesity, Inflammation Markers, and Disease Severity in Pediatric Patients with Obstructive Sleep Apnea Before and After Adenotonsillectomy. *J. Clin. Med.* **2020**, *9*, 579. [CrossRef] [PubMed]
16. Eltzschig, H.K.; Carmeliet, P. Hypoxia and inflammation. *N. Engl. J. Med.* **2011**, *364*, 656–665. [CrossRef]
17. Wu, B.G.; Sulaiman, I.; Wang, J.; Shen, N.; Clemente, J.C.; Li, Y.; Laumbach, R.J.; Lu, S.E.; Udasin, I.; Le-Hoang, O.; et al. Severe Obstructive Sleep Apnea Is Associated with Alterations in the Nasal Microbiome and an Increase in Inflammation. *Am. J. Respir. Crit. Care Med.* **2019**, *199*, 99–109. [CrossRef]
18. Dirain, C.O.; Silva, R.C.; Collins, W.O.; Antonelli, P.J. The Adenoid Microbiome in Recurrent Acute Otitis Media and Obstructive Sleep Apnea. *J. Int. Adv. Otol.* **2017**, *13*, 333–339. [CrossRef] [PubMed]
19. Johnston, J.; Hoggard, M.; Biswas, K.; Astudillo-Garcia, C.; Waldvogel-Thurlow, S.; Radcliff, F.J.; Mahadevan, M.; Douglas, R.G. The bacterial community and local lymphocyte response are markedly different in patients with recurrent tonsillitis compared to obstructive sleep apnoea. *Int. J. Pediatric Otorhinolaryngol.* **2018**, *113*, 281–288. [CrossRef]
20. Yang, W.; Shao, L.; Heizhati, M.; Wu, T.; Yao, X.; Wang, Y.; Wang, L.; Li, N. Oropharyngeal Microbiome in Obstructive Sleep Apnea: Decreased Diversity and Abundance. *J. Clin. Sleep Med. JCSM Off. Publ. Am. Acad. Sleep Med.* **2019**, *15*, 1777–1788. [CrossRef] [PubMed]
21. Xu, H.; Li, X.; Zheng, X.; Xia, Y.; Fu, Y.; Li, X.; Qian, Y.; Zou, J.; Zhao, A.; Guan, J.; et al. Pediatric Obstructive Sleep Apnea is Associated With Changes in the Oral Microbiome and Urinary Metabolomics Profile: A Pilot Study. *J. Clin. Sleep Med.* **2018**, *14*, 1559–1567. [CrossRef]
22. Lu, D.; Yao, X.; Abulimiti, A.; Cai, L.; Zhou, L.; Hong, J.; Li, N. Profiling of lung microbiota in the patients with obstructive sleep apnea. *Medicine (Baltimore)* **2018**, *97*, e11175. [CrossRef] [PubMed]
23. Kim, K.S.; Min, H.J. Correlation between adenotonsillar microbiome and clinical characteristics of pediatrics with snoring. *Clin. Exp. Otorhinolaryngol.* **2020**. [CrossRef]
24. Chuang, H.H.; Hsu, J.F.; Chuang, L.P.; Chen, N.H.; Huang, Y.S.; Li, H.Y.; Chen, J.Y.; Lee, L.A.; Huang, C.G. Differences in Anthropometric and Clinical Features among Preschoolers, School-Age Children, and Adolescents with Obstructive Sleep Apnea-A Hospital-Based Study in Taiwan. *Int. J. Environ. Res. Public Health* **2020**, *17*, 4663. [CrossRef]
25. Johnston, J.J.; Douglas, R. Adenotonsillar microbiome: An update. *Postgrad. Med. J.* **2018**, *94*, 398–403. [CrossRef] [PubMed]
26. Verma, D.; Garg, P.K.; Dubey, A.K. Insights into the human oral microbiome. *Arch. Microbiol.* **2018**, *200*, 525–540. [CrossRef] [PubMed]
27. Baugh, R.F.; Archer, S.M.; Mitchell, R.B.; Rosenfeld, R.M.; Amin, R.; Burns, J.J.; Darrow, D.H.; Giordano, T.; Litman, R.S.; Li, K.K.; et al. Clinical practice guideline: Tonsillectomy in children. *Otolaryngol. Head Neck Surg.* **2011**, *144*, S1–S30. [CrossRef]
28. Kaditis, A.; Kheirandish-Gozal, L.; Gozal, D. Algorithm for the diagnosis and treatment of pediatric OSA: A proposal of two pediatric sleep centers. *Sleep Med.* **2012**, *13*, 217–227. [CrossRef]
29. de Onis, M.; Onyango, A.W.; Borghi, E.; Siyam, A.; Nishida, C.; Siekmann, J. Development of a WHO growth reference for school-aged children and adolescents. *Bull. World Health Organ.* **2007**, *85*, 660–667. [CrossRef]
30. Burton, M.J.; Glasziou, P.P.; Chong, L.Y.; Venekamp, R.P. Tonsillectomy or adenotonsillectomy versus non-surgical treatment for chronic/recurrent acute tonsillitis. *Cochrane Database Syst. Rev.* **2014**, CD001802. [CrossRef] [PubMed]
31. Franco, R.A., Jr.; Rosenfeld, R.M.; Rao, M. First place—Resident clinical science award 1999. Quality of life for children with obstructive sleep apnea. *Otolaryngol. Head Neck Surg. Off. J. Am. Acad. Otolaryngol. Head Neck Surg.* **2000**, *123*, 9–16. [CrossRef] [PubMed]
32. Huang, Y.-S.; Hwang, F.-M.; Lin, C.-H.; Lee, L.-A.; Huang, P.-Y.; Chiu, S.-T. Clinical manifestations of pediatric obstructive sleep apnea syndrome: Clinical utility of the Chinese-version Obstructive Sleep Apnea Questionaire-18. *Psychiatry Clin. Neurosci.* **2015**, *69*, 752–762. [CrossRef] [PubMed]
33. Brodsky, L. Modern Assessment of Tonsils and Adenoids. *Pediatric Clin. N. Am.* **1989**, *36*, 1551–1569. [CrossRef]
34. Fujioka, M.; Young, L.W.; Girdany, B.R. Radiographic evaluation of adenoidal size in children: Adenoidal-nasopharyngeal ratio. *AJR Am. J. Roentgenol.* **1979**, *133*, 401–404. [CrossRef]

35. Berry, R.B.; Budhiraja, R.; Gottlieb, D.J.; Gozal, D.; Iber, C.; Kapur, V.K.; Marcus, C.L.; Mehra, R.; Parthasarathy, S.; Quan, S.F.; et al. Rules for scoring respiratory events in sleep: Update of the 2007 AASM Manual for the Scoring of Sleep and Associated Events. Deliberations of the Sleep Apnea Definitions Task Force of the American Academy of Sleep Medicine. *J. Clin. Sleep Med.* **2012**, *8*, 597–619. [CrossRef] [PubMed]
36. Dehlink, E.; Tan, H.L. Update on paediatric obstructive sleep apnoea. *J. Thorac. Dis.* **2016**, *8*, 224–235. [CrossRef] [PubMed]
37. Lu, C.T.; Li, H.Y.; Lee, G.S.; Huang, Y.S.; Huang, C.G.; Chen, N.H.; Lee, L.A. Snoring sound energy as a potential biomarker for disease severity and surgical response in childhood obstructive sleep apnoea: A pilot study. *Clin. Otolaryngol.* **2019**, *44*, 47–52. [CrossRef]
38. The fourth report on the diagnosis, evaluation, and treatment of high blood pressure in children and adolescents. *Pediatrics* **2004**, *114*, 555–576. [CrossRef]
39. Flynn, J.T.; Kaelber, D.C.; Baker-Smith, C.M.; Blowey, D.; Carroll, A.E.; Daniels, S.R.; de Ferranti, S.D.; Dionne, J.M.; Falkner, B.; Flinn, S.K.; et al. Clinical Practice Guideline for Screening and Management of High Blood Pressure in Children and Adolescents. *cPediatrics* **2017**, *140*, e20171904. [CrossRef] [PubMed]
40. Chang, C.C.; Huang, Y.S.; Lin, Y.M.; Lin, C.J.; Jeng, J.C.; Liu, S.M.; Ho, T.L.; Chang, R.T.; Changou, C.A.; Ho, C.C.; et al. The role of sentrin-specific protease 2 substrate recognition in TGF-beta-induced tumorigenesis. *Sci. Rep.* **2018**, *8*, 9786. [CrossRef]
41. Wu, T.R.; Lin, C.S.; Chang, C.J.; Lin, T.L.; Martel, J.; Ko, Y.F.; Ojcius, D.M.; Lu, C.C.; Young, J.D.; Lai, H.C. Gut commensal Parabacteroides goldsteinii plays a predominant role in the anti-obesity effects of polysaccharides isolated from Hirsutella sinensis. *Gut* **2019**, *68*, 248–262. [CrossRef]
42. Magoc, T.; Salzberg, S.L. FLASH: Fast length adjustment of short reads to improve genome assemblies. *Bioinformatics* **2011**, *27*, 2957–2963. [CrossRef]
43. Caporaso, J.G.; Kuczynski, J.; Stombaugh, J.; Bittinger, K.; Bushman, F.D.; Costello, E.K.; Fierer, N.; Pena, A.G.; Goodrich, J.K.; Gordon, J.I.; et al. QIIME allows analysis of high-throughput community sequencing data. *Nat. Methods* **2010**, *7*, 335–336. [CrossRef]
44. Edgar, R.C.; Haas, B.J.; Clemente, J.C.; Quince, C.; Knight, R. UCHIME improves sensitivity and speed of chimera detection. *Bioinformatics* **2011**, *27*, 2194–2200. [CrossRef] [PubMed]
45. Edgar, R.C. UPARSE: Highly accurate OTU sequences from microbial amplicon reads. *Nat. Methods* **2013**, *10*, 996–998. [CrossRef] [PubMed]
46. McDonald, D.; Price, M.N.; Goodrich, J.; Nawrocki, E.P.; DeSantis, T.Z.; Probst, A.; Andersen, G.L.; Knight, R.; Hugenholtz, P. An improved Greengenes taxonomy with explicit ranks for ecological and evolutionary analyses of bacteria and archaea. *ISME J.* **2012**, *6*, 610–618. [CrossRef] [PubMed]
47. Caporaso, J.G.; Bittinger, K.; Bushman, F.D.; DeSantis, T.Z.; Andersen, G.L.; Knight, R. PyNAST: A flexible tool for aligning sequences to a template alignment. *Bioinformatics* **2010**, *26*, 266–267. [CrossRef]
48. Asnicar, F.; Weingart, G.; Tickle, T.L.; Huttenhower, C.; Segata, N. Compact graphical representation of phylogenetic data and metadata with GraPhlAn. *PeerJ* **2015**, *3*, e1029. [CrossRef] [PubMed]
49. Wu, I.W.; Lin, C.Y.; Chang, L.C.; Lee, C.C.; Chiu, C.Y.; Hsu, H.J.; Sun, C.Y.; Chen, Y.C.; Kuo, Y.L.; Yang, C.W.; et al. Gut Microbiota as Diagnostic Tools for Mirroring Disease Progression and Circulating Nephrotoxin Levels in Chronic Kidney Disease: Discovery and Validation Study. *Int. J. Biol. Sci.* **2020**, *16*, 420–434. [CrossRef] [PubMed]
50. Clarke, K.R. Non-parametric multivariate analyses of changes in community structure. *Austral Ecol.* **1993**, *18*, 117–143. [CrossRef]
51. Schloss, P.D.; Gevers, D.; Westcott, S.L. Reducing the effects of PCR amplification and sequencing artifacts on 16S rRNA-based studies. *PLoS ONE* **2011**, *6*, e27310. [CrossRef]
52. Lozupone, C.A.; Hamady, M.; Kelley, S.T.; Knight, R. Quantitative and qualitative beta diversity measures lead to different insights into factors that structure microbial communities. *Appl. Environ. Microbiol.* **2007**, *73*, 1576–1585. [CrossRef]
53. Cornejo-Pareja, I.; Ruiz-Limon, P.; Gomez-Perez, A.M.; Molina-Vega, M.; Moreno-Indias, I.; Tinahones, F.J. Differential Microbial Pattern Description in Subjects with Autoimmune-Based Thyroid Diseases: A Pilot Study. *J. Pers. Med.* **2020**, *10*, 192. [CrossRef] [PubMed]
54. Jensen, A.; Fago-Olsen, H.; Sorensen, C.H.; Kilian, M. Molecular mapping to species level of the tonsillar crypt microbiota associated with health and recurrent tonsillitis. *PLoS ONE* **2013**, *8*, e56418. [CrossRef]
55. Eichorst, S.A.; Trojan, D.; Roux, S.; Herbold, C.; Rattei, T.; Woebken, D. Genomic insights into the Acidobacteria reveal strategies for their success in terrestrial environments. *Environ. Microbiol.* **2018**, *20*, 1041–1063. [CrossRef] [PubMed]
56. Liu, S.; Li, E.; Sun, Z.; Fu, D.; Duan, G.; Jiang, M.; Yu, Y.; Mei, L.; Yang, P.; Tang, Y.; et al. Altered gut microbiota and short chain fatty acids in Chinese children with autism spectrum disorder. *Sci. Rep.* **2019**, *9*, 287. [CrossRef] [PubMed]
57. Tiihonen, K.; Ouwehand, A.C.; Rautonen, N. Effect of overweight on gastrointestinal microbiology and immunology: Correlation with blood biomarkers. *Br. J. Nutr.* **2010**, *103*, 1070–1078. [CrossRef] [PubMed]
58. Tzanetakis, G.N.; Azcarate-Peril, M.A.; Zachaki, S.; Panopoulos, P.; Kontakiotis, E.G.; Madianos, P.N.; Divaris, K. Comparison of Bacterial Community Composition of Primary and Persistent Endodontic Infections Using Pyrosequencing. *J. Endod.* **2015**, *41*, 1226–1233. [CrossRef]
59. Ley, R.E.; Turnbaugh, P.J.; Klein, S.; Gordon, J.I. Microbial ecology: Human gut microbes associated with obesity. *Nature* **2006**, *444*, 1022–1023. [CrossRef] [PubMed]

60. Moreno-Indias, I.; Torres, M.; Montserrat, J.M.; Sanchez-Alcoholado, L.; Cardona, F.; Tinahones, F.J.; Gozal, D.; Poroyko, V.A.; Navajas, D.; Queipo-Ortuno, M.I.; et al. Intermittent hypoxia alters gut microbiota diversity in a mouse model of sleep apnoea. *Eur. Respir. J.* **2015**, *45*, 1055–1065. [CrossRef] [PubMed]
61. Moreno-Indias, I.; Torres, M.; Sanchez-Alcoholado, L.; Cardona, F.; Almendros, I.; Gozal, D.; Montserrat, J.M.; Queipo-Ortuno, M.I.; Farre, R. Normoxic Recovery Mimicking Treatment of Sleep Apnea Does Not Reverse Intermittent Hypoxia-Induced Bacterial Dysbiosis and Low-Grade Endotoxemia in Mice. *Sleep* **2016**, *39*, 1891–1897. [CrossRef] [PubMed]
62. Ko, C.Y.; Fan, J.M.; Hu, A.K.; Su, H.Z.; Yang, J.H.; Huang, L.M.; Yan, F.R.; Zhang, H.P.; Zeng, Y.M. Disruption of sleep architecture in Prevotella enterotype of patients with obstructive sleep apnea-hypopnea syndrome. *Brain Behav.* **2019**, *9*, e01287. [CrossRef] [PubMed]
63. Albenberg, L.; Esipova, T.V.; Judge, C.P.; Bittinger, K.; Chen, J.; Laughlin, A.; Grunberg, S.; Baldassano, R.N.; Lewis, J.D.; Li, H.; et al. Correlation between intraluminal oxygen gradient and radial partitioning of intestinal microbiota. *Gastroenterology* **2014**, *147*, 1055–1063.e8. [CrossRef]
64. Li, H.Y.; Lee, L.A. Sleep-disordered breathing in children. *Chang Gung Med. J.* **2009**, *32*, 247–257. [PubMed]
65. Lai, C.C.; Lin, P.W.; Lin, H.C.; Friedman, M.; Chang, H.W.; Salapatas, A.M.; Lin, M.C.; Wang, P.C. Clinical Predictors of Pediatric Obstructive Sleep Apnea Syndrome. *Ann. Otol. Rhinol. Laryngol.* **2018**, *127*, 608–613. [CrossRef] [PubMed]
66. Tally, F.P.; Stewart, P.R.; Sutter, V.L.; Rosenblatt, J.E. Oxygen tolerance of fresh clinical anaerobic bacteria. *J. Clin. Microbiol.* **1975**, *1*, 161–164. [CrossRef] [PubMed]

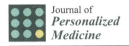

Article

Rifaximin as a Potential Treatment for IgA Nephropathy in a Humanized Mice Model

Vincenzo Di Leo [1,2,3,4,5], Patrick J. Gleeson [1,2,3,4], Fabio Sallustio [5], Carine Bounaix [1,2,3,4], Jennifer Da Silva [1,2,3,4], Gesualdo Loreto [5,*,†], Sanae Ben Mkaddem [1,2,3,4,*,†] and Renato C. Monteiro [1,2,3,4,6,*,†]

1. INSERM U1149, Centre de Recherche sur l'Inflammation, 75018 Paris, France; vincenzodileo88@yahoo.it (V.D.L.); james.gleeson@inserm.fr (P.J.G.); bounaix.carine@gmail.com (C.B.); jennifer.da-silva@inserm.fr (J.D.S.)
2. CNRS ERL8252, 75018 Paris, France
3. Faculté de Médecine, Université Paris Diderot, Sorbonne Paris Cité, Site Xavier Bichat, 75018 Paris, France
4. Inflamex Laboratory of Excellence, 75018 Paris, France
5. Division of Nephrology, Dialysis, and Transplantation, Department of Emergency and Organ Transplantation, University of Bari, 70124 Bari, Italy; fabio.sallustio@uniba.it
6. Service d'Immunologie, DHU Fire, Assistance Publique de Paris, Hôpital Bichat-Claude Bernard, 75018 Paris, France
* Correspondence: loretoge60@gmail.com (G.L.); sanae.benmkaddem@inserm.fr or sanae.benmkaddem@gmail.com (S.B.M.); renato.monteiro@inserm.fr (R.C.M.)
† Contributed equally to this study.

Abstract: Abstract: Background IgA Nephropathy (IgAN) is the most common glomerulonephritis worldwide, characterized by the mesangial deposition of abnormally glycosylated IgA1 (Gd-IgA). The production of Gd-IgA occurs in mucose-associated lymphoid tissue (MALT). The microbiota plays a role in MALT modulation. Rifaximin (NORMIX®), a non-absorbable oral antibiotic, induces positive modulation of the gut microbiota, favoring the growth of bacteria beneficial to the host. Here, we evaluate the effect of rifaximin on a humanized mice model of IgAN ($\alpha1^{KI}$-CD89^{Tg}). **Methods:** The $\alpha1^{KI}$-CD89^{Tg} mice were treated by the vehicle (olive oil) or rifaximin (NORMIX®). Serum levels of hIgA, hIgA1–sCD89, and mIgG–hIgA1 immune complexes were determined. Glomerular hIgA1 deposit and CD11b+ cells recruitment were revealed using confocal microscopy. Furthermore, the mRNA of the B-Cell Activating Factor (BAFF), polymeric immunoglobulin receptor (pIgR), and Tumor Necrosing Factor-α (TNF-α) in gut samples were detected by qPCR. **Results:** Rifaximin treatment decreased the urinary protein-to-creatinine ratio, serum levels of hIgA1–sCD89 and mIgG–hIgA1 complexes, hIgA1 glomerular deposition, and CD11b+ cell infiltration. Moreover, rifaximin treatment decreased significantly BAFF, pIgR, and TNF-α mRNA expression. **Conclusions:** Rifaximin decreased the IgAN symptoms observed in $\alpha1^{KI}$-CD89^{Tg} mice, suggesting a possible role for it in the treatment of the disease.

Keywords: IgA Nephropathy; rifaximin; microbiota; $\alpha1^{KI}$-CD89^{Tg} mice

Citation: Di Leo, V.; Gleeson, P.J.; Sallustio, F.; Bounaix, C.; Da Silva, J.; Loreto, G.; Ben Mkaddem, S.; Monteiro, R.C. Rifaximin as a Potential Treatment for IgA Nephropathy in a Humanized Mice Model. *J. Pers. Med.* **2021**, *11*, 309. https://doi.org/10.3390/jpm11040309

Academic Editor: Lucrezia Laterza

Received: 20 February 2021
Accepted: 11 April 2021
Published: 16 April 2021

Publisher's Note: MDPI stays neutral with regard to jurisdictional claims in published maps and institutional affiliations.

Copyright: © 2021 by the authors. Licensee MDPI, Basel, Switzerland. This article is an open access article distributed under the terms and conditions of the Creative Commons Attribution (CC BY) license (https://creativecommons.org/licenses/by/4.0/).

1. Introduction

IgA Nephropathy (IgAN) is a frequent cause of end-stage renal failure (about 20–40% of cases) [1] and it is characterized by dominant mesangial IgA deposition [2]. Microscopic hematuria and proteinuria are the most common clinical presentations [3]. Abnormally glycosylated IgA1 (Gd-IgA1) has a central role in the multi-hit process in IgAN patients [4]. Moreover, it has been demonstrated that there are two IgA receptors involved in IgAN pathogenicity: the FcαRI (CD89), expressed by blood myeloid cells and the transferrin receptor (CD71), expressed by mesangial cells [5]. Gd-IgA1-CD89 interaction induces the release of the extracellular portion of CD89 (soluble form of CD89) leading to the formation of circulating CD89-IgA immune complexes, which bind to CD71 leading to IgA1 deposits and mesangial cells proliferation in IgAN patients [6]. In patients with progressive disease, the IgA-CD89 complex has a role in the pathogenesis of IgAN and it seems to be positively correlated with proteinuria, microalbuminuria, and with some features of the Oxford score (endocapillary and extracapillary proliferation) [7].

Moreover, genetic variants, lifestyle, diet, and environmental factors contribute to disease onset [8]. The mucose-associated lymphoid tissue (MALT) is largely involved in the pathogenesis of the disease and, considering that it is influenced by antigenic stimulation from the commensal microflora, in recent years, scientific efforts have focused on the possible role of the microbiota and its modulation on the development and progression of IgAN [9]. Using antibiotics to manipulate the gut microbiota may represent a potentially effective treatment option for IgAN. A previous study by Chemouny et al. [10] has demonstrated that antibiotic treatment (ampicillin, vancomycin, neomycin, and metronidazole) of an IgAN mice model ($\alpha 1^{KI}$-CD89^{Tg} mice) reverses the IgAN phenotype without affecting serum IgA levels.

Rifaximin is a non-absorbable oral antibiotic that inhibits the synthesis of bacterial RNA by binding the β subunit of bacterial DNA-dependent RNA polymerase. It demonstrates bactericidal and bacteriostatic activity against both Gram-positive and Gram-negative aerobic and anaerobic bacteria. It has been proven to be safe and well-tolerated. Previous studies have shown that rifaximin can alter intestinal flora, inhibit bacterial attachment, prevent intestinal inflammation, and modulate gut barrier function [11]. This special feature distinguishes rifaximin from other systemic antibiotics. However, it is not clear whether orally administered rifaximin can prevent the development of IgAN by down-regulation of the inflammatory response triggered by gut microbes.

In this study, we investigated the effect of rifaximin on the IgAN progression, using a humanized mouse model of IgAN ($\alpha 1$KI-CD89^{Tg} mice). Rifaximin decreased the IgAN phenotype in a humanized mouse model of IgAN opening new therapeutic avenues for this disease.

2. Materials and Methods

2.1. In Vivo Experiments

Twelve-week-old $\alpha 1^{KI}$-CD89^{Tg} mice (n = 24) were raised and maintained in a specific pathogen-free mouse facility at the Centre for Research on Inflammation, Paris, France. All experiments were performed in accordance with the National Ethics Guidelines and with the approval of the Local Ethics Committee. These 12-week-old mice were divided into two groups to receive, by oral gavage, olive oil (n = 12) or rifaximin (NORMIX®) 100 mg/kg/die dissolved in olive oil (n = 12) [APAFIS number: #14265] for two weeks. We used olive oil because rifaximin is water-insoluble.

Urine was collected before starting, every four days, and at the end of the treatment experiment. Blood was collected by retro-orbital bleeding and the mice were sacrificed by cervical dislocation; the blood samples were centrifuged at $1500\times g$ rpm for 10 min at room temperature. The serum was collected and kept frozen at -80 °C until use. Kidneys and part of the ileum (2 cm above the ileocecal valve) were collected. Organs were conserved in OCT (CellPath Ltd., Newtown, Powys, UK).

2.2. Histopathology Procedures

For immunohistochemistry, 4 µm sections of cryostat frozen kidney were fixed in acetone for 30 min. Immunofluorescence staining was performed with goat anti-hIgA FITC (1/50, Southern Biotech, Birmingham, AL, USA) and Phalloidin (1/100, Invitrogen, Carlsbad, CA, USA) or anti-mouse CD11b antibody (M1/70) FITC (1/100, Abcam, Cambridge, UK) and Phalloidin (1/100, Invitrogen). Slides were mounted with Immuno-mount (Thermo Scientific, Waltham, MA, USA) and read with an immunofluorescent microscope (Zeiss, Oberkochen, Germany, LSM 780). Mean fluorescence intensity area positive for hIgA1 or for CD11b was measured using ImageJ and it was normalized for the total glomerular area.

2.3. Enzyme-Linked Immunosorbent Assay

Serum levels of hIgA were determined with a sandwich enzyme-linked immunosorbent assay (ELISA). Goat anti-hIgA (Bethyl Laboratories, Montgomery, TX, USA, A80–120A, 1:500 dilution) was used for coating. Sera (1:3000 diluted) were then added and revealed with goat anti-hIgA antibody HRP conjugated (Bethyl Laboratories, A80–120P, 1:50,000 dilution). The optic density (OD) was measured at 450 nm.

The hIgA1–sCD89 and mIgG–hIgA1 complexes were determined with ELISA [12]. A3 mAb anti-human CD89 (5 µg/mL, homemade [13]) or goat anti-hIgA (Bethyl Laboratories, 1:500 diluted) were used for coating.

Sera (1:10 diluted) were then added and revealed with goat anti-hIgA (Southern Biotech, 1:2000 dilution) or goat anti-mouse IgG (Southern Biotech, 1:5000 dilution) coupled with alkaline phosphatase (Southern Biotech, Birmingham, AL, USA). The OD at 405 nm was measured after 4 h from the addition of alkaline phosphatase substrate (Sigma-Aldrich, St. Louis, MO, USA). The complex levels were expressed as OD.

2.4. Real-Time PCR

Total RNA from mouse small intestine (four mice for each group) was isolated with RNABle (Eurobio laboratories, Les Ulis, France), according to the manufacturer's instructions, and complementary DNA was synthesized using Moloney-Murine Leukemia Virus reverse transcriptase (M-MLV RT, Invitrogen). cDNA was subjected to quantitative real-time PCR using a Chromo4 Real-Time PCR Detection System (Bio-Rad Laboratories, Marnes-la-Coquette, France). The mouse TNF-α, pIgR, BAFF, and ß-actin primers used and the corresponding Taqman probes are listed in Table S1 (Supplementary data 1).

The data from the qPCR were converted to 2-Ct, where Ct represents the threshold cycle. The mean Ct value of the duplicate PCRs was determined, and the mean 2-$\Delta\Delta$Ct was calculated from the duplicate cDNAs. PCR data were reported as the relative increase in mRNA transcripts versus that found in the pool of RNA of olive-oil-treated mice and corrected using the respective levels of ß-actin mRNA.

2.5. Statistical Analysis

Statistical analyses were performed with GraphPad Prism 6.0 (GraphPad Software, Inc., San Diego, CA, USA). We compared the results of the treatment and control group using the Mann–Whitney U test. The qPCR data were reported as the relative increase in mRNA transcripts versus that found in respective tissues from vehicle mice, corrected by the respective levels of β-actin mRNA, used as an internal standard. All the values of olive-oil-tested mice are 1. Statistical analyses were performed using the Wilcoxon test. Differences between groups were considered to be significant at a p-value of <0.05.

3. Results

3.1. Rifaximin Reduces the Disease Phenotype in IgAN Mice Model

Twelve-week-old α1KI-CD89Tg mice spontaneously present mesangial hIgA1 deposition, associated with proteinuria, mimicking IgAN in humans as described previously [13]. Mice treated with rifaximin for two weeks had a reduction in proteinuria (initial and final uPCR mean: 3.09 g/mmol and 2.39 g/mmol, respectively) compared to the mice treated with just the vehicle (olive oil) which showed an increase in proteinuria (initial and final uPCR mean in the oil group: 2.72 g/mmol and 2.87 g/mmol, respectively). There was no statistically significant difference in uPCR between the groups at T0 ($p > 0,05$; Figure 1B), while we found a significant difference between uPCR at T0 and uPCR after 14 days [delta T4–T0 ($p^* = 0.0172$; Figure 1C)]. Moreover, anti-hIgA immunostaining of mouse kidneys revealed that hIgA1 deposition was significantly reduced in antibiotic mice compared to the olive oil group ($p^{**} = 0.0014$, Figure 1D). To explore whether rifaximin affects the level of the total circulating hIgA1, we measured the serum IgA1 level by ELISA. Serum levels of hIgA1 were similar in the rifaximin group and the vehicle group ($p > 0.05$, Figure 1E).

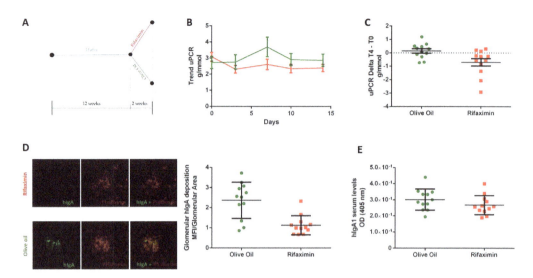

Figure 1. (**A**) Twelve-week-old mice were given 100 mg/kg of Rifaximin or of olive oil by oral gavage for two weeks before sacrifice. (**B**) Trend of uPCR from 12 weeks to sacrifice. (**C**) uPCR Delta t3-t0, where t3 is the uPCR after two weeks of treatment and t0 is uPCR before starting antibiotic or vehicle. (**D**) Representative sections of kidneys after immunostaining with anti-hIgA-FITC antibody and Phalloidin–Alexaflour 564 to underline glomerular structures (green anti-hIgA1, red phalloidin) and the ratio between the glomerular area positive for hIgA1 and total area of the glomerulus, measured using ImageJ. (**E**) hIgA serum level measured by ELISA in mice that received antibiotics or vehicle and compared using the Mann–Whitney test.

In contrast, mice in the antibiotic group showed less hIgA1-CD89 (Figure 2A, $p^* = 0.0145$) and mIgG-hIgA1 complexes (Figure 2B, $p^* = 0.0447$) than the control group. To evaluate the effect of rifaximin on kidney inflammation in the IgAN mice model, we assessed the immunofluorescence to analyze whether rifaximin affects CD11b+ renal infiltration. The antibiotic reduced the development of glomerular inflammation as illustrated by less CD11b-positive area normalized for the total glomerular area (Figure 2C, $p^* = 0.0317$).

3.2. Rifaximin Group Showed Less TNF-α, BAFF, and pIgR mRNA Gut Expression Levels

It has been shown that epithelial-derived BAFF is the major modulator of B cell development and it has a key role in IgA class switching and plasma cell survival in the MALT [14,15]. Consistent with the effect of rifaximin on renal inflammation, mice treated with this antibiotic present a significant decrease of TNF-α, BAFF, and pIgR mRNA gut expression when compared to the control group (respectively $p^* = 0.0369$, $p^* = 0.0490$, $p^* = 0.0271$). TNF-α, BAFF, and pIgR mRNA expression levels are illustrated in Figure 3.

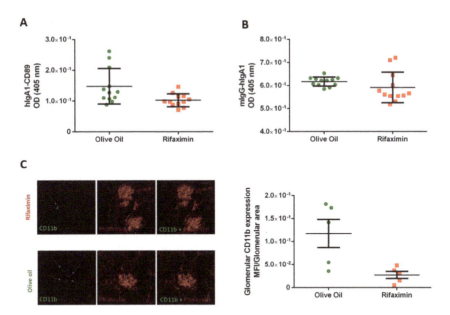

Figure 2. Antibiotic treatment decreases the formation of hIgA1–sCD89 and of mIgG–hIgA1 complexes but not the hIgA1 serum level. (**A**) hIgA-CD89 complexes in mice that received rifaximin or olive oil. (**B**) Levels of mIgG-hIgA complexes in mice that received antibiotics or vehicle. Anti-hIgA or A3 monoclonal-antibody anti-human CD89 was used for coating. Polyethylene glycol precipitated sera were then added; detection with anti-hIgG or anti-hIgA-HRP. Serum hIgA1 and mIgG levels were measured by ELISA. Statistical analyses were performed using Mann–Whitney test. (**C**) Quantification of glomerular cells was performed by counting the area positive for CD11b measured using ImageJ. Representative sections of kidneys after immunostaining with anti-CD11b-FITC antibody and Phalloidin–Alexaflour 564 to underline glomerular structures (green anti CD11b, red phalloidin) and the ratio between the glomerular fluorescence area positive for CD11b and total area of the glomerulus, measured using ImageJ.

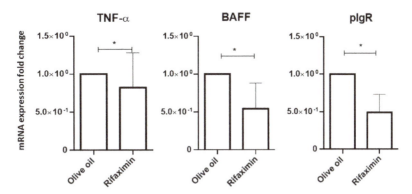

Figure 3. Antibiotic treatment reduced the expression of TNF-α, BAFF, and pIgR mRNA in small intestine samples, compared with the control. The qPCR data were reported as the relative increase in mRNA transcripts versus that found in respective tissues from vehicle mice, corrected by the respective levels of β-actin mRNA, used as an internal standard. All the values of olive oil tested mice were 1. Statistical analyses performed using the Wilcoxon test.

4. Discussion

Although IgAN seems to be a final common endpoint of different pathological processes, numerous studies indicate that it is closely associated with perturbed homeostasis of intestinal-activated B cells and intestinal IgA class switch and, at the same time, with alterations of the gut microbiota and of intestinal-barrier, in humans and animal models [9,16,17].

The intestinal-activated B cells play a central role in pathogens and mucosal inflammatory diseases [18,19]. Epithelium-derived BAFF is the major modulator of B cell development and it has a key role in IgA class switching and plasma cell survival in the MALT. Moreover, the gut microbiota, through toll-like receptor (TLR) ligation on mucosal dendritic cells, can induce inflammation and production of proinflammatory cytokines, inducing the overexpression of BAFF mRNA in mucosal epithelial cells [20]. The upregulation of BAFF is associated with hyper-IgA syndrome in the gut and the deposition of IgA immune complexes in the glomerular mesangium [16]. Given these findings, over the last few years, the need to test new interventions in IgAN patients and new therapeutic strategies, such as the administration of antibiotics or dietary implementation with prebiotics and/or probiotics, or through fecal microbiota transplantation (FMT) [21,22], has earned high demand, especially following the latest results from trials of gut-targeted corticosteroids [23,24].

Here we investigated the effects of rifaximin, a broad-spectrum, non-absorbable, oral antibiotic, on α1KI-CD89Tg mice. Rifaximin inhibits microbe-induced immune response, acts on intestinal barrier integrity, and has a direct anti-inflammatory property through binding to the Pregnane X Receptor (PXR) and modulating gut microbiota [11,25–27]. In particular, it is already demonstrated that rifaximin increases the relative abundance of beneficial intestinal bacteria, such as *Lactobacillus* and *Bifidobacterium* [28], reduces activation of T helper 17 cells [29], and attenuates TLR-4/NF-kB pathway activation in the gut [30].

However, the therapeutic effect of rifaximin has not yet been studied in IgAN. In this study, through a combination of ELISAs, confocal microscopy, and qPCR, we analyzed the characteristic features of α1KI-CD89Tg mice and the impact of rifaximin.

Our hypothesis is that, in IgAN, the leaky gut syndrome and the dysbiosis can lead, through the production of pro-inflammatory cytokines and an increased bacterial translocation, to gut inflammation, activation of dendritic cells (DCs) and, via T-cell-independent pathway (BAFF mediated), overproduction of Gd-IgA1 [14]. These are secreted, in the form of IgA1 dimers, across intestinal epithelial cells by transcytosis, in which pIgR facilitates the release of secretory IgA (sIgA) into the gut lumen. Rifaximin, through restoring symbiosis (including increased *Bacteroidetes/Firmicutes* ratio, as well as selective promotion of probiotic populations) and by binding PXR, is able to restore intestinal barrier function and inhibit the TLR-4/NF-kB signaling pathway in the small intestine [30], leading to decreased TNF-α synthesis [26]. Since the expression of BAFF and pIgR genes is regulated by TNF-α [31,32], the reduction of the latter causes the down-regulation of pIgR, BAFF and, consequently, of Gd-IgA1 (the proposal mechanism of rifaximin action in IgAN is represented in Supplementary data 2). Indeed, under gene expression profiling, our findings support reduced gut inflammation following rifaximin treatment, showed by a downregulation of TNF-α and BAFF gene transcription. Moreover, although we did not find any difference in IgA serum levels between the two groups, we found a reduction of hIgA1–mIgG, hIgA1–sCD89 complexes serum levels (the main serum markers of disease in this animal model), and of IgA mesangial deposition that could be explained by a greater availability and ability of IgA to bind CD89 or mIgG or mesangial cells in the control group compared to the treated group.

Although the "eubiotic" effect of rifaximin on gut microbiota is established [27], the exact mechanism of action in IgAN requires further investigations. Indeed, there were some limitations to this study, particularly the lack of the analysis of microbiota, that did not allow us to state whether our results are due to the modulation of the intestinal microbiota or if they are due to other effects of rifaximin on the gut.

In conclusion, the present study demonstrated that rifaximin reduces the progression and the severity of IgAN observed in humanized mice ($\alpha 1^{KI}$-CD89^{Tg}) and showed that rifaximin might open a new therapeutic avenue for IgAN. However, more detailed research is required to establish the precise molecular mechanism involved and the exact role of microbiota in this pathway.

Supplementary Materials: The following are available online at https://www.mdpi.com/article/10.3390/jpm11040309/s1, Supplementary data 1 Table S1; Supplementary data 2 Proposal mechanism.

Author Contributions: V.D.L. and S.B.M. performed experiments and analyzed data. R.C.M. generated $\alpha 1^{KI}$-CD89^{Tg} mice. P.J.G. and F.S. contributed to science discussion. C.B., J.D.S. performed experiments and analyzed data. V.D.L., G.L., R.C.M., and S.B.M. contributed to the analysis of the data and editing of the manuscript. V.D.L. and S.B.M. designed the research, analyzed data, and wrote the manuscript. All authors have read and agreed to the published version of the manuscript.

Funding: This work was supported by grants from INSERM, ANR JC (ANR-17-CE17-0002-01).

Institutional Review Board Statement: Animal protocol #APAFIS number: 14265-21 November 2018# was reviewed and approved by the Institutional Animal Care Committee.

Informed Consent Statement: Not applicable.

Data Availability Statement: Data is contained within the article.

Conflicts of Interest: The authors declare no conflict of interest.

References

1. Rodrigues, J.C.; Haas, M.; Reich, H.N. IgA Nephropathy. *Clin. J. Am. Soc. Nephrol.* **2017**, *12*, 677–686. [CrossRef]
2. Suzuki, H.; Kiryluk, K.; Novak, J.; Moldoveanu, Z.; Herr, A.B.; Renfrow, M.B.; Wyatt, R.J.; Scolari, F.; Mestecky, J.; Gharavi, A.G.; et al. The pathophysiology of IgA nephropathy. *J. Am. Soc. Nephrol.* **2011**, *22*, 1795–1803. [CrossRef]
3. Tan, M.; Fang, J.; Xu, Q.; Zhang, C.; Zou, G.; Wang, M.; Li, W. Outcomes of normotensive IgA nephropathy patients with mild proteinuria who have impaired renal function. *Ren. Fail.* **2019**, *41*, 875–882. [CrossRef]
4. Maixnerova, D.; Ling, C.; Hall, S.; Reily, C.; Brown, R.; Neprasova, M.; Suchanek, M.; Honsova, E.; Zima, T.; Novak, J.; et al. Galactose-deficient IgA1 and the corresponding IgG autoantibodies predict IgA nephropathy progression. *PLoS ONE* **2019**, *14*, e0212254. [CrossRef] [PubMed]
5. Launay, P.; Grossetete, B.; Arcos-Fajardo, M.; Gaudin, E.; Torres, S.P.; Beaudoin, L.; Patey-Mariaud de Serre, N.; Lehuen, A.; Monteiro, R.C. Fcalpha receptor (CD89) mediates the development of immunoglobulin A (IgA) nephropathy (Berger's disease). Evidence for pathogenic soluble receptor-Iga complexes in patients and CD89 transgenic mice. *J. Exp. Med.* **2000**, *191*, 1999–2009. [CrossRef] [PubMed]
6. Monteiro, R.C. Recent advances in the physiopathology of IgA nephropathy. *Nephrol. Ther.* **2018**, *14* (Suppl. S1), S1–S8. [CrossRef] [PubMed]
7. Cambier, A.; James, G.; Lillia, A.; Georges, D.; Hogan, J.; Laureline, B.; Sanaa, B.M.; Marion, R.; Michel, P.; Olivia, G.B.; et al. Soluble CD89-IgA1 complexes and galactose deficient-IgA1 are biomarkers associated with histologic inflammation in children IgA nephropathy. *Nephrol. Dial. Transplant.* **2019**, *34*. [CrossRef]
8. Sallustio, F.; Curci, C.; Di Leo, V.; Gallone, A.; Pesce, F.; Gesualdo, L. A New Vision of IgA Nephropathy: The Missing Link. *Int. J. Mol. Sci.* **2019**, *21*, 189. [CrossRef] [PubMed]
9. De Angelis, M.; Montemurno, E.; Piccolo, M.; Vannini, L.; Lauriero, G.; Maranzano, V.; Gozzi, G.; Serrazanetti, D.; Dalfino, G.; Gobbetti, M.; et al. Microbiota and metabolome associated with immunoglobulin A nephropathy (IgAN). *PLoS ONE* **2014**, *9*, e99006. [CrossRef] [PubMed]
10. Chemouny, J.M.; Gleeson, P.J.; Abbad, L.; Lauriero, G.; Boedec, E.; Le Roux, K.; Monot, C.; Bredel, M.; Bex-Coudrat, J.; Sannier, A.; et al. Modulation of the microbiota by oral antibiotics treats immunoglobulin A nephropathy in humanized mice. *Nephrol. Dial. Transplant. Off. Publ. Eur. Dial. Transpl. Assoc. Eur. Ren. Assoc.* **2018**. [CrossRef]
11. Lopetuso, L.R.; Napoli, M.; Rizzatti, G.; Gasbarrini, A. The intriguing role of Rifaximin in gut barrier chronic inflammation and in the treatment of Crohn's disease. *Expert Opin. Investig. Drugs* **2018**, *27*, 543–551. [CrossRef]
12. Lechner, S.M.; Abbad, L.; Boedec, E.; Papista, C.; Le Stang, M.B.; Moal, C.; Maillard, J.; Jamin, A.; Bex-Coudrat, J.; Wang, Y.; et al. IgA1 Protease Treatment Reverses Mesangial Deposits and Hematuria in a Model of IgA Nephropathy. *J. Am. Soc. Nephrol.* **2016**, *27*, 2622–2629. [CrossRef] [PubMed]
13. Berthelot, L.; Papista, C.; Maciel, T.T.; Biarnes-Pelicot, M.; Tissandie, E.; Wang, P.H.; Tamouza, H.; Jamin, A.; Bex-Coudrat, J.; Gestin, A.; et al. Transglutaminase is essential for IgA nephropathy development acting through IgA receptors. *J. Exp. Med.* **2012**, *209*, 793–806. [CrossRef] [PubMed]
14. Cerutti, A. The regulation of IgA class switching. *Nat. Rev. Immunol.* **2008**, *8*, 421–434. [CrossRef] [PubMed]

15. Zhang, Y.M.; Zhang, H. Insights into the Role of Mucosal Immunity in IgA Nephropathy. *Clin. J. Am. Soc. Nephrol. CJASN* **2018**, *13*, 1584–1586. [CrossRef] [PubMed]
16. McCarthy, D.D.; Kujawa, J.; Wilson, C.; Papandile, A.; Poreci, U.; Porfilio, E.A.; Ward, L.; Lawson, M.A.; Macpherson, A.J.; McCoy, K.D.; et al. Mice overexpressing BAFF develop a commensal flora-dependent, IgA-associated nephropathy. *J. Clin. Investig.* **2011**, *121*, 3991–4002. [CrossRef]
17. Zhou, N.; Shen, Y.; Fan, L.; Sun, Q.; Huang, C.; Hao, J.; Lan, J.; Yan, H. The Characteristics of Intestinal-Barrier Damage in Rats With IgA Nephropathy. *Am. J. Med. Sci.* **2020**, *359*, 168–176. [CrossRef] [PubMed]
18. Sallustio, F.; Curci, C.; Chaoul, N.; Fonto, G.; Lauriero, G.; Picerno, A.; Divella, C.; Di Leo, V.; De Angelis, M.; Ben Mkaddem, S.; et al. High levels of gut-homing immunoglobulin A-positive+B lymphocytes support the pathogenic role of intestinal mucosal hyperresponsiveness in immunoglobulin A nephropathy patients. *Nephrol. Dial. Transplant. Off. Publ. Eur. Dial. Transpl. Assoc. Eur. Ren. Assoc.* **2020**. [CrossRef]
19. Trimarchi, H.; Barratt, J.; Monteiro, R.C.; Feehally, J. IgA nephropathy: "State of the art": A report from the 15th International Symposium on IgA Nephropathy celebrating the 50th anniversary of its first description. *Kidney Int.* **2019**, *95*, 750–756. [CrossRef]
20. Do, K.H.; Choi, H.J.; Kim, J.; Park, S.H.; Kim, K.H.; Moon, Y. SOCS3 regulates BAFF in human enterocytes under ribosomal stress. *J. Immunol.* **2013**, *190*, 6501–6510. [CrossRef]
21. Papista, C.; Lechner, S.; Ben Mkaddem, S.; LeStang, M.B.; Abbad, L.; Bex-Coudrat, J.; Pillebout, E.; Chemouny, J.M.; Jablonski, M.; Flamant, M.; et al. Gluten exacerbates IgA nephropathy in humanized mice through gliadin-CD89 interaction. *Kidney Int.* **2015**, *88*, 276–285. [CrossRef]
22. Caggiano, G.; Cosola, C.; Di Leo, V.; Gesualdo, M.; Gesualdo, L. Microbiome modulation to correct uremic toxins and to preserve kidney functions. *Curr. Opin. Nephrol. Hypertens.* **2020**, *29*, 49–56. [CrossRef] [PubMed]
23. Lv, J.; Zhang, H.; Wong, M.G.; Jardine, M.J.; Hladunewich, M.; Jha, V.; Monaghan, H.; Zhao, M.; Barbour, S.; Reich, H.; et al. Effect of Oral Methylprednisolone on Clinical Outcomes in Patients with IgA Nephropathy: The TESTING Randomized Clinical Trial. *JAMA* **2017**, *318*, 432–442. [CrossRef]
24. Rauen, T.; Eitner, F.; Fitzner, C.; Sommerer, C.; Zeier, M.; Otte, B.; Panzer, U.; Peters, H.; Benck, U.; Mertens, P.R.; et al. Intensive Supportive Care plus Immunosuppression in IgA Nephropathy. *N. Engl. J. Med.* **2015**, *373*, 2225–2236. [CrossRef] [PubMed]
25. Bajaj, J.S.; Barbara, G.; DuPont, H.L.; Mearin, F.; Gasbarrini, A.; Tack, J. New concepts on intestinal microbiota and the role of the non-absorbable antibiotics with special reference to rifaximin in digestive diseases. *Dig. Liver Dis. Off. J. Ital. Soc. Gastroenterol. Ital. Assoc. Study Liver* **2018**, *50*, 741–749. [CrossRef] [PubMed]
26. Mohandas, S.; Vairappan, B. Role of pregnane X-receptor in regulating bacterial translocation in chronic liver diseases. *World J. Hepatol.* **2017**, *9*, 1210–1226. [CrossRef] [PubMed]
27. Ponziani, F.R.; Zocco, M.A.; D'Aversa, F.; Pompili, M.; Gasbarrini, A. Eubiotic properties of rifaximin: Disruption of the traditional concepts in gut microbiota modulation. *World J. Gastroenterol.* **2017**, *23*, 4491–4499. [CrossRef] [PubMed]
28. Jin, Y.; Ren, X.; Li, G.; Li, Y.; Zhang, L.; Wang, H.; Qian, W.; Hou, X. Beneficial effects of Rifaximin in post-infectious irritable bowel syndrome mouse model beyond gut microbiota. *J. Gastroenterol. Hepatol.* **2018**, *33*, 443–452. [CrossRef] [PubMed]
29. Pagliari, D.; Gambassi, G.; Piccirillo, C.A.; Cianci, R. The Intricate Link among Gut "Immunological Niche", Microbiota, and Xenobiotics in Intestinal Pathology. *Mediat. Inflamm.* **2017**, *2017*, 8390595. [CrossRef]
30. Yang, L.; Liu, B.; Zheng, J.; Huang, J.; Zhao, Q.; Liu, J.; Su, Z.; Wang, M.; Cui, Z.; Wang, T.; et al. Rifaximin Alters Intestinal Microbiota and Prevents Progression of Ankylosing Spondylitis in Mice. *Front. Cell Infect. Microbiol.* **2019**, *9*, 44. [CrossRef]
31. Bruno, M.E.; Frantz, A.L.; Rogier, E.W.; Johansen, F.E.; Kaetzel, C.S. Regulation of the polymeric immunoglobulin receptor by the classical and alternative NF-kappaB pathways in intestinal epithelial cells. *Mucosal Immunol.* **2011**, *4*, 468–478. [CrossRef] [PubMed]
32. Xu, J.; Luo, X.; Qu, S.; Yang, G.; Shen, N. B cell activation factor (BAFF) induces inflammation in the human fallopian tube leading to tubal pregnancy. *BMC Pregnancy Childbirth* **2019**, *19*, 169. [CrossRef] [PubMed]

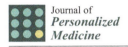

Review

Gut Microbiota and Acute Diverticulitis: Role of Probiotics in Management of This Delicate Pathophysiological Balance

Andrea Piccioni [1,*], Laura Franza [2], Mattia Brigida [3], Christian Zanza [2], Enrico Torelli [2], Martina Petrucci [2], Rebecca Nicolò [2], Marcello Covino [1], Marcello Candelli [1], Angela Saviano [2], Veronica Ojetti [1,2] and Francesco Franceschi [1,2]

[1] Emergency Medicine, Fondazione Policlinico Universitario A. Gemelli IRCCS, 1-00168 Rome, Italy; marcello.covino@policlinicogemelli.it (M.C.); marcello.candelli@policlinicogemelli.it (M.C.); veronica.ojetti@unicatt.it (V.O.); francesco.franceschi@unicatt.it (F.F.)
[2] Università Cattolica del Sacro Cuore, 1-00168 Rome, Italy; laura.franza@policlinicgemelli.it (L.F.); christian.zanza@live.it (C.Z.); rikho88@gmail.com (E.T.); martina.petrucci@policlinicogemelli.it (M.P.); rebecca.nicolo@policlinicogemelli.it (R.N.); saviange@libero.it (A.S.)
[3] Unit of Gastroenterology, Department of Systems Medicine, Tor Vergata University, 2-00133 Rome, Italy; mattiabrigida@hotmail.it
* Correspondence: andrea.piccioni@policlinicogemelli.it

Abstract: How can the knowledge of probiotics and their mechanisms of action be translated into clinical practice when treating patients with diverticular disease and acute diverticulitis? Changes in microbiota composition have been observed in patients who were developing acute diverticulitis, with a reduction of taxa with anti-inflammatory activity, such as Clostridium cluster IV, Lactobacilli and Bacteroides. Recent observations supported that a dysbiosis characterised by decreased presence of anti-inflammatory bacterial species might be linked to mucosal inflammation, and a vicious cycle results from a mucosal inflammation driving dysbiosis at the same time. An alteration in gut microbiota can lead to an altered activation of nerve fibres, and subsequent neuronal and muscular dysfunction, thus favoring abdominal symptoms' development. The possible role of dysbiosis and mucosal inflammation in leading to dysmotility is linked, in turn, to bacterial translocation from the lumen of the diverticulum to perivisceral area. There, a possible activation of Toll-like receptors has been described, with a subsequent inflammatory reaction at the level of the perivisceral tissues. Being aware that bacterial colonisation of diverticula is involved in the pathogenesis of acute diverticulitis, the rationale for the potential role of probiotics in the treatment of this disease becomes clearer. For this review, articles were identified using the electronic PubMed database through a comprehensive search conducted by combining key terms such as "gut microbiota", "probiotics and gut disease", "probiotics and acute diverticulitis", "probiotics and diverticular disease", "probiotics mechanism of action". However, the amount of data present on this matter is not sufficient to draw robust conclusions on the efficacy of probiotics for symptoms' management in diverticular disease.

Keywords: gut microbiota; probiotics and gut disease; probiotics and acute diverticulitis; probiotics and diverticular disease; probiotics mechanism of action

Citation: Piccioni, A.; Franza, L.; Brigida, M.; Zanza, C.; Torelli, E.; Petrucci, M.; Nicolò, R.; Covino, M.; Candelli, M.; Saviano, A.; et al. Gut Microbiota and Acute Diverticulitis: Role of Probiotics in Management of This Delicate Pathophysiological Balance. *J. Pers. Med.* **2021**, *11*, 298. https://doi.org/10.3390/jpm11040298

Academic Editor: Lucrezia Laterza

Received: 20 February 2021
Accepted: 11 April 2021
Published: 14 April 2021

Publisher's Note: MDPI stays neutral with regard to jurisdictional claims in published maps and institutional affiliations.

Copyright: © 2021 by the authors. Licensee MDPI, Basel, Switzerland. This article is an open access article distributed under the terms and conditions of the Creative Commons Attribution (CC BY) license (https://creativecommons.org/licenses/by/4.0/).

1. Introduction—Microbiota in Health and Disease

Over the last three decades, the importance of gut microbiota in determining health and disease has become increasingly clear.

Already in the late 1800s, researchers were warning the public that the bacteria living in our intestine could be "pathological" [1] even though the concept of dysbiosis had yet to be formulated.

Microbiota has proven to be an important player in the pathogenesis of many different diseases, ranging from more "obvious" disorders, for instance small intestine bacterial overgrowth (SIBO) [2], to more complicated diseases, such as immune deficits, thyroid disorders, neurodegenerative diseases [3–5], and have also been linked to mood disorders [6].

In this review, our aim was to discuss the potential role of probiotics for the treatment of diverticular disease and acute diverticulitis, with particular attention to their possible mechanisms of action.

The most important mechanisms through which microbiota can influence systemic health is through immune/inflammatory mechanisms [7,8]. The presence of certain bacterial strains can exert regulatory functions, improving immune-tolerance and stimulating regulatory T-cell (T-reg) expression [9]. This activity was observed, for instance, in *Bacteroides fragilis* [10] and in some Clostridium species [11].

Immune modulation also takes place through the production of short-chain fatty acids (SCFAs). Indeed, when digesting fibre, bacteria produce a vast array of SCFAs. Butyrate is particularly important among them, as it directly modulates the expression of histone deacetylase (HDAC), consequently increasing the expression of T-regs. Moreover, its role in obesity and metabolic control is not yet clear [12].

Additionally, a "healthy" microbiota works as a physical barrier against pathogens, stopping them from overcoming the gut mucosa and spreading systemically [13]. Indeed, beneficial species compete for nutrients and can produce antimicrobial substances which do not allow the growth of other microorganisms. Yet, it is worth noting that a certain microbial population can shift from protective to harmful even in the same individual based on circumstance.

In Table 1 there is a short summary of the relevant literature we discussed.

2. Materials and Methods

For this review, articles were identified using the electronic PubMed database through a comprehensive search conducted by combining key terms such as "probiotics", "gut microbiota", "probiotics and gut disease", "probiotics and acute diverticulitis", "probiotics and diverticular disease", "probiotics mechanism of action", "gut immunology and probiotics". English-language articles were screened for relevance. A full review of publications for the relevant studies was conducted, including additional publications that were identified from individual article reference lists. At first, the literature search was conducted individually by the single authors, who then compared their results, to include in the review only the most recent and relevant papers.

3. What Is a Healthy Microbiota?

As discussed above, the role of microbiota in determining health and disease, via immune modulation, is becoming increasingly clear. Some microbes have been identified as definitely pathogenic, for instance *Clostridium difficile*, yet there still are some grey areas, in particular when it comes to determine what defines a healthy microbiota [14].

An example of this comes from studies on microbiota and cancer: *Helicobacter pylori* is a known risk factor for the development of gastric cancer, but it has a protective effect against oesophageal cancer [15]. Similarly, *Escherichia coli* protects against pancreatic cancer, but favours colorectal and liver tumours [16]. In these cases, the ambivalent role of these bacteria was determined by the site of colonisation.

It is, indeed, important to underline that, even though it is common to refer to "gut microbiota", this does change widely throughout the gastrointestinal tract. In the oral cavity, for instance, it is common to find *Neisseria spp.*, which is instead difficult to find in other sites [17]. The stomach has a completely different microbiota than all the other parts of the gastrointestinal tract in healthy patients, but resembles oesophageal or intestinal microbiota in those with gastric cancer [18]. The small intestine even has a different composition based on which tract is being studied, and its composition is different from that of the colon.

Even considering specific parts of the gastrointestinal tract, microbiota changes with age [19], and even depending on geographic localisation, diet and ethnicity [20].

Yet, even though it is not possible to precisely define what species compose a healthy microbiota, it is worth noting that some general characteristics have been observed: a healthy microbiota is made up of a dynamic and diverse community of microbes, which is able to self-regulate [21].

While these do seem to be vague concepts, it is interesting to notice that the modern, western diet directly affects microbiota diversity, reducing its capacity to bounce back when frankly pathogenic species start colonising the gut [22].

4. Gut Disease and Microbiota

While gut microbiota influences all aspects of human health, its action on the gastrointestinal system is particularly important.

Indeed, gut microbiota directly modulates gastrointestinal homeostasis, through a variety of mechanisms. The presence of pathogens at the intestinal barrier, for instance, can directly damage the gastrointestinal mucosa and determine inflammation. This is the mechanism through which *C. difficile*, *Salmonella spp* and others can create direct intestinal damage [23].

Direct damage also activates immunologic pathways, particularly through the activation of the inflammasome. IL-1β and IL-18 are a direct consequence of its activation, causing pyroptosis, a particular form of immune-mediated cellular death [24]. Meanwhile, the activation of the inflammasome is important to maintain gut homeostasis, as it helps restore microbiota eubiosis, and it can also lead to chronic gut inflammation, which in turn promotes an inflammatory gut microbiota, in a difficult-to-break vicious circle.

It was observed that *Bifidobacterium adolescentis, Lactobacillus, Phascolarctobacterium, Akkermansia muciniphila* are all reduced in patients with intestinal inflammation. Interestingly, when present, they are capable of reducing inflammation, particularly acting on C-reactive protein (CRP), IL-6, and tumour necrosis factor (TNF)-α [25]. The action on these inflammatory mediators partly explains how gut microbiota can influence systemic health.

In the gut, the action of these mediators has direct consequences in terms of permeability and inflammation, both extremely important in the pathogenesis of different gastrointestinal disorders [26]. The presence of dysbiosis can trigger the development of inflammatory bowel disease (IBD) and irritable bowel syndrome (IBS). The role of microbiota has been particularly underlined in the pathogenesis of IBDs, in which dysbiosis is marked by the presence of *Mycobacterium avium* subsp. *paratuberculosis, Fusobacterium nucleatum,* adherent–invasive *E. coli* [27].

Inflammation caused by microbiota dysbiosis is also responsible of liver disorders, particularly non-alcoholic liver steatosis. In this case, there is a direct colonisation of the bile ducts, which adds up to the action of bacterial metabolic products. Interestingly, the capacity of bacteria to metabolise biliary salts is also linked to dysbiosis [28].

Inflammation is also a well-known risk factor for the development of cancer, and it is no different in the intestine; the impact of microbiota composition in modulating the intestinal immunologic niche has proven essential in different forms of cancer [16].

5. Microbiota Modulation: The Case for Probiotics

Given the importance of microbiota in human health, the possibility of modulating it to obtain benefits is an interesting potential therapeutic target.

Microbiota modulation can take place in two different ways, either through the use of antibiotics or through the use of probiotics.

Antibiotic use can target specific pathological bacteria in the gut, eliminating it, as in the case of vancomycin in *C. difficile* infection [29]. Some antibiotics, such as rifaximin, can instead be used to target a larger number of pathogens, improving conditions such as IBS, SIBO and preventing encephalopathy in patients suffering from liver disease [30]. Ozone, for instance, also seems to have a similar capacity to reduce inflammation in the gut, also through microbiota modulation [31,32].

Yet the use of antibiotics can be tricky. The use of antibiotics can reduce taxonomic diversity of gut microbiota and induce resistance mechanisms in pathogenic species, while also favouring the development of *C. difficile* infection and other dangerous pathogens [33].

Using probiotics can provide similar positive effects to antibiotics, in reducing pathogens, but at the same time avoiding many of the side effects [34]. Probiotics have been used with different degrees of success in patients suffering from IBS, gastroenteritis and even in *C. difficile*-associated diarrhoea [35]. Probiotics have also been used in neonatal sepsis and necrotising enterocolitis [36].

Probiotic use has also been discussed in extra-gut conditions, such as autism and acute respiratory infections [37,38].

Some authors even suggest that microbiota modulation through probiotics could be beneficial in preventing cancer [39] and improving response to chemotherapy, reducing gastrointestinal side effects [40].

6. Microbiota and Acute Diverticulitis: What We Know, What We Can Do

Diverticulitis is usually merely considered an inflammation of a herniation of colonic mucosa and submucosa, through the muscle layer. While it is obvious that the inflammatory process is driven by the resident microbiota, it is not as clear whether the microbial population may play a role in promoting the herniation in the first place [41].

It is known that dietary factors are key in determining the onset of diverticular disorder and they also determine changes in microbiota composition. It is difficult to determine whether the changes in the composition of the microbiota may act as an enhancing factor in the development of diverticulitis, but it is worth noting that the microbial species associated with diverticular disease are *Enterobacteriaceae, Streptococcus* and *Bacteroides*, while reducing the expression of "good" bacteria, such *Bifidobacteria* and *Lactobacilli* [42].

The role of microbiota in determining diverticular inflammation is instead far clearer. Recurring diverticulitis not susceptible to surgery has, indeed, been treated with faecal transplant, leading to complete remission [43]. Additionally, it has been reported that a patient, with moderate diverticular disease, who underwent faecal transplant for *C. difficile* infection, developed her first ever episode of diverticulitis after the procedure, further proving that, while it may not take part in the first, more mechanical stages of the disease, microbiota is not a bystander during the inflammatory phase [44].

Changes in microbiota composition have been observed in patients who were developing acute diverticulitis, with a reduction of taxa with anti-inflammatory activity, such as *Clostridium* cluster IV, Lactobacilli and Bacteroides. At the same time, overgrowth of Bifidobacteria, Enterobacteriaceae and *Akkermansia* have been reported [41]. This diversity, also characterised by an increase in Proteobacteria, has proven significant and could be used for an early diagnosis of the disease [45].

Overall, the importance of microbiota in diverticular disease has been demonstrated indirectly by the therapies used to treat the disorder. Indeed, the use of rifaximin and probiotics has proven interesting, even though mostly through clinical trials.

Rifaximin has been used to treat Symptomatic Uncomplicated Diverticular Disease in a clinical trial and results were encouraging, not only in terms of symptom control but also as far as faecal microbiota composition, with a reduction of *Roseburia, Veillonella, Streptococcus* and *Haemophilus* [46]. In another study, there was also a reduction in *Akkermansia* [47].

Lactobacilli have been demonstrated to reduce Symptomatic Uncomplicated Diverticular Disease, particularly in reducing bloating and abdominal pain [48], while *Lactobacillus salivarius, Lactobacillus acidophilus* and *Bifidobacterium lactis* have proven effective in managing acute diverticulitis [49]. A double-blind randomised control trial was recently published by Ojetti et al., in which the authors tested the efficacy of *L. reuteri* 4659 in treating patients affected by acute uncomplicated diverticular diseases (AUD). Supplementation of the standard AUD therapy with this specific probiotic with an anti-inflammatory effect significantly reduced abdominal pain and inflammatory markers compared to those who were not taking the same supplementation [50]. These data were also observed in another paper, published in 2019, in which the authors demonstrated that in patients affected by AUD supplementation with a mix of probiotics *B. lactis* LA 304, *L. salivarius* LA302 and *L. acidophilus* LA 201, with a well-known capacity for reducing TNF levels, in combination with the standard antibiotic therapy reduced PCR level and the abdominal pain compared to patients with the disease who did not receive the supplementation [51].

Table 1. Summary of the most relevant research.

Title	Topic	Reference Number
Belkaid Y, Hand TW. "Role of the microbiota in immunity and inflammation". Cell. 2014	Microbiota-driven immune responses	[8]
Iebba V, Totino V, Gagliardi A, Santangelo F, Cacciotti F, Trancassini M, et al. "Eubiosis and dysbiosis: the two sides of the microbiota". New Microbiol. 2016	Dysbiosis and eubiosis in defining a "healthy" gut microbiota	[14]
Cianci R, Franza L. "The Interplay between Immunity and Microbiota at Intestinal Immunological Niche: The Case of Cancer". 2019	The intestinal niche in health and disease	[16]
Lange K, Buerger M, Stallmach A, Bruns T. "Effects of Antibiotics on Gut Microbiota". Dig Dis. 2016	The role of antibiotics in shaping the microbiota	[33]
Suez J, Zmora N, Segal E. "The pros, cons, and many unknowns of probiotics". 2019	The role of probiotics in shaping the microbiota	[35]
Kim SK, Guevarra RB, Kim YT, Kwon J, Kim H, Cho JH, et al. "Role of Probiotics in Human Gut Microbiome-Associated Diseases". J Microbiol Biotechnol. 2019	Probiotics in gut-microbiota associated diseases	[38]
Ticinesi A, Nouvenne A, Corrente V, Tana C, Di Mario F, Meschi T. "Diverticular Disease: a Gut Microbiota Perspective. Journal of gastrointestinal and liver diseases". JGLD. 2019	The role of microbiota in diverticular disease	[41]
Ojetti V, Petruzziello C, Cardone S, Saviano L, Migneco A, Santarelli L, et al. "The Use of Probiotics in Different Phases of Diverticular Disease. Reviews on recent clinical trials". 2018	Action of probiotics in diverticular disease	[49]
Petruzziello C, Migneco A, Cardone S, Covino M, Saviano A, Franceschi F, et al. Supplementation with Lactobacillus reuteri ATCC PTA 4659 in patients affected by acute uncomplicated diverticulitis: a randomised double-blind placebo controlled trial. 2019	Action of probiotics in diverticular disease	[50]
Petruzziello C, Marannino M, Migneco A, Brigida M, Saviano A, Piccioni A, et al. The efficacy of a mix of three probiotic strains in reducing abdominal pain and inflammatory biomarkers in acute uncomplicated diverticulitis. European review for medical and pharmacological sciences. 2019	Action of probiotics in diverticular disease	[51]

In Figure 1, the described mechanisms are shown.

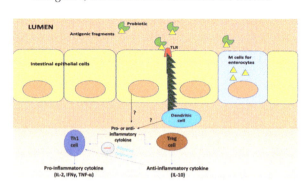

Figure 1. The immunomodulatory properties of probiotics.

The immunomodulatory properties of probiotics are also associated with cytokine release, in particular tumour necrosis factors (TNF), transforming growth factor (TGF), interleukins (IL), interferons (IFN) and chemokines derived from immune cells that regulate the innate and adaptive compartments of the immune system. Some cell wall components of Lactobacilli and Bifidobacteria, such as lipoteichoic acid, stimulate nitric oxide (NO) synthesis, which is key in pathogen-infected cell death mechanisms, induced by macrophages via TNF-α secretion. Furthermore, two surface receptors involved in phagocytosis, namely FcγRIII and toll-like receptors (TLR), are also upregulated by NO.

Probiotics have been proven to interact with enterocytes, Th1, Th2, Treg cells and dendritic cells in the gut and also regulate the adaptive immunity.

7. Probiotics in Diverticulitis: Mechanisms of Action

To better understand how probiotics exert an impact on diverticular disease and diverticulitis, attention should be focused on some aspects of pathophysiology linked to microbiota.

Recent observations support that a dysbiosis characterised by decreased presence of anti-inflammatory bacterial species might be linked to mucosal inflammation, and a vicious cycle results from a mucosal inflammation driving dysbiosis at the same time [51].

Another key element is the possible role of dysbiosis and mucosal inflammation in leading to dysmotility: an alteration in gut microbiota, indeed, can lead to altered nerve fibre activation and subsequent neuronal and muscular dysfunction, thus favouring the development of diverticulosis, while also possibly inducing abdominal symptoms [52]. Altered motility is linked, in turn, to bacterial translocation from the lumen of the diverticulum to perivisceral area. There, a possible activation of Toll-like receptors (TLR) [53] has been described, with a subsequent inflammatory reaction at the level of the perivisceral tissues [54].

Moreover, Foligne and colleagues [55] have studied, in the context of IBD, thirteen strains of probiotics in terms of anti-inflammatory properties and, among these, *L. acidophilus* and *L. salivarius* Ls33 seemed to be the best-performing concerning increased induction of IL-10 and decreased induction of IL-12.

Data coming from in vitro and in vivo studies, concerning *L. salivarius* Ls33, suggest that its administration is linked to an improved recovery of inflamed tissue in a rat colitis model [56].

This evidence has led researchers to consider changes in peri-diverticular bacterial flora as a critical element in acute diverticulitis pathogenesis, and a similar model was applied to explain acute appendicitis pathogenesis. Basically, stasis of faecal material within diverticula can be favoured by a prolonged colonic transit, which in turn predisposes to altered microflora and bacterial overgrowth. Mucosal barrier function can be consequently impaired and provoke an inflammatory reaction by means of cytokine release; a low-grade, localised microscopic colitis may result, which can evolve towards microperforation and show the clinical features of acute diverticulitis [57].

Being aware that bacterial colonisation of diverticula is involved in the pathogenesis of acute diverticulitis, the rationale for the potential role of probiotics in the treatment of this disease becomes clearer. As Quigley reports, probiotics may be able to modify the localised and persistent inflammation, present in some patients who are between acute bouts of diverticulitis. Acting on inflammation they may also act on symptom development, in individuals affected by uncomplicated diverticular disease [58].

In addition, the intestinal bacterial flora produces the outer membrane vesicles which play an important role in microbiota-host communication, the interaction of which takes place thanks to the action of adhesins, sulfatases and proteases and pathways such as micropinocytosis, clathrin- and lipid raft-dependent endocytosis [59].

These outer membrane vesicles have a positive impact on mucosal immunity and its signaling pathways. This would therefore seem to be another mechanism of action that can be exploited through the administration of probiotics in the context of various intestinal diseases, including diverticulitis. However, there is still scarcity of literature on the exact mechanisms of vesicles secreted by various species of microbiota and probiotics [57,60].

In a paper published by Brandimarte et al. [61], the pros and cons were discussed regarding evidence of probiotic action in diverticular disease. Recognising that overgrowth and alteration of gut microbiota can play a role in the development of inflammation related to diverticular disease, there is a clear rationale for administering probiotics with the aim to restore a healthy microenvironment in the colon. Different mechanisms have been discussed, such as a decrease in bacterial translocation, competitive inhibition of pathogenic and proinflammatory bacterial strains overgrowth, down-regulation of inflammatory cytokines, together with an improvement in mucosal defence, due to enhanced tight junction integrity [48,62,63].

However, the amount of data present on this matter is not sufficient to draw robust conclusions on the efficacy of probiotics for symptom management in diverticular disease, and this was confirmed by a recent expert consensus with a submaximal level of agreement [64].

Indeed, concerning therapy with probiotics, there are no established protocols defining which strain, what dosage and for how long to use them, and this reflects the absence of reliable meta-analyses in this regard [61].

Literature should be broadened as new mechanisms of action come to light from the many investigations being currently conducted in numerous centres around the globe, and new protocols should be established in order to study how exactly probiotic administration could make the difference in the management of diverticular disease and acute diverticulitis.

Author Contributions: Conceptualization, A.P., F.F. and V.O.; methodology, C.Z., E.T., M.P.; software, M.C. (Marcello Covino); validation, F.F., V.O.; formal analysis, A.P., L.F.; investigation, M.C. (Marcello Candelli), R.N.; resources, M.B.; data curation, A.S.; writing—original draft preparation, M.B., A.P., L.F.; writing—review and editing, A.P.; supervision, V.O., F.F. All authors have read and agreed to the published version of the manuscript.

Funding: This research received no external funding.

Institutional Review Board Statement: The study was conducted according to the guidelines of the Declaration of Helsinki. Ethical review and approval were waived for this study, because it is a review.

Conflicts of Interest: The authors declare no conflict of interest.

References

1. Metchnikoff, E. Etudes sur la flore intestinale: Putrefaction intestinale. *Ann. Int. Pasteur.* **1908**, *22*, 930–955.
2. Quigley, E.M.M. The Spectrum of Small Intestinal Bacterial Overgrowth (SIBO). *Curr. Gastroenterol. Rep.* **2019**, *21*, 3. [CrossRef] [PubMed]
3. Franza, L.; Carusi, V.; Altamura, S.; Gasbarrini, A.; Caraffa, A.; Kritas, S.K.; Ronconi, G.; E Gallenga, C.; Di Virgilio, F.; Pandolfi, F. Gut microbiota and immunity in common variable immunodeficiency: Crosstalk with pro-inflammatory cytokines. *J. Biol. Regul. Homeost. Agents* **2019**, *33*, 315–319. [PubMed]
4. Fröhlich, E.; Wahl, R. Microbiota and Thyroid Interaction in Health and Disease. *Trends Endocrinol. Metab.* **2019**, *30*, 479–490. [CrossRef] [PubMed]
5. Quigley, E.M.M. Microbiota-Brain-Gut Axis and Neurodegenerative Diseases. *Curr. Neurol. Neurosci. Rep.* **2017**, *17*, 94. [CrossRef] [PubMed]
6. Huang, T.-T.; Lai, J.-B.; Du, Y.-L.; Xu, Y.; Ruan, L.-M.; Hu, S.-H. Current Understanding of Gut Microbiota in Mood Disorders: An Update of Human Studies. *Front. Genet.* **2019**, *10*, 98. [CrossRef] [PubMed]
7. Foligne, B.; Dewulf, J.; Breton, J.; Claisse, O.; Lonvaud-Funel, A.; Pot, B. Probiotic properties of non-conventional lactic acid bacteria: Immunomodulation by Oenococcus oeni. *Int. J. Food Microbiol.* **2010**, *140*, 136–145. [CrossRef] [PubMed]
8. Belkaid, Y.; Hand, T.W. Role of the Microbiota in Immunity and Inflammation. *Cell* **2014**, *157*, 121–141. [CrossRef]
9. Sefik, E.; Geva-Zatorsky, N.; Oh, S.; Konnikova, L.; Zemmour, D.; McGuire, A.M. Mucosal Immunology. Individual intestinal symbionts induce a distinct population of RORγ$^+$ regulatory T cells. *Science* **2015**, *349*, 993–997. [CrossRef]
10. Round, J.L.; Lee, S.M.; Li, J.; Tran, G.; Jabri, B.; Chatila, T.A.; Mazmanian, S.K. The Toll-Like Receptor 2 Pathway Establishes Colonization by a Commensal of the Human Microbiota. *Science* **2011**, *332*, 974–977. [CrossRef]
11. Atarashi, K.; Tanoue, T.; Shima, T.; Imaoka, A.; Kuwahara, T.; Momose, Y.; Cheng, G.; Yamasaki, S.; Saito, T.; Ohba, Y.; et al. Induction of colonic regulatory T cells by indigenous clostridium species. *Science* **2011**, *331*, 337–341. [CrossRef]
12. Liu, H.; Wang, J.; He, T.; Becker, S.; Zhang, G.; Li, D.; Ma, X. Butyrate: A Double-Edged Sword for Health? *Adv. Nutr.* **2018**, *9*, 21–29. [CrossRef]
13. Takiishi, T.; Fenero, C.I.M.; Câmara, N.O.S. Intestinal barrier and gut microbiota: Shaping our immune responses throughout life. *Tissue Barriers* **2017**, *5*, e1373208. [CrossRef]
14. Iebba, V.; Totino, V.; Gagliardi, A.; Santangelo, F.; Cacciotti, F.; Trancassini, M.; Mancini, C.; Cicerone, C.; Corazziari, E.; Pantanella, F.; et al. Eubiosis and dysbiosis: The two sides of the microbiota. *New Microbiol.* **2016**, *39*, 1–12.
15. Castro, C.; Peleteiro, B.; Lunet, N. Modifiable factors and esophageal cancer: A systematic review of published meta-analyses. *J. Gastroenterol.* **2017**, *53*, 37–51. [CrossRef]
16. Cianci, R.; Franza, L.; Schinzari, G.; Rossi, E.; Ianiro, G.; Tortora, G.; Gasbarrini, A.; Gambassi, G.; Cammarota, G. The Interplay between Immunity and Microbiota at Intestinal Immunological Niche: The Case of Cancer. *Int. J. Mol. Sci.* **2019**, *20*, 501. [CrossRef]
17. Ruan, W.; Engevik, M.A.; Spinler, J.K.; Versalovic, J. Healthy Human Gastrointestinal Microbiome: Composition and Function After a Decade of Exploration. *Dig. Dis. Sci.* **2020**, *65*, 695–705. [CrossRef]
18. Yu, G.; Torres, J.; Hu, N.; Medrano-Guzman, R.; Herrera-Goepfert, R.; Humphrys, M.S.; Wang, L.; Wang, C.; Ding, T.; Ravel, J.; et al. Molecular Characterization of the Human Stomach Microbiota in Gastric Cancer Patients. *Front. Cell. Infect. Microbiol.* **2017**, *7*, 302. [CrossRef]
19. Takagi, T.; Naito, Y.; Inoue, R.; Kashiwagi, S.; Uchiyama, K.; Mizushima, K.; Tsuchiya, S.; Dohi, O.; Yoshida, N.; Kamada, K.; et al. Differences in gut microbiota associated with age, sex, and stool consistency in healthy Japanese subjects. *J. Gastroenterol.* **2019**, *54*, 53–63. [CrossRef]
20. Dehingia, M.; Adak, A.; Khan, M.R. Ethnicity-Influenced Microbiota: A Future Healthcare Perspective. *Trends Microbiol.* **2019**, *27*, 191–193. [CrossRef]
21. Lloyd-Price, J.; Abu-Ali, G.; Huttenhower, C. The healthy human microbiome. *Genome Med.* **2016**, *8*, 1–11. [CrossRef] [PubMed]
22. Bibbò, S.; Ianiro, G.; Giorgio, V.; Scaldaferri, F.; Masucci, L.; Gasbarrini, A.; Cammarota, G. The role of diet on gut microbiota composition. *Eur. Rev. Med. Pharmacol. Sci.* **2016**, *20*, 4742–4749. [PubMed]
23. Kc, D.; Sumner, R.; Lippmann, S. Gut microbiota and health. *Postgrad. Med.* **2019**, *132*, 274. [CrossRef] [PubMed]
24. Man, S.M. Inflammasomes in the gastrointestinal tract: Infection, cancer and gut microbiota homeostasis. *Nat. Rev. Gastroenterol. Hepatol.* **2018**, *15*, 721–737. [CrossRef]
25. Al Bander, Z.; Nitert, M.D.; Mousa, A.; Naderpoor, N. The Gut Microbiota and Inflammation: An Overview. *Int. J. Environ. Res. Public Health.* **2020**, *17*, 7618. [CrossRef]
26. Tilg, H.; Zmora, N.; Adolph, T.E.; Elinav, E. The intestinal microbiota fuelling metabolic inflammation. *Nat. Rev. Immunol.* **2020**, *20*, 40–54. [CrossRef]
27. Ni, J.; Wu, G.D.; Albenberg, L.; Tomov, V.T. Gut microbiota and IBD: Causation or correlation? *Nat. Rev. Gastroenterol. Hepatol.* **2017**, *14*, 573–584. [CrossRef]
28. Shen, T.-C.D.; Pyrsopoulos, N.; Rustgi, V.K.V.K. Microbiota and the liver. *Liver Transplant.* **2018**, *24*, 539–550. [CrossRef]
29. Brown, C.C.; Manis, M.M.; Bohm, N.M.; Curry, S.R. Oral Vancomycin for Secondary Prophylaxis of Clostridium difficile Infection. *Ann. Pharmacol.* **2019**, *53*, 396–401. [CrossRef]
30. Pimentel, M. Review of rifaximin as treatment for SIBO and IBS. *Expert Opin. Investig. Drugs* **2009**, *18*, 349–358. [CrossRef]

31. Villani, E.R.; Ranaldi, G.T.; Franza, L. Rationale for ozone-therapy as an adjuvant therapy in COVID-19: A narrative review. *Med. Gas Res.* **2020**, *10*, 134–138. [CrossRef]
32. Lange, K.; Buerger, M.; Stallmach, A.; Bruns, T. Effects of Antibiotics on Gut Microbiota. *Dig. Dis.* **2016**, *34*, 260–268. [CrossRef]
33. Delcenserie, V.; Martel, D.; Lamoureux, M.; Amiot, J.; Boutin, Y.; Roy, D. Immunomodulatory effects of probiotics in the intestinal tract. *Curr. Issues Mol. Biol.* **2008**, *10*, 37–54.
34. Suez, J.; Zmora, N.; Segal, E.; Elinav, E. The pros, cons, and many unknowns of probiotics. *Nat. Med.* **2019**, *25*, 716–729. [CrossRef]
35. Patel, R.M.; Underwood, M.A. Probiotics and necrotizing enterocolitis. *Semin. Pediatr. Surg.* **2018**, *27*, 39–46. [CrossRef]
36. Doenyas, C. Gut Microbiota, Inflammation, and Probiotics on Neural Development in Autism Spectrum Disorder. *Neuroscience* **2018**, *374*, 271–286. [CrossRef]
37. Sundararaman, A.; Ray, M.; Ravindra, P.V.; Halami, P.M. Role of probiotics to combat viral infections with emphasis on COVID-19. *Appl. Microbiol. Biotechnol.* **2020**, *104*, 1–16. [CrossRef]
38. Kim, S.-K.; Guevarra, R.B.; Kim, Y.-T.; Kwon, J.; Kim, H.; Cho, J.H.; Kim, H.B.; Lee, J.-H. Role of Probiotics in Human Gut Microbiome-Associated Diseases. *J. Microbiol. Biotechnol.* **2019**, *29*, 1335–1340. [CrossRef]
39. Gopalakrishnan, V.; Helmink, B.A.; Spencer, C.N.; Reuben, A.; Wargo, J.A. The Influence of the Gut Microbiome on Cancer, Immunity, and Cancer Immunotherapy. *Cancer Cell* **2018**, *33*, 570–580. [CrossRef]
40. Ticinesi, A.; Nouvenne, A.; Corrente, V.; Tana, C.; Di Mario, F.; Meschi, T. Diverticular Disease: A Gut Microbiota Perspective. *J. Gastrointest. Liver Dis.* **2019**, *28*, 327–337. [CrossRef]
41. Ma, N.; Tian, Y.; Wu, Y.; Ma, X. Contributions of the Interaction Between Dietary Protein and Gut Microbiota to Intestinal Health. *Curr. Protein Pept. Sci.* **2017**, *18*, 795–808. [CrossRef]
42. Meyer, D.C.; Hill, S.S.; Bebinger, D.M.; McDade, J.A.; Davids, J.S.; Alavi, K.; Maykel, J.A. Resolution of multiply recurrent and multifocal diverticulitis after fecal microbiota transplantation. *Tech. ColoProctol.* **2020**, *24*, 971–975. [CrossRef]
43. Mandalia, A.; Kraft, C.S.; Dhere, T. Diverticulitis after Fecal Microbiota Transplant for C. difficile Infection. *Am. J. Gastroenterol.* **2014**, *109*, 1956–1957. [CrossRef]
44. Daniels, L.; Budding, A.E.; De Korte, N.; Eck, A.; Bogaards, J.A.; Stockmann, H.B.; Consten, E.C.; Savelkoul, P.H.; Boermeester, M.A. Fecal microbiome analysis as a diagnostic test for diverticulitis. *Eur. J. Clin. Microbiol. Infect. Dis.* **2014**, *33*, 1927–1936. [CrossRef]
45. Ponziani, F.R.; Scaldaferri, F.; Petito, V.; Paroni Sterbini, F.; Pecere, S.; Lopetuso, L.R.; Palladini, A.; Gerardi, V.; Masucci, L.; Pompili, M.; et al. The Role of Antibiotics in Gut Microbiota Modulation: The Eubiotic Effects of Rifaximin. *Dig. Dis.* **2016**, *34*, 269–278. [CrossRef]
46. Tursi, A.; Mastromarino, P.; Capobianco, D.; Elisei, W.; Miccheli, A.; Capuani, G. Assessment of Fecal Microbiota and Fecal Metabolome in Symptomatic Uncomplicated Diverticular Disease of the Colon. *J. Clin. Gastroenterol.* **2016**, *50* (Suppl. 1), S9–S12. [CrossRef]
47. Lahner, E.; Bellisario, C.; Hassan, C.; Zullo, A.; Esposito, G.; Annibale, B. Probiotics in the Treatment of Diverticular Disease. A Systematic Review. *J. Gastrointest. Liver Dis.* **2016**, *25*, 79–86. [CrossRef]
48. Ojetti, V.; Petruzziello, C.; Cardone, S.; Saviano, L.; Migneco, A.; Santarelli, L.; Gabrielli, M.; Zaccaria, R.; Lopetuso, L.; Covino, M.; et al. The Use of Probiotics in Different Phases of Diverticular Disease. *Rev. Recent Clin. Trials* **2018**, *13*, 89–96. [CrossRef]
49. Petruzziello, C.; Migneco, A.; Cardone, S.; Covino, M.; Saviano, A.; Franceschi, F.; Ojetti, V. Supplementation with Lactobacillus reuteri ATCC PTA 4659 in patients affected by acute uncomplicated diverticulitis: A randomized double-blind placebo controlled trial. *Int. J. Color. Dis.* **2019**, *34*, 1087–1094. [CrossRef]
50. Petruzziello, C.; Marannino, M.; Migneco, A.; Brigida, M.; Saviano, A.; Piccioni, A.; Franceschi, F.; Ojetti, V. The efficacy of a mix of three probiotic strains in reducing abdominal pain and inflammatory biomarkers in acute uncomplicated diverticulitis. *Eur. Rev. Med. Pharmacol. Sci.* **2019**, *23*, 9126–9133.
51. Wedel, T.; Böttner, M. Anatomy and pathogenesis of diverticular disease. *Z. Alle Geb. Oper. Medizen* **2014**, *85*, 281–288. [CrossRef] [PubMed]
52. Schwandner, R.; Dziarski, R.; Wesche, H.; Rothe, M.; Kirschning, C.J. Peptidoglycan- and Lipoteichoic Acid-induced Cell Activation Is Mediated by Toll-like Receptor. *J. Biol. Chem.* **1999**, *274*, 17406–17409. [CrossRef] [PubMed]
53. Severi, C.; Carabotti, M.; Cicenia, A.; Pallotta, L.; Annibale, B. Recent advances in understanding and managing diverticulitis. *F1000Research* **2018**, *7*, 971. [CrossRef] [PubMed]
54. Foligne, B.; Nutten, S.; Grangette, C.; Dennin, V.; Goudercourt, D.; Poiret, S. Correlation between in vitro and in vivo immunomodulatory properties of lactic acid bacteria. *World J. Gastroenterol.* **2007**, *13*, 236–243. [CrossRef]
55. Peran, L.; Camuesco, D.; Comalada, M.; Nieto, A.; Concha, A.; Diaz-Ropero, M.P.; Olivares, M.; Xaus, J.; Zarzuelo, A.; Galvez, J. Preventative effects of a probiotic, *Lactobacillus salivarius* ssp. salivarius, in the TNBS model of rat colitis. *World J. Gastroenterol.* **2005**, *11*, 5185–5192.
56. Narula, N.; Marshall, J.K. Role of probiotics in management of diverticular disease. *J. Gastroenterol. Hepatol.* **2010**, *25*, 1827–1830. [CrossRef]
57. Quigley, E.M.M. Gut microbiota, inflammation and symptomatic diverticular disease. New insights into an old and neglected disorder. *J. Gastrointest. Liver Dis.* **2010**, *19*, 127–129.

58. Carvalho, A.L.; Fonseca, S.; Miquel-Clopés, A.; Cross, K.; Kok, K.-S.; Wegmann, U.; Gil-Cardoso, K.; Bentley, E.G.; Al Katy, S.H.; Coombes, J.L.; et al. Bioengineering commensal bacteria-derived outer membrane vesicles for delivery of biologics to the gastrointestinal and respiratory tract. *J. Extracell. Vesicles* **2019**, *8*, 1632100. [CrossRef]

59. Shen, Y.; Torchia, M.L.G.; Lawson, G.W.; Karp, C.L.; Ashwell, J.D.; Mazmanian, S.K. Outer Membrane Vesicles of a Human Commensal Mediate Immune Regulation and Disease Protection. *Cell Host Microbe* **2012**, *12*, 509–520. [CrossRef]

60. Brandimarte, G.; Bafutto, M.; Kruis, W.; Scarpignato, C.; Mearin, F.; Barbara, G.; Štimac, D.; Vranić, L.; Cassieri, C.; Lecca, P.G.; et al. Hot Topics in Medical Treatment of Diverticular Disease: Evidence Pro and Cons. *J. Gastrointest. Liver Dis.* **2020**, *28*, 23–29. [CrossRef]

61. Azad, A.K.; Sarker, M.; Wan, D. Immunomodulatory Effects of Probiotics on Cytokine Profiles. *Biomed. Res. Int.* **2018**, *2018*, 1–10. [CrossRef] [PubMed]

62. Guslandi, M. Medical treatment of uncomplicated diverticular disease of the colon: Any progress? *Minerva Gastroenterol. Dietol.* **2010**, *56*, 367–370. [PubMed]

63. Binda, G.A.; Cuomo, R.; Laghi, A.; Nascimbeni, R.; Serventi, A.; Bellini, D.; Gervaz, P.; Annibale, B. Practice parameters for the treatment of colonic diverticular disease: Italian Society of Colon and Rectal Surgery (SICCR) guidelines. *Tech. Coloproctology* **2015**, *19*, 615–626. [CrossRef] [PubMed]

64. Cuomo, R.; Barbara, G.; Pace, F.; Annese, V.; Bassotti, G.; Binda, G.A.; Casetti, T.; Colecchia, A.; Festi, D.; Fiocca, R.; et al. Italian consensus conference for colonic diverticulosis and diverticular disease. *United Eur. Gastroenterol. J.* **2014**, *2*, 413–442. [CrossRef]

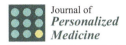

Article

Streptococcus australis and *Ralstonia pickettii* as Major Microbiota in Mesotheliomas

Rumi Higuchi [1,†], Taichiro Goto [1,*,†], Yosuke Hirotsu [2], Sotaro Otake [1], Toshio Oyama [3], Kenji Amemiya [2], Hitoshi Mochizuki [2] and Masao Omata [2,4]

[1] Lung Cancer and Respiratory Disease Center, Yamanashi Central Hospital, Yamanashi 400-8506, Japan; r-higuchi1504@ych.pref.yamanashi.jp (R.H.); ootake.sotaro.gx@mail.hosp.go.jp (S.O.)
[2] Genome Analysis Center, Yamanashi Central Hospital, Yamanashi 400-8506, Japan; hirotsu-bdyu@ych.pref.yamanashi.jp (Y.H.); amemiya-bdcd@ych.pref.yamanashi.jp (K.A.); h-mochiduki2a@ych.pref.yamanashi.jp (H.M.); m-omata0901@ych.pref.yamanashi.jp (M.O.)
[3] Department of Pathology, Yamanashi Central Hospital, Yamanashi 400-8506, Japan; t-oyama@ych.pref.yamanashi.jp
[4] Department of Gastroenterology, The University of Tokyo Hospital, Tokyo 113-8655, Japan
* Correspondence: taichiro@1997.jukuin.keio.ac.jp; Tel.: +81-55-253-7111
† These authors contributed equally to this work.

Abstract: The microbiota has been reported to be correlated with carcinogenesis and cancer progression. However, its involvement in the pathology of mesothelioma remains unknown. In this study, we aimed to identify mesothelioma-specific microbiota using resected or biopsied mesothelioma samples. Eight mesothelioma tissue samples were analyzed via polymerase chain reaction (PCR) amplification and 16S rRNA gene sequencing. The operational taxonomic units (OTUs) of the effective tags were analyzed in order to determine the taxon composition of each sample. For the three patients who underwent extra pleural pneumonectomy, normal peripheral lung tissues adjacent to the tumor were also included, and the same analysis was performed. In total, 61 OTUs were identified in the tumor and lung tissues, which were classified into 36 species. *Streptococcus australis* and *Ralstonia pickettii* were identified as abundant species in almost all tumor and lung samples. *Streptococcus australis* and *Ralstonia pickettii* were found to comprise mesothelioma-specific microbiota involved in tumor progression; thus, they could serve as targets for the prevention of mesothelioma.

Keywords: mesothelioma; microbiome; 16S RNA sequencing; species

Citation: Higuchi, R.; Goto, T.; Hirotsu, Y.; Otake, S.; Oyama, T.; Amemiya, K.; Mochizuki, H.; Omata, M. *Streptococcus australis* and *Ralstonia pickettii* as Major Microbiota in Mesotheliomas. *J. Pers. Med.* **2021**, *11*, 297. https://doi.org/10.3390/jpm11040297

Academic Editor: Jorge Luis Espinoza

Received: 9 March 2021
Accepted: 12 April 2021
Published: 14 April 2021

Publisher's Note: MDPI stays neutral with regard to jurisdictional claims in published maps and institutional affiliations.

Copyright: © 2021 by the authors. Licensee MDPI, Basel, Switzerland. This article is an open access article distributed under the terms and conditions of the Creative Commons Attribution (CC BY) license (https://creativecommons.org/licenses/by/4.0/).

1. Introduction

The field of microbiome research was primarily initiated to study gastrointestinal diseases, such as pseudomembranous enteritis and irritable bowel syndrome; however, as the human intestinal microbiota is involved in carcinogenesis and cancer progression, it has also begun to focus on this area [1–3]. Moreover, new sequencing technologies have revealed bacterial flora in the pancreatic, lung, and breast tissues, in addition to the intestinal tissue [4–8].

Described as "the worst type of malignancy", mesothelioma is a disease associated with extremely poor treatment outcomes and a 5-year overall survival of 3.4% [9]. Epidemiologically, mesothelioma is strongly correlated with asbestos inhalation and, since its onset, is usually observed approximately 40 years after asbestos inhalation. As of 2020, it is being increasingly reported worldwide [10]. Therefore, there is an urgent need to clarify its pathophysiology and establish methods for preventing its onset, as well as to introduce new treatments [11,12].

Several recent studies have reported the relationship between microbiota and carcinogenesis in colorectal cancer, oral cancer, pancreatic cancer, and lung cancer [13–17]; however, the significance of the microbiota in mesothelioma remains to be elucidated. Unlike previously studied oral, gastrointestinal and respiratory cancers, mesothelioma occurs in the thoracic cavity, and undergoes no direct interaction with external areas. Since the tumor environment of mesothelioma is presumably sterile, and since it is a rare disease, microbiome research on the involvement of the microbiota in the pathophysiology of this disease is lacking.

Here, the 16S rRNA of the bacterial genome of resected or biopsied mesothelioma specimens was amplified via polymerase chain reaction (PCR), followed by 16S sequence analysis via next-generation sequencing, to determine the composition of the microbiota and identify mesothelioma-specific bacterial flora. Furthermore, a predictive model for the onset of disease was developed based on these results, and the possibility of the prevention/control of mesothelioma onset was discussed.

2. Methods

2.1. Patients and Sample Preparation

In this study, eight patients who underwent surgical resection for mesothelioma at our hospital between January 2016 and August 2020 were enrolled unbiasedly. Since antibiotics treatment might modify bacterial composition, patients who had taken antibiotics orally or intravenously before surgery were excluded from this study. Written informed consent for genetic research was obtained from all the enrolled patients in compliance with the protocols of the Institutional Review Board at our hospital. The resected specimens were classified and staged according to WHO histological guidelines and the TNM (Tumor-Node-Metastasis) staging system, respectively [18]. Sections of formalin-fixed and paraffin-embedded tissues were stained with hematoxylin–eosin, followed by microdissection with the ArcturusXT laser-capture microdissection system (Thermo Fisher Scientific, Waltham, MA, USA), as previously reported [19–24]. For patients who underwent extra pleural pneumonectomy (EPP) and surgical resection of the lung, normal lung tissues, just under the visceral pleura, were also microdissected and examined. Since there were three surgical patients, eight patients and 11 specimens were analyzed. The GeneRead DNA FFPE Kit (Qiagen, Hilden, Germany) was utilized following the manufacturer's instructions, and the DNA quality was examined by the use of primers for ribonuclease P [25]. In the same manner, tumor DNA was extracted from the FFPE (formalin-fixed paraffin embedded) samples obtained from patients with thymoma, the other rare malignant neoplasm in the thorax, and used as a control ($n = 19$).

2.2. 16S rRNA Amplification and Targeted Sequencing

The 16S rDNA V4 region was amplified by PCR and sequencing as previously described with minor modifications [7]. FFPE DNA was amplified with the Platinum PCR SuperMix High Fidelity (Thermo Fisher Scientific, Waltham, MA, USA) with forward primer 5′-GTGYCAGCMGCCGCGGTAA-3′ (16S_rRNA_V4_515F) and reverse primer 5′-GGACTACNVGGGTWTCTAAT-3′ (16S_rRNA_V4_806R). PCR products were confirmed by agarose gel electrophoresis and purified with Agencourt AMPure XP reagents (Beckman Coulter, Brea, CA, USA). End repair and barcode adaptors were ligated with an Ion Plus Fragment Library Kit (Thermo Fisher Scientific, Waltham, MA, USA) in compliance with the manufacturer's instructions, and libraries were constructed. The library concentration was determined with an Ion Library Quantitation Kit (Thermo Fisher Scientific, Waltham, MA, USA), and the same quantity of libraries was set for each sequence. Emulsion PCR and chip loading were performed on the Ion Chef with an Ion PGM Hi-Q View Chef Kit, and sequencing was performed on the Ion PGM Sequencer (Thermo Fisher Scientific, Waltham, MA, USA). The sequence data were transferred to the IonReporter local server with the IonReporterUploader plugin. Data were analyzed with the Metagenomics Research Application using a custom primer set. The analytical parameter was set as the default.

2.3. Data Analysis

The original raw tags were obtained by merging paired-end reads using FLASH (v1.2.7), then they were filtered to obtain clean tags via Qiime (Version 1.9.1). The operational taxonomic units (OTUs) of the effective tags were classified and PCR chimeras were removed via Usearch (Uparse v7.0.1001) to identify the taxa composition of each sample with 97% identity. To obtain taxonomic assignments from phylum to species, the presentative sequence of each OTU was classified by taxonomy via the RDP (Ribosomal Database Project) classifier, with reference to the Silva (SSU123) 16S rRNA database, with confidence estimates of 80%.

2.4. Statistics

Continuous variables are described as the mean $\pm$ SD. One-way ANOVA (analysis of variance) and the Tukey–Kramer multiple comparison test were utilized to identify significant differences among groups. Statistical significance was defined as p-values below 0.05 in the two-tailed analyses.

3. Results

3.1. Patient Characteristics

In total, we analyzed 11 resected specimens from eight patients with mesotheliomas who had undergone surgery at our institution between January 2014 and August 2020. The clinicopathologic characteristics of the patients, including age, sex, histology, stage, smoking status, and performance of chemotherapy or extrapleural pneumonectomy (EPP), are shown in Table 1. Among the eight patients, all were males, seven were smokers and one was a non-smoker. According to the histological classification, there were six epithelioid, one sarcomatoid, and one biphasic mesotheliomas (Table 1). The eight patients enrolled in this study were classified according to TNM stage: stage IA ($n = 1$), IB ($n = 4$) and II ($n = 3$). The patients' ages ranged between 53 and 78 years (68.1 $\pm$ 8.5 years). Seven patients underwent chemotherapy, and three patients underwent EPP.

Table 1. Patient characteristics.

Parameter		Number of Patients	Overall Percentage
Total number		8	
Age (years), median (range)		71 (53–78)	
Sex			
	Male	8	100.0%
	Female	0	0.0%
Histology			
	Epithelioid mesothelioma	6	75.0%
	Sarcomatoid mesothelioma	1	12.5%
	Biphasic mesothelioma	1	12.5%
Stage			
	IA	1	12.5%
	IB	4	50.0%
	II	3	37.5%
Smoking Status (Pack year)			
	0	1	12.5%
	$0 < PY \leqq 30$	4	50.0%
	> 30	3	37.5%
Chemotherapy			
	Performed	7	87.5%
	Not performed	1	12.5%
EPP			
	Performed	3	37.5%
	Not performed	5	62.5%

3.2. OTU Analyses

Via OTU analysis, 61 OTUs were detected in 11 samples. The predominant (> 1% average relative abundance) classifiable OTUs involved two species, *Streptococcus australis* (abundance: 32.2 ± 29.6%) and *Ralstonia pickettii* (abundance: 24.4 ± 21.1%) (Figure 1). Both *Streptococcus australis* and *Ralstonia pickettii* were detected in the tumor tissues of six patients and in the lung tissues of all three patients who underwent EPP (Figure 1, Supplementary Figure S1), and both species were identified in all mesothelioma tissues (Figure 1).

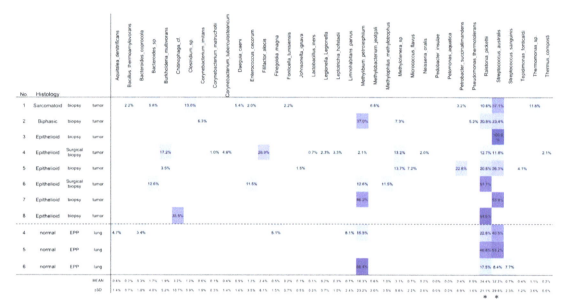

Figure 1. Composition and abundance of dominant species in all the samples. Heatmap visualizes the abundance of detected species. *, $p < 0.05$, compared with the other species except *Methylibium petroleiphilum*.

3.3. Differences in Microbiota between Mesotheliomas and Thymomas

To identify mesothelioma-specific microbiota, we compared the microbiota between mesothelioma and thymoma samples (Figure 2). The thymoma specimens showed no specific distribution of microbiota, and *Streptococcus australis* and *Ralstonia pickettii* were not detected either, suggesting that these species are specific to mesothelioma.

J. Pers. Med. **2021**, *11*, 297

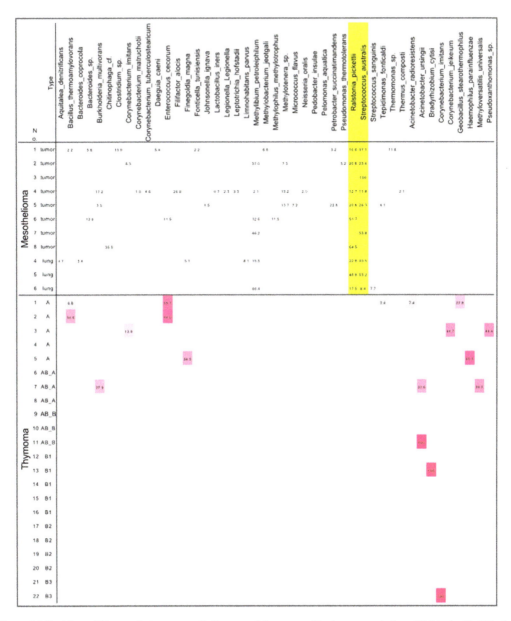

Figure 2. Microbiome differences between mesotheliomas and thymomas. *Streptococcus australis* and *Ralstonia pickettii* in the mesotheliomas are highlighted in yellow.

4. Discussion

The microbiota has recently been identified in some cancer tissues, including pancreatic and lung cancers, and its significance is attracting attention [4–8]; however, microbiome research focusing on mesothelioma is lacking. In this study, microbiome analysis was performed using resected mesothelioma specimens, and *Streptococcus australis* and *Ralstonia pickettii* were identified in almost all mesothelioma patients, with high levels of bacterial composition and abundance. Peripheral normal lung tissues adjacent to the tumor were also analyzed in patients who underwent EPP. *Streptococcus australis* and *Ralstonia pickettii* were detected in abundance in both the tumor and the adjacent lung tissues. Mesothelioma specimens and thymoma tissues (control) were analyzed simultaneously via the same process at the Genome Analysis Center in our institution, which determined that the specimens were not contaminated with these two bacterial species during the analysis process. By contrast, neither *Streptococcus australis* nor *Ralstonia pickettii* were detected in lung cancer tissues in recently published reviews of the microbiota [4,26–28]. Furthermore, the involvement of these two genera in the carcinogenesis of any organs has not been investigated. Since these two genera were detected in almost all mesothelioma patients, *Streptococcus australis* and *Ralstonia pickettii* may represent differential microbiome-related mechanisms in mesothelioma development.

Basic research on the lung microbiome has revealed that certain symbiotic bacteria form numerous micropores on the surface layer (visceral pleura) of the lungs of healthy individuals [29]. These micropores are formed by the secretion of cholesterol-dependent cytolysin (CDC), and there are five main types of CDC: pneumolysin, streptolysin, intermedilysin, mitilysin, and lectinolysin [30]. CDC, a pore-forming toxin, binds to the cholesterol on the cell surface and then polymerizes on the cell membrane to form transmembrane pores [29,31]. Furthermore, *Streptococcus pneumoniae*, *Streptococcus pyogenes*, *Streptococcus intermedius* and *Streptococcus mitis* are the major cause of CDC [30].

The *Streptococcus australis* identified in this study was first isolated from the saliva of children in Sydney, Australia, in 1991 [32]. During microbiological analyses of the saliva of children, Willcox et al. isolated strains of streptococci that could grow in media containing high concentrations of NaCl or KCl (up to 500 mM) [32]. These strains were initially identified as *Streptococcus mitis*, but were subsequently determined to be a separate species, according to DNA–DNA hybridization and biochemical analysis (Willcox, 1996) [33]. Nevertheless, based on 16S rRNA sequences, *Streptococcus australis* was shown to be clustered in the group corresponding to the *Streptococcus mitis* [32,34]. Based on the above information, it is likely that *Streptococcus australis* is present in the lung, particularly in the peripheral lung adjacent to the visceral pleura, in patients who develop mesothelioma, and it produces CDC in order to form numerous micropores in the visceral pleura on the lung surface. Furthermore, the pathophysiological hypothesis that asbestos microfibers pass through these micropores and reach the parietal pleura should also be considered. This hypothesis is consistent with the observation that ultra-thin fibers (about 0.02 μm in diameter) were the only asbestos fibers detected in the parietal pleura and mesothelioma tissues, and that the diameter of the micropores formed in the visceral pleura was estimated to be 250 Å (0.025 μm) [30]. However, there are many instances wherein mesothelioma does not occur even after asbestos inhalation. Differences in the composition of bacterial flora may contribute to individual differences in the occurrence of mesothelioma. This is a new hypothesis concerning the pathogenesis of mesothelioma, and further detailed investigation is urgently needed.

On the other hand, *Ralstonia pickettii* is a Gram-negative, rod-shaped bacterium [35]. *Ralstonia pickettii*, a Betaproteobacteria species, is a common microorganism inhabiting various environments, such as soils, rivers, and lakes. It is an oligotrophic organism, making it capable of surviving in nutrient-poor environments. The ability to use diverse organic compounds and survive in these harsh conditions makes *R. pickettii* useful for bioremediation [36]. *Ralstonia pickettii* is an emerging pathogen in clinical settings [37]. *R. pickettii* has come to be severely pathogenic in immunocompromised or fragile patients. Several medical institutions have reported outbreaks—patients with Crohn's disease and cystic fibrosis in particular were found to be infected with *R. picketti*. Among the 55 reported cases of *R. picketti*. infection, most were due to contaminated saline solutions and sterile drugs [38]. These solutions are supposed to be contaminated during the manufacturing procedure, because *R. pickettii* is theoretically able to pass through the 0.2 μm filters that are generally used to sterilize medicinal products.

There are many indigenous microorganisms in the epithelia of several human organs (oral and auricular cavities, respiratory organs, gastrointestinal tract, skin, and reproductive organs), which play various roles in the body and have symbiotic relationships [1,3]. Disturbances in the bacterial flora (dysbiosis) change the risk of disease onset. Moreover, intestinal bacterial flora are relevant to numerous diseases, such as allergies, cancer, multiple sclerosis, Parkinson's disease, depression, inflammatory bowel disease, and rheumatism [26]. Furthermore, the onset of these diseases has been alleviated and prevented via aseptic and specific pathogen-free processing in pathophysiological mouse models of the aforementioned diseases, and disease onset may also be prevented by improving the bacterial flora in humans [39]. If one or several organisms are the cause of disease, they may be a potential therapeutic target. In clinical practice for gastric cancer, carcinogenesis can be prevented by eradicating *Helicobacter pylori*, which is currently the standard treatment for the prevention of disease onset in infected patients [40]. Therefore, since the bacterial flora involved in the onset of mesothelioma has been identified, it may be possible to prevent the onset of mesothelioma in future clinical applications by controlling these two species. In particular, asbestos inhalation is a known cause of mesothelioma, and the prevention of mesothelioma is particularly important in high-risk populations exposed to asbestos [10]. The establishment of a probiosis model, with antimicrobial or vaccine therapy targeting the two target species identified in this study, may serve as a treatment regime for the prevention of the onset of mesothelioma.

This study has some limitations. First, the number of patients was small, owing to the extreme rarity of the tumor type, and the patients enrolled in this study were only Japanese. Second, no blood samples were analyzed for microbiota containing the two species *Streptococcus australis* and *Ralstonia pickettii*. The greater abundance of these two species in the tumor tissue may be associated with the impaired immunity of the tumor microenvironment, which may help these bacteria to proliferate in the blood, and thus they may be clinically applicable as serum biomarkers for mesothelioma. Third, it is unclear from our observational design whether the identified bacterial profiles are causally associated with oncogenesis, or are merely reflective of pathological processes in the mesothelioma. In this context, a larger series will be required to analyze the microbiome landscape of mesotheliomas more extensively, and to more clearly interpret the relevance of clinical variables via comprehensive multivariate analysis. However, since the major objective of this exploratory analysis was to identify the mesothelioma-specific microbiota that could be useful for clinical development, the modest sample size can still offer much insight.

5. Conclusions

This is the first study to examine the microbiota involved in mesothelioma, revealing two mesothelioma-specific species, *Streptococcus australis* and *Ralstonia pickettii*. Further research is required to reveal how the two species coexist with mesothelioma and how they are involved in the mechanism of carcinogenesis. In addition, by establishing probiosis models that can control these species, "precision medicine" can be developed for the prevention of the onset of mesothelioma. The results of this study might have clinical applicability, such as in preventing the onset of mesothelioma by controlling and enhancing the symbiotic bacterial flora through antibiotic or vaccine therapy, or in establishing a regular screening system in patients presumed to be at high risk for developing mesothelioma.

Supplementary Materials: The following are available online at https://www.mdpi.com/article/10.3390/jpm11040297/s1. Figure S1: Composition of detected species in all samples.

Author Contributions: T.G., R.H. and Y.H. wrote the manuscript. T.G., S.O. and R.H. performed the surgery. T.O., R.H. and K.A. carried out the pathological examination. Y.H., T.G., K.A., R.H., H.M., S.O. and M.O. participated in the genomic analyses. T.G. and M.O. edited the final manuscript. All authors have read and agreed to the final version of this manuscript.

Funding: This study was supported by a Grant-in-Aid for Genome Research Project from Yamanashi Prefecture (to M.O. and Y.H.).

Institutional Review Board Statement: The study was conducted according to the guidelines of the Declaration of Helsinki, and approved by the Institutional Review Board of Yamanashi Central Hospital.

Informed Consent Statement: Informed consent was obtained from all subjects involved in the study.

Acknowledgments: The authors greatly appreciate Yoshihiro Miyashita, Toshiharu Tsutsui, and Yumiko Kakizaki for their helpful scientific discussion.

Conflicts of Interest: The authors declare no conflict of interest. The funder had no role in the design of the study; in the collection, analyses, or interpretation of data; in the writing of the manuscript; or in the decision to publish the results.

References

1. Kovaleva, O.V.; Romashin, D.; Zborovskaya, I.B.; Davydov, M.M.; Shogenov, M.S.; Gratchev, A. Human Lung Microbiome on the Way to Cancer. *J. Immunol. Res.* **2019**, *2019*, 1–6. [CrossRef] [PubMed]
2. Mao, Q.; Jiang, F.; Yin, R.; Wang, J.; Xia, W.; Dong, G.; Ma, W.; Yang, Y.; Xu, L.; Hu, J. Interplay between the lung microbiome and lung cancer. *Cancer Lett.* **2018**, *415*, 40–48. [CrossRef]
3. Power, S.E.; O'Toole, P.W.; Stanton, C.; Ross, R.P.; Fitzgerald, G.F. Intestinal microbiota, diet and health. *Br. J. Nutr.* **2014**, *111*, 387–402. [CrossRef] [PubMed]
4. Goto, T. Airway Microbiota as a Modulator of Lung Cancer. *Int. J. Mol. Sci.* **2020**, *21*, 3044. [CrossRef]
5. Laborda-Illanes, A.; Sanchez-Alcoholado, L.; Dominguez-Recio, M.E.; Jimenez-Rodriguez, B.; Lavado, R.; Comino-Méndez, I.; Alba, E.; Queipo-Ortuño, M.I. Breast and Gut Microbiota Action Mechanisms in Breast Cancer Pathogenesis and Treatment. *Cancers* **2020**, *12*, 2465. [CrossRef]
6. Peters, B.A.; Hayes, R.B.; Goparaju, C.; Reid, C.; Pass, H.I.; Ahn, J. The Microbiome in Lung Cancer Tissue and Recurrence-Free Survival. *Cancer Epidemiol. Biomark. Prev.* **2019**, *28*, 731–740. [CrossRef]
7. Riquelme, E.; Zhang, Y.; Zhang, L.; Montiel, M.; Zoltan, M.; Dong, W.; Quesada, P.; Sahin, I.; Chandra, V.; San Lucas, A.; et al. Tumor Microbiome Diversity and Composition Influence Pancreatic Cancer Outcomes. *Cell* **2019**, *178*, 795–806.e712. [CrossRef] [PubMed]
8. Wei, M.Y.; Shi, S.; Liang, C.; Meng, Q.C.; Hua, J.; Zhang, Y.Y.; Liu, J.; Zhang, B.; Xu, J.; Yu, X.J. The microbiota and Microbiome in Pancreatic Cancer: More Influential than Expected. *Mol. Cancer* **2019**, *18*, 97. [CrossRef] [PubMed]
9. Asciak, R.; George, V.; Rahman, N.M. Update on biology and management of mesothelioma. *Eur. Respir. Rev.* **2021**, *30*, 200226. [CrossRef] [PubMed]
10. Cakiroglu, E.; Senturk, S. Genomics and Functional Genomics of Malignant Pleural Mesothelioma. *Int. J. Mol. Sci.* **2020**, *21*, 6342. [CrossRef] [PubMed]
11. Woodard, G.A.; Jablons, D.M. Surgery for pleural mesothelioma, when it is indicated and why: Arguments against surgery for malignant pleural mesothelioma. *Transl. Lung Cancer Res.* **2020**, *9*, S86–S91. [CrossRef] [PubMed]
12. Xu, D.; Yang, H.; Schmid, R.A.; Peng, R.W. Therapeutic Landscape of Malignant Pleural Mesothelioma: Collateral Vulnerabilities and Evolutionary Dependencies in the Spotlight. *Front. Oncol.* **2020**, *10*, 579464. [CrossRef] [PubMed]
13. Castellarin, M.; Warren, R.L.; Freeman, J.D.; Dreolini, L.; Krzywinski, M.; Strauss, J.; Barnes, R.; Watson, P.; Allen-Vercoe, E.; Moore, R.A.; et al. Fusobacterium nucleatum infection is prevalent in human colorectal carcinoma. *Genome. Res.* **2012**, *22*, 299–306. [CrossRef]
14. Gethings-Behncke, C.; Coleman, H.G.; Jordao, H.W.T.; Longley, D.B.; Crawford, N.; Murray, L.J.; Kunzmann, A.T. Fusobacterium nucleatum in the Colorectum and Its Association with Cancer Risk and Survival: A Systematic Review and Meta-analysis. *Cancer Epidemiol. Biomark. Prev.* **2020**, *29*, 539–548. [CrossRef]
15. Gur, C.; Ibrahim, Y.; Isaacson, B.; Yamin, R.; Abed, J.; Gamliel, M.; Enk, J.; Bar-On, Y.; Stanietsky-Kaynan, N.; Coppenhagen-Glazer, S.; et al. Binding of the Fap2 protein of Fusobacterium nucleatum to human inhibitory receptor TIGIT protects tumors from immune cell attack. *Immunity* **2015**, *42*, 344–355. [CrossRef]
16. Kostic, A.D.; Chun, E.; Robertson, L.; Glickman, J.N.; Gallini, C.A.; Michaud, M.; Clancy, T.E.; Chung, D.C.; Lochhead, P.; Hold, G.L.; et al. Fusobacterium nucleatum potentiates intestinal tumorigenesis and modulates the tumor-immune microenvironment. *Cell Host Microbe* **2013**, *14*, 207–215. [CrossRef]
17. Rubinstein, M.R.; Wang, X.; Liu, W.; Hao, Y.; Cai, G.; Han, Y.W. Fusobacterium nucleatum promotes colorectal carcinogenesis by modulating E-cadherin/beta-catenin signaling via its FadA adhesin. *Cell Host Microbe* **2013**, *14*, 195–206. [CrossRef]
18. Galateau-Salle, F.; Churg, A.; Roggli, V.; Travis, W.D. The 2015 World Health Organization Classification of Tumors of the Pleura: Advances since the 2004 Classification. *J. Thorac. Oncol.* **2016**, *11*, 142–154. [CrossRef]
19. Amemiya, K.; Hirotsu, Y.; Goto, T.; Nakagomi, H.; Mochizuki, H.; Oyama, T.; Omata, M. Touch imprint cytology with massively parallel sequencing (TIC-seq): A simple and rapid method to snapshot genetic alterations in tumors. *Cancer Med.* **2016**, *5*, 3426–3436. [CrossRef] [PubMed]
20. Goto, T.; Hirotsu, Y.; Amemiya, K.; Nakagomi, T.; Shikata, D.; Yokoyama, Y.; Okimoto, K.; Oyama, T.; Mochizuki, H.; Omata, M. Distribution of circulating tumor DNA in lung cancer: Analysis of the primary lung and bone marrow along with the pulmonary venous and peripheral blood. *Oncotarget* **2017**, *8*, 59268–59281. [CrossRef]

21. Higuchi, R.; Nakagomi, T.; Goto, T.; Hirotsu, Y.; Shikata, D.; Yokoyama, Y.; Otake, S.; Amemiya, K.; Oyama, T.; Mochizuki, H.; et al. Identification of Clonality through Genomic Profile Analysis in Multiple Lung Cancers. *J. Clin. Med.* **2020**, *9*, 573. [CrossRef] [PubMed]

22. Nakagomi, T.; Goto, T.; Hirotsu, Y.; Shikata, D.; Yokoyama, Y.; Higuchi, R.; Otake, S.; Amemiya, K.; Oyama, T.; Mochizuki, H.; et al. Genomic Characteristics of Invasive Mucinous Adenocarcinomas of the Lung and Potential Therapeutic Targets of B7-H3. *Cancers* **2018**, *10*, 478. [CrossRef]

23. Nakagomi, T.; Hirotsu, Y.; Goto, T.; Shikata, D.; Yokoyama, Y.; Higuchi, R.; Otake, S.; Amemiya, K.; Oyama, T.; Mochizuki, H.; et al. Clinical Implications of Noncoding Indels in the Surfactant-Encoding Genes in Lung Cancer. *Cancers* **2019**, *11*, 552. [CrossRef] [PubMed]

24. Oyama, T.; Goto, T.; Amemiya, K.; Hirotsu, Y.; Omata, M. Squamous Cell Carcinoma of the Lung with Micropapillary Pattern. *J. Thorac. Oncol.* **2020**, *15*, 1541–1544. [CrossRef] [PubMed]

25. Goto, T.; Hirotsu, Y.; Oyama, T.; Amemiya, K.; Omata, M. Analysis of tumor-derived DNA in plasma and bone marrow fluid in lung cancer patients. *Med. Oncol.* **2016**, *33*, 29. [CrossRef]

26. Maddi, A.; Sabharwal, A.; Violante, T.; Manuballa, S.; Genco, R.; Patnaik, S.; Yendamuri, S. The microbiome and lung cancer. *J. Thorac. Dis.* **2019**, *11*, 280–291. [CrossRef]

27. Ramirez-Labrada, A.G.; Isla, D.; Artal, A.; Arias, M.; Rezusta, A.; Pardo, J.; Galvez, E.M. The Influence of Lung Microbiota on Lung Carcinogenesis, Immunity, and Immunotherapy. *Trends Cancer* **2020**, *6*, 86–97. [CrossRef] [PubMed]

28. Xu, N.; Wang, L.; Li, C.; Ding, C.; Li, C.; Fan, W.; Cheng, C.; Gu, B. Microbiota dysbiosis in lung cancer: Evidence of association and potential mechanisms. *Transl. Lung Cancer Res.* **2020**, *9*, 1554–1568. [CrossRef]

29. Tweten, R.K. Cholesterol-dependent cytolysins, a family of versatile pore-forming toxins. *Infect. Immun.* **2005**, *73*, 6199–6209. [CrossRef]

30. Magouliotis, D.E.; Tasiopoulou, V.S.; Molyvdas, P.A.; Gourgoulianis, K.I.; Hatzoglou, C.; Zarogiannis, S.G. Airways microbiota: Hidden Trojan horses in asbestos exposed individuals? *Med. Hypotheses* **2014**, *83*, 537–540. [CrossRef]

31. Geny, B.; Popoff, M.R. Bacterial protein toxins and lipids: Pore formation or toxin entry into cells. *Biol. Cell* **2006**, *98*, 667–678. [CrossRef]

32. Willcox, M.D.; Zhu, H.; Knox, K.W. Streptococcus australis sp. nov., a novel oral streptococcus. *Int. J. Syst. Evol. Microbiol.* **2001**, *51*, 1277–1281. [CrossRef]

33. Willcox, M.D. Identification and classification of species within the Streptococcus sanguis group. *Aust. Dent. J.* **1996**, *41*, 107–112. [CrossRef]

34. Zheng, W.; Tan, T.K.; Paterson, I.C.; Mutha, N.V.; Siow, C.C.; Tan, S.Y.; Old, L.A.; Jakubovics, N.S.; Choo, S.W. StreptoBase: An Oral Streptococcus mitis Group Genomic Resource and Analysis Platform. *PLoS ONE* **2016**, *11*, e0151908. [CrossRef]

35. Yabuuchi, E.; Kosako, Y.; Yano, I.; Hotta, H.; Nishiuchi, Y. Transfer of two Burkholderia and an Alcaligenes species to Ralstonia gen. Nov.: Proposal of Ralstonia pickettii (Ralston, Palleroni and Doudoroff 1973) comb. Nov., Ralstonia solanacearum (Smith 1896) comb. Nov. and Ralstonia eutropha (Davis 1969) comb. Nov. *Microbiol. Immunol.* **1995**, *39*, 897–904. [CrossRef]

36. Ryan, M.P.; Pembroke, J.T.; Adley, C.C. Ralstonia pickettii in environmental biotechnology: Potential and applications. *J. Appl. Microbiol.* **2007**, *103*, 754–764. [CrossRef]

37. Ryan, M.P.; Adley, C.C. Ralstonia spp.: Emerging global opportunistic pathogens. *Eur. J. Clin. Microbiol. Infect. Dis.* **2014**, *33*, 291–304. [CrossRef] [PubMed]

38. Ryan, M.P.; Pembroke, J.T.; Adley, C.C. Ralstonia pickettii: A persistent gram-negative nosocomial infectious organism. *J. Hosp. Infect.* **2006**, *62*, 278–284. [CrossRef] [PubMed]

39. Sommariva, M.; Le Noci, V.; Bianchi, F.; Camelliti, S.; Balsari, A.; Tagliabue, E.; Sfondrini, L. The lung microbiota: Role in maintaining pulmonary immune homeostasis and its implications in cancer development and therapy. *Cell. Mol. Life Sci.* **2020**, *77*, 2739–2749. [CrossRef]

40. Liou, J.M.; Malfertheiner, P.; Lee, Y.C.; Sheu, B.S.; Sugano, K.; Cheng, H.C.; Yeoh, K.G.; Hsu, P.I.; Goh, K.L.; Mahachai, V.; et al. Screening and eradication of Helicobacter pylori for gastric cancer prevention: The Taipei global consensus. *Gut* **2020**, *69*, 2093–2112. [CrossRef]

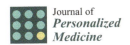

Article

Gut Microbiome in a Russian Cohort of Pre- and Post-Cholecystectomy Female Patients

Irina Grigor'eva [1,*], Tatiana Romanova [1], Natalia Naumova [2,*], Tatiana Alikina [2], Alexey Kuznetsov [3] and Marsel Kabilov [2]

[1] Research Institute of Internal and Preventive Medicine—Branch of the Institute of Cytology and Genetics, Siberian Branch of Russian Academy of Sciences, Novosibirsk 630089, Russia; tarom_75@mail.ru
[2] Institute of Chemical Biology and Fundamental Medicine, Siberian Branch of the Russian Academy of Sciences, Novosibirsk 630090, Russia; alikina@niboch.nsc.ru (T.A.); kabilov@niboch.nsc.ru (M.K.)
[3] Novosibirsk State Medical University, Novosibirsk 630091, Russia; 1xo2788353@mail.ru
* Correspondence: igrigorieva@ngs.ru (I.G.); naumova@niboch.nsc.ru (N.N.)

Abstract: The last decade saw extensive studies of the human gut microbiome and its relationship to specific diseases, including gallstone disease (GSD). The information about the gut microbiome in GSD-afflicted Russian patients is scarce, despite the increasing GSD incidence worldwide. Although the gut microbiota was described in some GSD cohorts, little is known regarding the gut microbiome before and after cholecystectomy (CCE). By using Illumina MiSeq sequencing of 16S rRNA gene amplicons, we inventoried the fecal bacteriobiome composition and structure in GSD-afflicted females, seeking to reveal associations with age, BMI and some blood biochemistry. Overall, 11 bacterial phyla were identified, containing 916 operational taxonomic units (OTUs). The fecal bacteriobiome was dominated by *Firmicutes* (66% relative abundance), followed by *Bacteroidetes* (19%), *Actinobacteria* (8%) and *Proteobacteria* (4%) phyla. Most (97%) of the OTUs were minor or rare species with ≤1% relative abundance. *Prevotella* and *Enterocossus* were linked to blood bilirubin. Some taxa had differential pre- and post-CCE abundance, despite the very short time (1–3 days) elapsed after CCE. The detailed description of the bacteriobiome in pre-CCE female patients suggests bacterial foci for further research to elucidate the gut microbiota and GSD relationship and has potentially important biological and medical implications regarding gut bacteria involvement in the increased GSD incidence rate in females.

Keywords: gallstone disease; 16S rDNA gene diversity; gut microbiota; blood biochemical characteristics

Citation: Grigor'eva, I.; Romanova, T.; Naumova, N.; Alikina, T.; Kuznetsov, A.; Kabilov, M. Gut Microbiome in a Russian Cohort of Pre- and Post-Cholecystectomy Female Patients. *J. Pers. Med.* **2021**, *11*, 294. https://doi.org/10.3390/jpm11040294

Academic Editor: Lucrezia Laterza

Received: 19 February 2021
Accepted: 8 April 2021
Published: 12 April 2021

Publisher's Note: MDPI stays neutral with regard to jurisdictional claims in published maps and institutional affiliations.

Copyright: © 2021 by the authors. Licensee MDPI, Basel, Switzerland. This article is an open access article distributed under the terms and conditions of the Creative Commons Attribution (CC BY) license (https://creativecommons.org/licenses/by/4.0/).

1. Introduction

Gallstone disease (GSD) has been, for many years, a significant public health problem worldwide, and its prevalence rate is expected to increase due to the ongoing changes in lifestyle and dietary habits. Gallstones are highly prevalent in Russia, with 100,000–200,000 cholecystectomies performed annually [1,2].

By now, there is little doubt about the multifaceted relationship between GSD and the microbiota [3], as some intestinal bacteria can promote gallstone formation [4–6], particularly by modifying the bile acid profile [7]. However, laparoscopic cholecystectomy (CCE), albeit currently a radical gold standard treatment, is not a neutral event and may increase the risk of some serious disorders and diseases, including metabolic syndrome, cardiovascular disease and cancers [4,8–10]. Post-cholecystectomy constant inflow of bile into the intestine and its metabolites can directly affect the intestinal microbiota [11], causing shifts in the gut–brain and gut–muscle axes and thus indirectly affecting the etiology and course of many related diseases and disorders. Although it is not yet possible to predict how particular perturbations will modify the microbiota, it is possible that different microbiome configurations might allow stratified treatment and diet recommendations in the future, becoming a novel and powerful candidate for personalized treatment of human diseases [4]. Among more than 500 oral drugs tested, 13% were discovered to be metabolized by the microbiome [12]. Another study identified 30 human gut microbiome-encoded enzymes responsible for the biotransformation of 20 drugs to 59 candidate metabolites [13]. Such findings strongly suggest the importance of including microbiomes into the framework of precision medicine. Although the pathogenesis of cholesterol gallstones is still not fully understood, gut microbiota dysbiosis plays an important role in their formation [14]. There is a paucity of studies describing fecal/gut bacteriobiome profiles in GSD-afflicted patients, both before and after surgery. The aim of our study was to inventory the fecal microbiota composition, as assessed by 16S rRNA gene sequencing, in a cohort of female patients with GSD and compare bacterial diversity before and after CCE.

2. Materials and Methods

2.1. Participants

Twenty-eight female patients with gallstone disease diagnosed by abdominal ultra-sonography were recruited for the study (Table 1). The older patients had a higher BMI (Pearson's correlation coefficient 0.66, $p < 0.001$). All patients underwent clinical examination to assess their gastrointestinal and gallbladder status and severity of their clinical condition; 21 patients had chronic disease, and the rest had acute disease. The patients had no history of treatment with antibiotics and proton pump inhibitors at least for 1 month prior to feces sampling, as well as no probiotics and/or prebiotics as special supplementation. Half of the patients had arterial hypertension, associated with increased BMI. The patients fasted for at least 12 h before the surgery. After the surgery, the patients received the antibiotic ceftriaxone. No specific diet was prescribed after the surgery.

Table 1. Demographics of the study cohort (N = 28, females).

	Mean	Median	Min	Max
Age, years	51.6	55.0	18.0	73.0
BMI $^{\$}$, kg/m^2	25.7	24.8	17.6	34.5

$^{\$}$ BMI stands for body mass index.

All patients were duly informed, gave their consent to the study and signed the informed consent form. The study observed all the relevant institutional and governmental regulations. The protocol of the study was approved by the Ethic Committee of the Research Institute of Internal and Preventive Medicine-Branch of the Institute of Cytology and Genetics, SB RAS. All clinical aspects of the study were supervised by a gastroenterologist.

2.2. Fecal and Blood Sample Collection

Fecal samples were collected 1 day prior to the CCE and 1–3 days after the surgery, i.e., as soon as patients had stool, into 10 mL sterile fecal specimen containers and stored at −80 °C until use for DNA extraction. Blood samples were taken twice on the same day as stool samples.

2.3. Blood Analyses

Collected blood samples were used to determine aspartate aminotransferase (AST, EC 2.6.1.1) and alanine aminotransferase (ALT, EC 2.6.1.2) by the kinetic method, as recommended by the International Federation of Clinical Chemistry and Laboratory Medicine (IFCC2), using a biochemical analyzer, "Konelab Prime 30i" (Thermo Fisher Scientific, Vantaa, Finland).

2.4. Extraction of Total Nucleic Acid from Feces

Total DNA was extracted from 50 to 100 mg of thawed patient fecal samples using the MetaHIT protocol [15]. The bead beating was performed using TissueLyser II (Qiagen,

Hilden, Germany), for 10 min at 30 Hz. No further purification of the DNA was needed. The quality of the DNA was assessed using agarose gel electrophoresis. No further purification of the DNA was needed.

2.5. 16S rRNA Gene Amplification and Sequencing

The 16S rRNA genes were amplified with the primer pair V3/V4, combined with Illumina adapter sequences [16]. PCR amplification was performed as described earlier [17]. A total of 200 ng of PCR product from each sample was pooled together and purified through MinElute Gel Extraction Kit (Qiagen, Hilden, Germany). The obtained amplicon libraries were sequenced with 2 × 300 bp paired-end reagents on MiSeq (Illumina, San Diego, USA) in the SB RAS Genomics Core Facility (ICBFM SB RAS, Novosibirsk, Russia). The read data reported in this study were submitted to GenBank under the study accession number PRJNA687360.

2.6. Bioinformatic and Statistical Analyses

Raw sequences were analyzed with the UPARSE pipeline [18] using Usearch v.11.0.667. The UPARSE pipeline included merging of paired reads; read quality filtering (-fastq_maxee_rate 0.005); length trimming (remove less than 350 nt); merging of identical reads (dereplication); discarding singleton reads; removing chimeras and OTU clustering using the UPARSE-OTU algorithm. The OTU sequences were assigned a taxonomy using SINTAX [19] on the RDP database. As a reference for bacteria, we used the 16S RDP training set v.16 [20]. Statistical analyses (descriptive statistics, Wilcoxon's test for dependent variables, principal component analysis, multiple regression and general linear model, GLM, analysis with repeated measures) were performed by using Statistica v.13.3. Principle coordinate analysis (PCoA) was performed by PAST software v.3.17 [21]. The individual rarefaction showed that the sampling effort reached saturation for all samples (Figure S1); therefore, α-biodiversity indices were calculated for complete datasets using PAST software v.3.17 [21]. Statistical significance was defined as $p < 0.05$.

3. Results

3.1. Overall Bacteriobiome Diversity

After quality filtering and chimera and non-bacterial sequence removal, a total of 916 OTUs were identified at the 97% sequence identity level. All these OTUs could not be ascribed to a species level. Overall, they clustered into 11 phyla, 24 classes (with 18 explicitly classified at the class level), 59 orders (with 50 explicitly classified at the order level), 72 families (with 54 explicitly classified at the family level) and 172 genera (with 132 explicitly classified at the genus level). Sixty-one OTUs, i.e., ca. 7% of the species richness and ca. 0.1% of the relative abundance, could not be ascribed below the domain level. *Firmicutes* with 635 OTUs was, by far, the most species-rich phylum, accounting for 69% of the total number of OTUs. *Bacteroidetes* ranked second richest with 96 OTUs (10.5%), followed by *Actinobacteria* (64 OTUs, 7%) and *Proteobacteria* with 45 (5%). Such phyla as *Synergistetes*, *Tenericutes* and *Verrucomicrobia* were represented by 3–5 OTUs each, whereas the rest of the identified phyla, i.e., *Spirochaetes*, *Fusobacteria*, *Lentisphaerae* and cand. *Saccharibacteria*, were represented by one OTU each. The *Firmicutes* phylum was also the ultimate dominant phylum, accounting, on average, for ca. 66% of the total number of sequence reads. The *Firmicutes/Bacteroidetes* ratio varied widely: from 0.4 to 6837 (median 5.0) before CCE and from 0.4 to 2918 (median 3.8) after CCE (Table S1), showing no CCE-related difference ($p = 0.39$, Wilcoxon's test) and no correlation with blood biochemistry (Spearman's, $p > 0.05$).

The dominant bacterial OTUs, i.e., OTUs contributing $\geq 1\%$ (mean abundance) to the total number of sequence reads obtained for a sample, amounted to 27, with 18 OTUs representing *Firmicutes*, and *Bacteroidetes* and *Actinobacteria* contributing four and three OTUs, respectively, whereas *Veruccomicrobia* and *Synergestetes* each contributed one OTU to the dominants' pool. Thus, the overwhelming majority (ca. 97%) of the OTUs in the study were minor or rare species.

3.2. Fecal Bacteriobiome Composition in GSD Patients before the CCE Surgery

The fecal microbiota of GSD patients was dominated by the *Firmicutes* phylum (66% relative abundance), followed by *Bacteroidetes* (19%), *Actinobacteria* (8%) and *Proteobacteria* (4%) phyla (Figure 1a). At the class level, the ultimate dominance of *Firmicutes* translated into the dominance of its classes *Clostridia* (47%), *Bacilli* (11%), *Negativicutes* (5%) and *Erysipelotrichia* (1.4%). *Bacteroidetes* was represented by the *Bacteroidia* class (19%), whereas *Actinobacteria* was represented solely by the *Actinobacteria* class. *Proteobacteria* was present mostly as *Gammaproteobacteria*, with *Alpha-, Beta-, Delta-* and *Epsilonproteobacteria* summarily contributing less than 1%. As for orders, *Clostridiales, Lactobacillales, Selenomonadales* and *Erysipelotrichales (Firmicutes), Bacteroidales (Bacteroidetes), Bifidobacteriales* and *Coriobacteriales (Actinobacteria)* and *Enterobacteriales (Gammaproteobacteria)* were found to prevail. Just three *Firmicutes* families, namely, *Ruminococcaceae, Lachnospiraceae* and *Enterococcaceae*, together accounted for half of the bacteriobiome abundance (Figure 1b). Most of the dominant OTUs (Figure 1c) belonged to the genera of the abovementioned families, i.e., *Enerococcus, Gemmiger, Faecalibacterium, Ruminococcus, Blautia, Roseburia* and *Streptococcus*. Other dominant OTUs represented *Bacteroidetes/Bacteroidia/Bacteroidales* (*Prevotella* sp. and *Bacteroides* sp.) and *Bifidobacteriaceae/Bifidobacteriales/Actinobacteria* (*Bifidobacterium* sp.).

Overall, fecal bacterial assemblages of GSD-afflicted subjects were characterized by high inter-individual variability of relative abundance and many outliers or extreme values at all taxonomic levels (Figure 1). Since we could not reasonably explain the outliers by errors in sampling collection and handling, nor by patients' characteristics and analytical procedures, we performed principal component (PC) analysis (based on covariance) of the data matrix with bacterial relative abundances as variables for analysis and patients as subjects in order to (a) obtain a better insight into the variance structure throughout the cohort, (b) find an association of the major PCs with patients' demographics and blood characteristics and then (c) implicate some bacterial taxa that contributed the most to the major PCs, as major players in such associations.

PC and multiple regression analyses showed that the core phyla, accounting for most of the data variance, showed a tendency for some association (PC2) with age, whereas some minor dominants (PC3, PC4) showed a correlation with blood glucose and bilirubin (Table 2).

Table 2. Statistical analyses' results: contribution of bacterial phyla to the principal components extracted from the matrix with relative abundance in feces of females with GSD before CCE (percentage of the total data variance in brackets) and p-values for multiple regression with age, BMI and blood biochemistry.

	Phyla: PCA [1]			
Main	PC 1	PC 2	PC 3	PC 4
contributors	(65%)	(18%)	(11%)	(5%)
Bacteroidetes	**0.49** [2] [−0.96] [3]	**0.29** [−0.23]	0.04	0.01
Firmicutes	**0.48** [0.91]	**0.29** [−0.39]	0.00	0.06
Proteobacteria	0.01	0.14	**0.25** [0.03]	**0.14** [0.98]
Actinobacteria	0.01	**0.23** [0.97]	**0.59** [−0.18]	0.00
Verrucomicrobia	0.00	0.05	0.04	**0.78** [−0.13]
	Phyla: Multiple regression			
R/R^2	0.54/0.29	0.53/0.28	0.61/0.37	0.57/0.33
Age	0.70	*0.09* [4]	0.38	0.16
BMI	0.39	0.21	0.37	0.21
Glucose	0.13	1.00	*0.07*	0.70
ALT	0.84	0.68	0.11	0.12
AST	0.51	0.61	0.80	0.17
Bilirubin	0.13	0.20	0.70	*0.10*

1 PCA stands for principle component analysis (based on covariance). Only those principal components that (a) account for the bigger fraction of the total data variance and/or (b) displayed a statistically significant correlation with patients' characteristics are shown. [2] The values in bold show the two topmost contributions. [3] Factor loadings for variables (taxon relative abundance) are given in square brackets. [4] The values in bold italics and underlined italics are at $p \leq 0.05$ and $p \leq 0.10$, respectively.

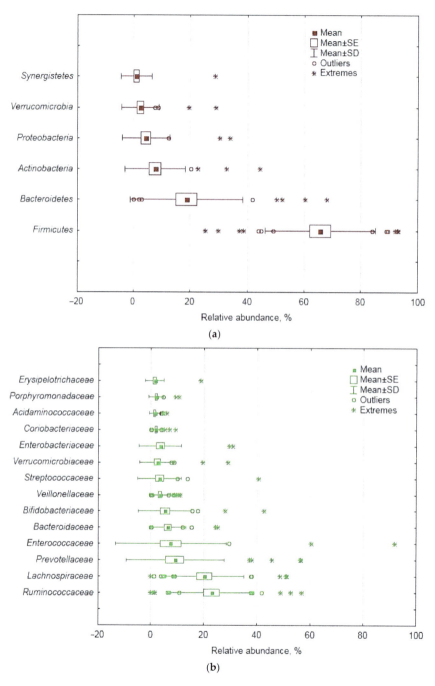

Figure 1. Cont.

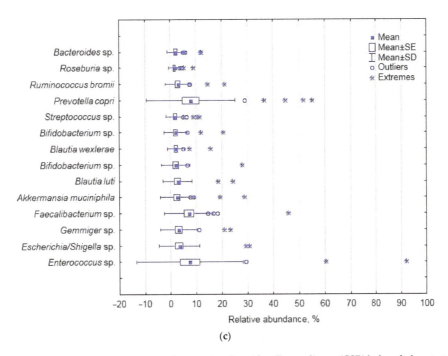

Figure 1. Relative abundance of the dominant bacterial taxa in females with gallstone disease (GSD) before cholecystectomy (CCE): (**a**) phyla, (**b**) families, (**c**) operational taxonomic units (OTUs).

As for the classes, the balance between the two core ones, i.e., *Clostridia* and *Bacteroidia* (PC2), was correlated with blood glucose, whereas the balance between two minor dominants, i.e., *Actinobacteria* and *Gammaproteobacteria* (PC4), was correlated with age (Table S2).

The core orders, i.e., *Clostridiales* and *Lactobacillales*, both belonging to the different classes of the *Firmicutes* phylum, accounted for half of the data variance at this taxonomical level, showing some age correlation tendency (Table S3).

At the family level, the balance between *Ruminococcaceae* and *Enterococcaceae* (PC1), both representing the ultimately dominating *Firmicutes* phylum, correlated strongly with the age and BMI of the studied cohort, whereas a tiny portion of the data variance (PC10), structured by the balance between *Veillonellaceae* and *Erysipelotrichaceae*, both also belonging to *Firmicutes*, was found to be associated with age, glucose and transaminase activity (Table S4).

At the genus level, the relative abundance was structured mainly by the balance between *Prevotella* (*Bacteroidetes*) and *Enterococcus* (*Firmicutes*), PC1 showing a correlation with blood bilirubin (Table 3). The balance between *Faecalibacterium* and *Bifidobacterium* showed some association with glucose, whereas the relationship between *Blautia* and some unclassified genus of the *Ruminococcaceae* family (PC6) had a statistically significant correlation with blood bilirubin and transaminase activity (Table 3).

As for the species level, the major part of the relative abundance variance was accounted for by the relationship between *Enterococcus sp.* (*Firmicutes*) and *Prevotella copri* (*Bacteroidetes*), correlating with age, BMI and, possibly, blood glucose (Table 4), whereas small portions of the data variance, attributed to the balance between *Blautia luti* (*Firmicutes*) and *Akkermansia muciniphila* (PC6) and between two *Bifidobacterium* OTUs (PC8), could be partially ascribed to blood bilirubin and transaminase activity (Table 4).

Table 3. Statistical analyses' results: contribution of bacterial genera to the principal components extracted from the matrix with relative abundance in feces of females with gallstone disease before CCE (percentage of total variance in brackets) and *p*-values for multiple regression with blood biochemistry (coefficients of determination in brackets).

	Genera: PCA [1]			
Main	PC 1	PC 2	PC 5	PC 6
contributors	(35%)	(21%)	(5%)	(5%)
Prevotella	**0.10** [2] [0.41] [3]	**0.79** [−0.90]	0.00	0.00
Enterococcus	**0.84** [−0.97]	**0.07** [0.22]	0.01	0.00
Faecalibacterium	0.02	0.00	**0.17** [−0.37]	0.02
Blautia	0.00	0.03	0.01	**0.21** [0.50]
Bifidobacterium	0.01	0.04	**0.30** [−0.49]	0.00
Gemmiger	0.00	0.02	0.15 [0.45]	0.00
Ruminococcus	0.00	0.01	0.01	0.07 [−0.39]
un. *Ruminococcaceae*	0.00	0.01	0.01	**0.21** [−0.57]
		Genera: Multiple regression		
R/R[2]	0.72/0.51	0.56/0.32	0.64/0.41	0.71/0.50
Age	0.16	0.92	0.13	0.12
BMI	0.29	0.72	*0.09* [3]	0.42
Glucose	0.71	0.25	***0.03*** [4]	0.76
ALT	0.55	0.22	0.12	***0.03***
AST	0.73	0.48	*0.10*	***0.03***
Bilirubin	***0.04***	0.55	0.17	***0.04***

[1] PCA stands for principle component analysis (based on covariance). Only those principal components that (a) account for the bigger fraction of the total data variance and/or (b) displayed a statistically significant correlation with patients' characteristics are shown. [2] The values in bold show the two topmost contributions. [3] Factor loadings for variables (taxon relative abundance) are given in square brackets. [4] The values in bold italics and underlined italics are at $p \leq 0.05$ and $p \leq 0.10$, respectively.

Table 4. Statistical analyses' results: contribution of bacterial OTUs into the principal components extracted from the matrix with relative abundance in feces of females with gallstone disease before CCE (percentage of total variance in brackets) and *p*-values for multiple regression with age, BMI and blood biochemistry (coefficients of determination in brackets).

	OTUs: PCA [1]				
Main	PC 1	PC 3	PC 4	PC 6	PC 8
contributors	(40%)	(9%)	(7%)	(3%)	(2%)
Enterococcus sp.	**0.86** [2] [0.96] [3]	0.00	0.00	0.00	0.00
Escherichia/Shigella sp.	0.00	**0.25** [−0.65]	**0.25** [−0.57]	0.07	0.01
Gemmiger	0.00	0.01	**0.28** [0.67]	0.00	0.00
Faecalibacterium prausnitzii	0.01	**0.63** [0.86]	0.16 [−0.38]	0.06	0.02
Akkermansia muciniphila	0.00	0.02	0.09 [0.41]	**0.22** [−0.45]	0.09
Blautia luti	0.00	0.01	0.05	**0.26** [−0.56]	0.02
Bifidobacterium sp.	0.00	0.03	0.02	0.07 [−0.30]	**0.35** [−0.49]
Bifidobacterium sp.	0.00	0.00	0.00	0.19 [0.60]	**0.27** [−0.52]
Streptococcus sp.	0.00	0.00	0.00	0.02	0.13 [0.48]
Prevotella copri	**0.12** [−0.42]	0.00	0.00	0.01	0.00
		OTUs: Multiple regression			
R/R[2]	0.71/0.50	0.39/0.15	0.40/0.16	0.73/0.53	0.54/0.29
Age	***0.05*** [4]	0.16	0.34	0.55	0.11
BMI	***0.03***	*0.10*	0.92	*0.09*	0.35
Glucose	*0.07* [3]	0.58	*0.07*	0.39	0.76
ALT	0.52	0.65	0.92	***0.00***	***0.03***
AST	0.68	0.74	0.98	***0.00***	***0.03***
Bilirubin	0.16	0.95	0.64	***0.02***	***0.05***

[1] PCA stands for principle component analysis (based on covariance). Only those principal components that (a) account for the bigger fraction of the total data variance and/or (b) displayed a statistically significant correlation with patients' characteristics are shown. [2] The values in bold show the two topmost contributions. [3] Factor loadings for variables (taxon relative abundance) are given in square brackets. [4] The values in bold italics and underlined italics are at $p \leq 0.05$ and $p \leq 0.10$, respectively.

3.3. Changes in Fecal Bacteriobiome Composition in GSD Patients after the CCE Surgery

At the phylum level, CCE did not show any effect, whereas an effect was revealed for the *Clostridia* class and the *Clostridiales* and *Coriobacteriales* orders (Table 5). Further down the taxonomical hierarchy, the effect was displayed by the differential surgery-related abundance of the *Clostridiaceae_1*, *Lachnospiraceae* and *Peptoniphilaceae* families (all belonging to *Clostridiales*) and *Coriobacteriaceae* of the namesake order of the *Actinobacteria* phylum (Table 6). *Lachnospiraceae*, being the predominating family with 129 OTUs in the studied cohort, accounted for 20% of the total number of *Firmicutes* OTUs and ranked the top family in abundance (with ca. 20%); its decreased post-CCE abundance was manifested by *Blautia*, *Roseburia* and some unclassified representatives of the family at the genus level (Table 6).

Table 5. The relative abundance of some higher bacterial taxa in patients' feces before and after CCE.

	Before CCE		After CCE		*p*-Value
	Median	Mean ± SD	Median	Mean ± SD	
	Phyla (dominant)				
Firmicutes	66.7	65.7 ± 19.6	64.7	65.4 ± 21.4	0.34
Bacteroidetes	12.2	18.6 ± 19.8	11.0	19.2 ± 21.4	0.53
Actinobacteria	3.8	7.7 ± 10.6	4.0	7.2 ± 9.8	0.96
Proteobacteria	0.5	4.4 ± 8.4	0.8	2.8 ± 4.9	0.55
Verrucomicrobia	0.0	2.4 ± 6.6	0.0	3.8 ± 9.4	0.09
un. [1] *Bacteria*	0.1	0.14 ± 0.27	0.1	0.12 ± 0.23	0.20
	Classes (dominant)				
Clostridia [2]	49.3	46.8 ± 23.1	42.9	40.7 ± 23.1	0.01
Bacteroidia	12.2	18.6 ± 19.8	10.9	19.2 ± 21.4	0.47
Bacilli	1.2	11.1 ± 23.0	0.5	16.8 ± 30.0	0.51
Actinobacteria	3.8	7.7 ± 10.6	4.0	7.2 ± 9.8	0.97
Negativicutes	4.5	4.9 ± 3.9	3.0	5.2 ± 6.3	0.84
Verrucomicrobiae	0.0	2.4 ± 6.6	0.0	3.8 ± 9.4	0.09
Gammaproteobacteria	0.0	3.5 ± 8.2	0.0	2.1 ± 5.0	0.43
un. *Firmicutes*	0.3	1.5 ± 3.2	0.5	1.4 ± 1.9	0.70
Erysipelotrichia	0.5	1.4 ± 3.5	0.4	1.4 ± 2.6	0.29
	Orders (dominant)				
Clostridiales	43.3	44.8 ± 23.5	40.5	39.0 ± 23.2	0.01
Bacteroidales	12.5	20.4 ± 20.4	14.6	21.3 ± 22.2	0.47
Lactobacillales	1.2	12.0 ± 22.5	0.9	16.9 ± 28.9	0.50
Selenomonadales	4.5	5.2 ± 4.5	3.2	5.7 ± 6.7	0.84
Bifidobacteriales	0.7	4.9 ± 9.6	0.0	4.4 ± 8.8	0.53
Verrucomicrobiales	0.0	2.3 ± 6.4	0.0	3.5 ± 9.1	0.09
Enterobacteriales	0.0	3.3 ± 7.7	0.0	1.9 ± 4.7	0.39
Coriobacteriales	0.8	1.9 ± 2.2	1.0	2.4 ± 2.7	0.03
Erysipelotrichales	0.5	1.4 ± 3.4	0.4	1.3 ± 2.5	0.25

[1] un. stands for unclassified. [2] Gray-shadowed lines have *p*-values ≤ 0.05.

Table 6. The relative abundance of some bacterial families, genera and OTUs in patients' feces before and after CCE.

Taxon	Before CCE		After CCE		p-Value
	Median	Mean ± SD	Median	Mean ± SD	
		Families			
Clostridiaceae_1 [4]		0.2 ± 0.4		0.3 ± 0.5	0.010
Lachnospiraceae		20.3 ± 14.8		16.6 ± 14.0	0.032
Coriobacteriaceae		1.9 ± 2.3		2.4 ± 2.8	0.033
Peptoniphilaceae		0.005 ± 0.013		0.002 ± 0.007	0.036
Peptostreptococcaceae		0.4 ± 0.6		0.6 ± 1.0	0.054
Ruminococcaceae		22.9 ± 15.9		19.5 ± 13.8	0.056
Rhodospirillaceae		0.1 ± 0.4		0.01 ± 0.05	0.059
Enterococcaceae		7.4 ± 20.8		13.6 ± 26.4	0.080
		Genera			
Clostridium s.s.		0.2 ± 0.4		0.3 ± 0.5	0.010
Gordonibacter		0.01 ± 0.04		0.01 ± 0.07	0.036
Peptoniphilus		0.005 ± 0.013		0.002 ± 0.007	0.036
un [1]. Rhodospirillaceae		0.08 ± 0.36		0.01 ± 0.05	0.059
Gemmiger		4.3 ± 7.4		3.2 ± 4.8	0.065
Collinsella		1.0 ± 1.8		1.3 ± 2.1	0.066
Blautia		6.4 ± 8.8		4.9 ± 7.3	0.067
Enterococcus		7.4 ± 20.8		13.6 ± 26.4	0.080
Faecalibacterium		7.7 ± 9.8		6.1 ± 8.6	0.089
Roseburia		2.8 ± 4.9		1.6 ± 2.5	0.089
Dialister		1.5 ± 2.5		1.0 ± 2.1	0.093
Peptostreptococcus		0.018 ± 0.063		0.024 ± 0.077	0.093
Lachnospiracea i.s.		2.1 ± 2.0		1.5 ± 1.6	0.094
		OTUs			
un.Lachnospiraceae		0.09 ± 0.17		0.04 ± 0.11	0.003
un.Clostridium s.s. [2]		0.14 ± 0.43		0.3 ± 0.5	0.005
un.Clostridium XIVa		0.01 ± 0.03		0.03 ± 0.05	0.021
un.Clostridiales		0.02 ± 0.06		0.09 ± 0.19	0.023
Clostridium leptum		0.05 ± 0.10		0.03 ± 0.07	0.025
un.Blautia		0.02 ± 0.06		0.03 ± 0.08	0.029
Ruminococcus faecis		0.4 ± 1.4		0.6 ± 1.5	0.030
un.Bacteroides		2.1 ± 3.4		1.0 ± 2.0	0.033
Dialister invisus		1.0 ± 2.1		0.4 ± 1.0	0.035
un.Ruminococcus		0.15 ± 0.37		0.07 ± 0.24	0.036
un.Ruminococcus		0.2 ± 0.6		0.07 ± 0.29	0.042
un.Lachnospiracea i.s. [3]		0.5 ± 0.8		0.2 ± 0.4	0.050
un.Coriobacteriaceae		0.04 ± 0.09		0.14 ± 0.40	0.059
un.Ruminococcaceae		0.09 ± 0.16		0.18 ± 0.30	0.068
un.Ruminococcaceae		0.0008 ± 0.0017		0.0002 ± 0.001	0.076
un.Enterococcus		7.4 ± 20.8		13.6 ± 26.4	0.080
un.Lachnospiraceae		0.01 ± 0.02		0.002 ± 0.007	0.080
un.Clostridiales		0.01 ± 0.03		0.03 ± 0.08	0.083
un.Collinsella		1.0 ± 1.8		1.3 ± 2.1	0.093
Peptostreptococcus stomatis		0.02 ± 0.06		0.02 ± 0.08	0.093

[1] un. stands for unclassified; [2] s.s. stands for *sensu stricto*; [3] i.s. stands for *incertae sedis*. [4] Gray-shadowed lines have p-values ≤ 0.05.

As for other genera, *Clostridium sensu stricto* increased, whereas *Peptoniphilus* decreased their presence in the fecal bacteriobiome of the studied cohort. Although *Coriobacteriaceae* increased their post-CCE abundance and were among the predominating families, at the genus level, they were represented by eight genera, only one of which (*Gordonibacter*) had a differential CCE-related abundance ($p \leq 0.05$), albeit at the very low level, and *Collinsella* with its post-CCE increased abundance at the $p \leq 0.10$ level (Table 6). At the species level, 20 OTUs manifested surgery-related differences in their relative abundance at the $p \leq 0.10$ level of statistical significance, with 17 OTUs attributed to *Firmicutes*, two OTUs to *Actinobacteria* and one OTU to the *Bacteroidetes* phylum. *Enterococcus* sp. of *Firmicutes* was the leading dominant, increasing its abundance almost two-fold after the surgery (Table 6). *Bacteroides* sp. and *Collinsella* sp. were minor dominants with relative abundance around 1%. The rest of the OTUs with differential CCE-related abundance were minor or rare species.

The results of GLM analysis with repeated measures (before and after CCE) and age and BMI as continuous factors (covariates) show that residuals complied with a normal distribution only for the *Firmicutes* taxa; nevertheless, this statistical approach revealed no CCE-associated effect on the phylum and its lower taxa abundance.

3.4. Fecal Bacteriobiome α-Diversity before and after the CCE Surgery

No differences in α-diversity indices at the $p \leq 0.05$ level were found in the studied cohort before and after CCE (Table 7). However, at the $p \leq 0.10$ level, evenness slightly decreased, whereas the maximal relative abundance (as shown by the Berger–Parker index) slightly increased. The location of samples in the plane of the first two principal coordinates (based on Bray–Curtis distance) did not reveal any distinct CCE-related pattern (Figure 2).

Table 7. Alpha-diversity indices estimated for patients' fecal bacterial assemblages before and after CCE.

Index	Before CCE Median	Before CCE Mean ± SD	After CCE Median	After CCE Mean ± SD	*p*-Value
OTUs' richness	90	93 ± 41	78	92 ± 46	0.89
Chao-1	100	104 ± 51	85	104 ± 55	0.75
Berger–Parker	0.24	0.29 ± 0.19	0.27	0.33 ± 0.21	0.07
Dominance (D)	0.12	0.16 ± 0.16	0.12	0.19 ± 0.17	0.11
Simpson (1-D)	0.88	0.84 ± 0.16	0.88	0.81 ± 0.17	0.11
Shannon	2.8	2.8 ± 0.8	2.7	2.7 ± 0.9	0.21
Evenness	0.23	0.22 ± 0.08	0.20	0.20 ± 0.09	0.09
Equitability	0.67	0.63 ± 0.13	0.62	0.60 ± 0.15	0.13

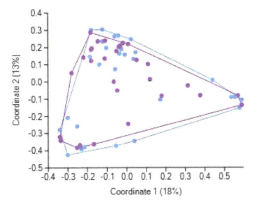

Figure 2. Location of patients' samples taken before (violet markers) and after (blue markers) CCE in the plane of the first two principal coordinates (Bray–Curtis distance).

3.5. Blood Biochemical Characteristics before and after the CCE Surgery

After CCE, both aspartate and alanine transaminase activity mean values increased 1.7 and 1.6 times, with bilirubin levels being unaffected (Table 8). Age and BMI as continuous predictors in GLM analysis with repeated measures decreased the p-value for glucose content comparison ($p = 0.06$) while increasing it for direct bilirubin content ($p = 0.80$) (residuals for only these two dependent variables showed a normal distribution).

Table 8. Blood biochemical test results before and after CCE.

Property	Before CCE		After CCE		p-Value
	Median	Mean $\pm$ SD	Median	Mean $\pm$ SD	
Glucose, mmol/L	5.25	5.24 $\pm$ 0.88	5.45	5.51 $\pm$ 0.82	0.107
Alanine transaminase, U/L	20.2	36.0 $\pm$ 68.5	29.0	57.4 $\pm$ 75.7	0.001
Aspartate transaminase, U/L	19.9	34.4 $\pm$ 47.9	32.3	56.8 $\pm$ 68.4	0.001
Bilirubin total, mcmol/L	15.1	18.8 $\pm$ 21.1	16.3	18.4 $\pm$ 7.0	0.168
Bilirubin direct, mcmol/L	11.8	12.4 $\pm$ 6.0	13.3	12.7 $\pm$ 5.7	0.186
Bilirubin indirect, mcmol/L	3.5	6.4 $\pm$ 16.7	3.6	3.7 $\pm$ 1.7	0.190

4. Discussion

4.1. Fecal Bacteriobiome Composition in GSD Patients before the CCE Surgery

In the studied cohort of GSD-afflicted female patients, the *Firmicutes* phylum was the ultimate dominant in the fecal bacteriobiome, with *Bacteroidetes* and *Actinobacteria* being second and third in the ranking of abundance. In this aspect, our cohort differed from a Chinese one, where *Proteobacteria*, instead of *Actinobacteria*, were found to be third in abundance, and *Bacteroidetes* were almost twice as abundant as in our cohort [22]. Moreover, in our cohort, the *Firmicutes* relative abundance was markedly higher, as compared with the Chinese cohorts [5,21]. The apparent discrepancy is most likely due to the fact that one third of the Chinese cohort were males, whereas ours was a purely female one; and to the difference in diet [23]. As for the biodiversity indices, however, the ones calculated in our study agree well with the indices describing the fecal bacteriobiome of a Chinese cohort of GSD patients [21].

High inter-individual variation in bacterial sequence reads is quite common in fecal bacteriobiome studies in cohorts of healthy human subjects and of those afflicted by various diseases, including GSD [21]. Even in cases when the authors [21] claimed that their results "showed that the individual differences within the group were small", the huge standard deviations for the OTUs' relative abundance in their study proved the opposite. Therefore, by structuring down the data variance in our study by principal component analysis, we identified some age- and BMI-related taxa within the studied cohort, as well as some taxa that showed a correlation with blood glucose, bilirubin and transaminase activity.

Some genera of *Lachnospiraceae* are known to be important for bile acid metabolism, having 7α-dehydroxylation activity: in the pre-CCE bacteriobiome of the studied cohort, the family accounted for one fifth of the total number of sequence reads, along with *Ruminocccaceae* ultimately prevailing at the family level and together accounting for almost half of the abundance; in a Chinese cohort, however, the family with less than 0.3% was not even close to any dominating position [21]. The latter study also found the relative abundance of *Clostridium* to be 0.01%, whereas in our study, the presence of *Clostridium sensu stricto* was an order of magnitude more pronounced (Table 6). The differences are plentiful and most likely attributable to racial, dietary, sex and other characteristics of the cohorts.

Principal component analysis based on covariance allows dealing with the original variance of the data, without standardizing them, easily structuring the variance by extracted principal components, featuring the contribution of the original variables to the new ones (PCs) and reducing the original plethora of variables to fewer ones (PCs), but accounting for most of the original variance in the data. Subjection of the extracted PCs as dependent variables in multiple regression analysis allowed finding links with patients' demographics and blood biochemical properties and bacterially interpreting them on the basis of a taxon contribution in the respective PC. We believe this approach to be informative for such kind of descriptive study.

The balance between two *Firmicutes* classes, namely, *Clostridia* and *Bacilli*, accounted for almost half of the abundance variance at this taxonomic level, being positively correlated with age at the $p \leq 0.10$ level; the situation was translated in a similar manner at the order level, i.e., *Clostridiales* and *Lactobacillales*. Then, at the family level, the balance between *Ruminococcaceae* (*Clostridiales*) and *Enterococcaceae* (*Lactobacillales*), accounting for one third of the total data variance (PC1), displayed a statistically significant positive correlation with age. This finding complies with the knowledge that the gut microbiota diversity changes with age [24,25], with *Firmicutes* taxa increasing. Thus, the increased abundance of the core gut bacterial taxa with age in GSD-compromised subjects seems quite a natural occurrence, not overshadowed by changed bile acid metabolism and other factors. Interestingly, at the genus level, the structure of the data variance shifted, with the *Prevotella* (*Bacteroidetes*) and *Enterococcus* (*Firmicutes*) relationship accounting for half of the total data variance at this taxonomic level; the finding underscores the importance of these two core taxa relationships in structuring the gut bacteriome in general and GSD-compromised female patients in particular. As increased plasma levels of bilirubin (secondary to the breakdown of free hemoglobin) were shown to be associated with an increased risk of gallstone disease [26], the statistically significant positive correlation of the *Prevotella–Enterococcus* balance with blood bilirubin, found in our study, necessitates further investigation of the role of the genera in gallstone formation, both pigmented and cholesterol ones [27].

The finding that the balance between *Faecalibacterium, Bifidobacterium* and *Gemminer* determined 10% of the total data variance and was correlated with blood glucose ($p \leq 0.05$) and BMI ($p \leq 0.10$) may be indicative of the indirect association of the genera with glucose metabolism and insulin sensitivity in overweight patients [28], but we cannot currently suggest the putative cause–effect mechanism. The joint variation in *Blautia, Ruminococcus* and some unclassified *Ruminococcaceae* correlated with blood ALT, AST and bilirubin, and the mechanism of the involvement of these genera has to be comprehensively examined.

Further down the hierarchy at the species level, the *Prevotella–Enterococcus* relationship was manifested by the balance between *Prevotella copri* and *Enterococcus* sp. (with 40% of the total data variance), which was positively correlated with the cohort's demographics, i.e., age and BMI ($p \leq 0.05$), and glucose ($p \leq 0.10$) and therefore may be related to glucose metabolism in overweight patients. Interestingly, *Akkermansia muciniphila* was found to contribute a small portion of the data variance associated with blood biochemistry (at $p \leq 0.05$) and, hence, generally with the disease-compromised status of the subjects. The increased relative abundance of this mucin-degrading bacterium is often found to be associated with disease [29,30]; however, as a propionogenic bacterium, *A. muciniphila* is also believed to have several health benefits in humans [31].

However, as the blood characteristics are far from being specific for gallstone disease diagnostics, it is not possible to implicate the taxa in the changed bile acid metabolism and gallstone formation based on the results of multiple regression analysis, despite the comprehensive outline of the GSD bacteriobiome variation as related to the common blood biochemical properties. The bile acid profiles of the studied patients, if they had been determined, might have been more suggestive in this respect, and we acknowledge this as a drawback in the study.

4.2. Changes in Fecal Bacteriobiome Composition in GSD Patients after the CCE Surgery

In the studied cohort of GSD-afflicted female patients, mainly members of the *Firmicutes* phylum displayed CCE-related differential abundance.

As for the *Bacteroidetes* phylum, its relative abundance did not change after CCE; the result does not agree with the finding of Israeli researchers, for example, when the phylum abundance was shown to be increased in the post-CCE cohort of subjects [32]. However, the time factor, i.e., the duration of the time span elapsed between CCE and feces sampling, is a critical factor affecting bacterial composition [33] and may, at least partially, explain the discrepancy between results.

The decreased abundance of *Clostridia* (by 7%) and *Clostridiales* (by 3–5%), found after CCE in our study, was not reported before. As these taxa are the most species-rich and physiologically diverse components of the fecal bacteriobiome, the CCE-associated shifts in their relative abundance cannot be unequivocally regarded as beneficial or not for human health. *Lachnospiraceae*, the most predominant family in the human gut, displayed decreased abundance in the post-CCE bacteriobiome, which is, however, difficult to interpret as (a) most of the OTU-level clusters (69), ascribed to the family in our study (129), could not be taxonomically attributed below the family level, and (b) some genera and species of this family might support/contribute to healthy functions, whereas other genera and species were found to be increased in diseases [34]. For example, *Blautia* and *Roseburia* species, often associated with a healthy state, are some of the main short-chain fatty acid producers [35,36]; therefore, their post-CCE decreased abundance ($p \leq 0.10$) may hardly be indicative of the better state of the gut bacteriobiome after surgery.

We could not find any information about the effect of CCE on *Actinobacteria/Coriobacteriales/Coriobacteriaceae* representatives, the latter known as pathobionts. As for *Collinsella*, the dominant genus in the *Coriobacteriaceae* family and the minor dominant in the studied cohort, its increased abundance after CCE (albeit at the $p \leq 0.10$ level) suggests negative implications after such shift [37–40]. As for another representative of the family with differential pre- and post-CCE abundance, i.e., the *Gordonibacter* genus with just ca. 0.01% of the total number of sequence reads, it is difficult to suggest any ecophysiological significance at such abundance rate, although some genus representatives are known to participate in primary bile acid transformation [41] or be involved in dietary polyphenol transformations generating more bioactive metabolites [42].

Interestingly, although specific bacterial species such as *Helicobacter* and *Salmonella* were shown to be involved in the pathogenesis of cholesterol gallstones [43], we did not find *Helicobacter* at all, and found only one *Salmonella* OTU with 0.3 and 0.6% abundance in pre- and post-CCE subcohorts, respectively; the finding infers potentially different bacterial involvement in GSD etiology in cohorts of different sex and ethnicity.

The actual number of OTUs per sample observed in our study was practically the same as the number obtained by the same methodology for post-CCE patients in Korea [44]. However, as the latter study did not report whether the control group, i.e., non-CCE control patients, was also diagnosed with GSD, it is not possible to compare our results about the CCE effect on the fecal bacteriobiome with those results in their entirety, only for the post-CCE subcohort. For instance, in our study, CCE did not affect the gut bacteriobiome species richness, whereas compared with the independent control group, CCE decreased it [43]. Notably, the α-biodiversity index (Shannon) reported in the aforementioned study was much higher than the one reported here (4.9 vs. 2.8): in our view, the discrepancy may be attributed to both the sex composition of the Korean cohort and the dietary habits, etc. At the same time, for the Israeli cohort of GDS patients, the pre- and post-CCE values of the Shannon index did not differ [31], being close to, but slightly lower than, those in our study (2.1 vs. 2.8, respectively). We cannot help but emphasize that often the studies claiming to reveal the effect of CCE on the gut microbiota performed comparisons between the post-CCE patients with GSD and the healthy subjects without a GSD history [33,43,44]. We believe such approach does not seem to be adequate for aiming to examine the effect of CCE per se, as only a direct comparison between pre- and post-CCE conditions of one and the same cohort of GSD-affected subjects is pertinent for the goal of revealing microbiome shifts associated with the surgery and potential biomarkers of the latter.

It was shown that CCE did not markedly affect the bile acid profile in the GSD patients [31], leading the authors to conclude that the modified fecal bile acid composition results from inherently aberrant bile acid metabolism, leading, in turn, to gallstone formation. In general, our finding that the pre- and post-CCE fecal bacteriobiome profiles were not overall differentially distinct (as revealed by principal coordinate analysis) apparently complies with this conclusion. It should be emphasized that the repeated collection of feces samples was performed 1–3 days after the surgery, i.e., quite soon. Therefore, we are inclined to believe that it was a very short time to interpret the observed differential abundance of some bacterial taxa as solely resultant from the changed inflow of bile acids; the overall post-surgery condition most likely contributed significantly, if not primarily and predominantly, to the observed short-term CCE-related shifts in fecal bacterial assemblages. It should be noted that the overall post-surgery condition included ceftriaxone treatment of all patients. This beta-lactam antibiotic is able to kill a broad spectrum of bacteria [45], thus potentially shaping the gut bacteriobiome [46], especially when administered orally. Therefore, despite the very short time between the surgery and stool collection in this study, and hence the short time of antibiotic treatment, the revealed changes in the fecal bacteriobiome might have resulted, in part, due to the antibiotic per se. However, we should also emphasize that our study did not aim at discriminating between the effects of post-CCE altered bile profiles and antibiotic therapy; we aimed at profiling the gut bacteriobiome, referring to post-CCE as a single factor, as such embracing many factors, aspects, nuances, etc. We described the fecal bacteriobiome just at the starting point of patients embarking on the rest of life without a gallbladder. Whether the longer-term shifts in the gut microbiota after CCE will occur and to what degree and at what rate remain to be determined in future studies, which, hopefully, will also elucidate if gut microbes can act as the main character in the broad scenery of liver diseases [47].

5. Conclusions

Our study provides the first detailed inventory of the fecal bacteriobiome in a Russian cohort of female patients with gallstone disease. It will help to construct a global picture of the disease-related bacteriobiome and eventually focus on specific bacterial taxa involved in gallstone formation, thus facilitating the development of non-invasive therapeutic tools for preventing and treating gallstone disease. The shifts found in the fecal microbiota just a few days after CCE did not distinctly discriminate between the pre- and post-surgery bacterial diversity profiles. Therefore, the shifts can be mostly attributed to the surgery effect on the entire status of the patients, including the initial stages of the changing bile inflow and metabolism, as well as cellular and molecular modifications in the gut. The presented pre- and post-cholecystectomy microbiota profiles in one and the same cohort of patients may improve the insight into the relationship between the fecal, gut and bile microbiota, contributing to future larger-scale studies of altered human bile metabolism/profiles and associated disorders.

Supplementary Materials: The following are available online at https://www.mdpi.com/article/10.3390/jpm11040294/s1, Figure S1: Rarefaction curves based on bacterial OTUs for the patients with gallstone disease before (a) and after (b) the cholecystectomy. The numbers in blue indicate patients' codes; Table S1: The ratio of Firmicutes/Bacteroidetes relative abundance in patients' feces before and after CCE.: Table S2: Statistical analyses' results: contribution of bacterial classes into the principal components extracted from the matrix with relative abundance in feces of females with gallstone disease before the CCE (percentage of total variance in brackets) and p-values for multiple regression with age, BMI and blood biochemistry; Table S3: Statistical analyses' results: contribution of bacterial orders into the principal components extracted from the matrix with relative abundance in feces of females with gallstone disease before the CCE (percentage of total variance in brackets) and p-values for multiple regression with age, BMI and blood biochemistry; Table S4: Statistical analyses' results: contribution of bacterial families into the principal components extracted from the matrix with relative abundance in feces of females with gallstone disease before the CCE (percentage of total variance in brackets) and p-values for multiple regression with age, BMI and blood biochemistry (coefficients of determination in brackets).

Author Contributions: Conceptualization, I.G.; methodology, I.G. and M.K.; software, M.K.; validation, M.K.; formal analysis, I.G. and T.A.; investigation, T.R. and A.K.; resources, I.G. and M.K.; data curation, N.N., T.R. and T.A.; writing—original draft preparation, N.N. and T.R.; writing—review and editing, I.G.; visualization, A.K.; supervision, I.G.; project administration, I.G. and M.K.; funding acquisition, I.G. All authors have read and agreed to the published version of the manuscript.

Funding: This research was funded by Russian State funded budget projects AAAA-A17-117112850280-2 and AAAA-A17-117020210021-7 with the financial support of the Biocodex MICROBIOTA Foundation, France.

Institutional Review Board Statement: The study was conducted according to the guidelines of the Declaration of Helsinki, and approved by the Institutional Review Board of the Research Institute of Internal and Preventive Medicine–Branch of the Institute of Cytology and Genetics SB RAS, Novosibirsk, Russia (protocol 38/1, approved 5 June 2018).

Informed Consent Statement: Informed consent was obtained from all subjects involved in the study.

Data Availability Statement: The read data reported in this study were submitted to GenBank under the study accession number PRJNA687360 (https://www.ncbi.nlm.nih.gov/bioproject/?term=PRJNA687360).

Acknowledgments: The authors are very thankful to Semyon Chastnykh (Municipal Clinical Hospital No. 2, Novosibirsk, Russia) for his superb technical assistance.

Conflicts of Interest: The authors declare no conflict of interest. The funders had no role in the design of the study; in the collection, analyses, or interpretation of data; in the writing of the manuscript, or in the decision to publish the results.

References

1. Ilchenko, A.A. *Diseases of the Gallbladder and Bile Ducts: Manual for Physicians*, 2nd ed.; Medical Information Agency Publishers LLC: Moscow, Russia, 2011; 458p. (In Russian)
2. Vinnik, Y.S.; Serova, E.V.; Andreev, R.I.; Leyman, A.V.; Struzik, A.S. Conservative and surgical treatment of gallstone disease. *Fudamental Res.* **2013**, *9*, 954–958. (In Russian)
3. Grigor'eva, I.N.; Romanova, T.I. Gallstone Disease and Microbiome. *Microorganisms* **2020**, *8*, 835. [CrossRef] [PubMed]
4. Rezasoltani, S.; Sadeghi, A.; Radinnia, E.; Naseh, A.; Gholamrezaei, Z.; Azizmohammad Looha, M.; Yadegar, A. The association between gut microbiota, cholesterol gallstones, and colorectal cancer. *Gastroenterol. Hepatol. Bed Bench* **2019**, *12* (Suppl. 1), S8–S13.
5. Wu, T.; Zhang, Z.; Liu, B.; Hou, D.; Liang, Y.; Zhang, J.; Shi, P. Gut microbiota dysbiosis and bacterial community assembly associated with cholesterol gallstones in large-scale study. *BMC Genom.* **2013**, *14*, 669. [CrossRef] [PubMed]
6. Wang, Q.; Jiao, L.; He, C.; Sun, H.; Cai, Q.; Han, T.; Hu, H. Alteration of gut microbiota in association with cholesterol gallstone formation in mice. *BMC Gastroenterol.* **2017**, *17*, 74. [CrossRef] [PubMed]
7. Chen, W.; Wei, Y.; Xiong, A.; Li, Y.; Guan, H.; Wang, Q.; Miao, Q.; Bian, Z.; Xiao, X.; Lian, M.; et al. Comprehensive Analysis of Serum and Fecal Bile Acid Profiles and Interaction with Gut Microbiota in Primary Biliary Cholangitis. *Clin. Rev. Allergy Immunol.* **2020**, *58*, 25–38. [CrossRef]
8. Di Ciaula, A.; Wang, D.Q.; Portincasa, P. Cholesterol cholelithiasis: Part of a systemic metabolic disease, prone to primary prevention. *Expert Rev. Gastroenterol. Hepatol.* **2019**, *13*, 157–171. [CrossRef]
9. Upala, S.; Sanguankeo, A.; Jaruvongvanich, V. Gallstone Disease and the Risk of Cardiovascular Disease: A Systematic Review and Meta-Analysis of Observational Studies. *Scand. J. Surg.* **2017**, *106*, 21–27. [CrossRef]
10. Fairfield, C.J.; Wigmore, S.J.; Harrison, E.M. Gallstone Disease and the Risk of Cardiovascular Disease. *Sci. Rep.* **2019**, *9*, 5830. [CrossRef]
11. Ramírez-Pérez, O.; Cruz-Ramón, V.; Chinchilla-López, P.; Méndez-Sánchez, N. The Role of the Gut Microbiota in Bile Acid Metabolism. *Ann. Hepatol.* **2017**, *16* (Suppl. 1), s15–s20. [CrossRef]
12. Chankhamjon, P.; Javdan, B.; Lopez, J.; Hull, R.; Chatterjee, S.; Donia, M.S. Systematic mapping of drug metabolism by the human gut microbiome. *bioRxiv* **2019**. bioRxiv:538215.
13. Zimmermann, M.; Zimmermann-Kogadeeva, M.; Wegmann, R.; Goodman, A.L. Mapping human microbiome drug metabolism by gut bacteria and their genes. *Nature* **2019**, *570*, 462–467. [CrossRef]
14. Grigor'eva, I.N. Gallstone Disease, Obesity and the Firmicutes/Bacteroidetes Ratio as a Possible Biomarker of Gut Dysbiosis. *J. Pers. Med.* **2021**, *11*, 13. [CrossRef]

15. Godon, J.J.; Zumstein, E.; Dabert, P.; Habouzit, F.; Moletta, R. Molecular microbial diversity of an anaerobic digestor as determined by small-subunit rDNA sequence analysis. *Appl. Environ. Microbiol.* **1997**, *63*, 2802–2813. [CrossRef]
16. Fadrosh, D.W.; Ma, B.; Gajer, P.; Sengamalay, N.; Ott, S.; Brotman, R.M.; Ravel, J. An improved dual-indexing approach for multiplexed 16S rRNA gene sequencing on the Illumina MiSeq platform. *Microbiome* **2014**, *2*, 1–6. [CrossRef]
17. Igolkina, A.A.; Grekhov, G.A.; Pershina, E.V.; Samosorov, G.G.; Leunova, V.M.; Semenov, A.N.; Baturina, O.A.; Kabilov, M.R.; Andronov, E.E. Identifying components of mixed and contaminated soil samples by detecting specific signatures of control 16S rRNA libraries. *Ecol. Ind.* **2018**, *94*, 446–453. [CrossRef]
18. Edgar, R.C. UPARSE: Highly accurate OTU sequences from microbial amplicon reads. *Nat. Meth.* **2013**, *10*, 996–998. [CrossRef]
19. Edgar, R.C. SINTAX, a Simple Non-Bayesian Taxonomy Classifier for 16S and ITS Sequences. *bioRxiv* **2016**. [CrossRef]
20. Wang, Q.; Garrity, G.M.; Tiedje, J.M.; Cole, J.R. Na ve Bayesian Classifier for Rapid Assignment of rRNA Sequences into the New Bacterial Taxonomy. *Appl. Environ. Microbiol.* **2007**, *73*, 5261–5267. [CrossRef]
21. Hammer, O.; Harper, D.A.T.; Ryan, P.D. PAST: Paleontological Statistics Software Package for Education and Data Analysis. *Palaeontol. Electron.* **2001**, *4*, 9.
22. Wang, Q.; Hao, C.; Yao, W.; Zhu, D.; Lu, H.; Li, L.; Ma, B.; Sun, B.; Xue, D.; Zhang, W. Intestinal flora imbalance affects bile acid metabolism and is associated with gallstone formation. *BMC Gastroenterol.* **2020**, *20*, 59. [CrossRef]
23. Gutiérrez-Díaz, I.; Molinero, N.; Cabrera, A.; Rodríguez, J.I.; Margolles, A.; Delgado, S.; González, S. Diet: Cause or Consequence of the Microbial Profile of Cholelithiasis Disease? *Nutrients* **2018**, *10*, 1307. [CrossRef]
24. Vaiserman, A.; Romanenko, M.; Piven, L.; Moseiko, V.; Lushchak, O.; Kryzhanovska, N.; Guryanov, V.; Koliada, A. Differences in the gut Firmicutes to Bacteroidetes ratio across age groups in healthy Ukrainian population. *BMC Microbiol.* **2020**, *20*, 221. [CrossRef]
25. Rinninella, E.; Cintoni, M.; Raoul, P.; Lopetuso, L.R.; Scaldaferri, F.; Pulcini, G.; Miggiano, G.A.D.; Gasbarrini, A.; Mele, M.C. Food Components and Dietary Habits: Keys for a Healthy Gut Microbiota Composition. *Nutrients* **2019**, *11*, 2393. [CrossRef] [PubMed]
26. Vítek, L.; Carey, M.C. New pathophysiological concepts underlying pathogenesis of pigment gallstones. *Clin. Res. Hepatol. Gastroenterol.* **2012**, *36*, 122–129. [CrossRef]
27. Stender, S.; Frikke-Schmidt, R.; Nordestgaard, B.G.; Tybjærg-Hansen, A. Extreme Bilirubin Levels as a Causal Risk Factor for Symptomatic Gallstone Disease. *JAMA Intern. Med.* **2013**, *173*, 1222–1228. [CrossRef]
28. Di Ciaula, A.; Wang, D.Q.; Portincasa, P. An update on the pathogenesis of cholesterol gallstone disease. *Curr. Opin. Gastroenterol.* **2018**, *34*, 71–80. [CrossRef]
29. Gandy, K.; Zhang, J.; Nagarkatti, P.; Nagarkatti, M. The role of gut microbiota in shaping the relapse-remitting and chronic-progressive forms of multiple sclerosis in mouse models. *Sci. Rep.* **2019**, *9*, 6923. [CrossRef]
30. Kozhieva, M.; Naumova, N.; Alikina, T.; Boyko, A.; Vlassov, V.; Kabilov, M. Primary progressive multiple sclerosis in a Russian cohort: Relationship with gut bacterial diversity. *BMC Microbiol.* **2019**, *19*, 309. [CrossRef]
31. Jayachandran, M.; Chung, S.S.M.; Xu, B. A critical review of the relationship between dietary components, the gut microbe *Akkermansia muciniphila*, and human health. *Crit. Rev. Food Sci. Nutr.* **2019**, *60*, 1–12. [CrossRef]
32. Keren, N.; Konikoff, F.M.; Paitan, Y.; Gabay, G.; Reshef, L.; Naftali, T.; Gophna, U. Interactions between the intestinal microbiota and bile acids in gallstones patients. *Environ. Microbiol. Rep.* **2015**, *7*, 874–880. [CrossRef] [PubMed]
33. Ren, X.; Xu, J.; Zhang, Y.; Chen, G.; Zhang, Y.; Huang, Q.; Liu, Y. Bacterial Alterations in Post-Cholecystectomy Patients Are Associated with Colorectal Cancer. *Front. Oncol.* **2020**, *10*, 1418. [CrossRef] [PubMed]
34. Vacca, M.; Celano, G.; Calabrese, F.M.; Portincasa, P.; Gobbetti, M.; de Angelis, M. The Controversial Role of Human Gut *Lachnospiraceae*. *Microorganisms* **2020**, *8*, 573. [CrossRef] [PubMed]
35. Koh, A.; de Vadder, F.; Kovatcheva-Datchary, P.; Bäckhed, F. From Dietary Fiber to Host Physiology: Short-Chain Fatty Acids as Key Bacterial Metabolites. *Cell* **2016**, *165*, 1332–1345. [CrossRef]
36. La Rosa, S.L.; Leth, M.L.; Michalak, L.; Hansen, M.E.; Pudlo, N.A.; Glowacki, R.; Pereira, G.; Workman, C.T.; Arntzen, M.Ø.; Pope, P.B.; et al. The human gut Firmicute Roseburia intestinalis is a primary degrader of dietary β-mannans. *Nat. Comm.* **2019**, *10*, 905. [CrossRef]
37. Chow, J.; Tang, H.; Mazmanian, S.K. Pathobionts of the gastrointestinal microbiota and inflammatory disease. *Curr. Opin. Immunol.* **2011**, *23*, 473–480.
38. Chen, J.; Wright, K.; Davis, J.M.; Jeraldo, P.; Marietta, E.V.; Murray, J.; Nelson, H.; Matteson, E.L.; Taneja, V. An expansion of rare lineage intestinal microbes characterizes rheumatoid arthritis. *Genome Med.* **2016**, *8*, 43. [CrossRef]
39. Gomez-Arango, L.F.; Barrett, H.L.; Wilkinson, S.A.; Callaway, L.K.; McIntyre, H.D.; Morrison, M.; Dekker Nitert, M. Low dietary fiber intake increases Collinsella abundance in the gut microbiota of overweight and obese pregnant women. *Gut Microbes* **2018**, *9*, 189–201. [CrossRef]
40. Astbury, S.; Atallah, E.; Vijay, A.; Aithal, G.P.; Grove, J.I.; Valdes, A.M. Lower gut microbiome diversity and higher abundance of proinflammatory genus Collinsella are associated with biopsy-proven nonalcoholic steatohepatitis. *Gut Microbes* **2020**, *11*, 569–580. [CrossRef]
41. Heinken, A.; Ravcheev, D.A.; Baldini, F.; Heirendt, L.; Fleming, R.M.; Thiele, I. Systematic assessment of secondary bile acid metabolism in gut microbes reveals distinct metabolic capabilities in inflammatory bowel disease. *Microbiome* **2019**, *7*, 75. [CrossRef]

42. Corrêa, T.; Rogero, M.M.; Hassimotto, N.; Lajolo, F.M. The Two-Way Polyphenols-Microbiota Interactions and Their Effects on Obesity and Related Metabolic Diseases. *Front. Nutr.* **2019**, *6*, 188. [CrossRef]
43. Wang, W.; Wang, J.; Li, J.; Yan, P.; Jin, Y.; Zhang, R.; Yue, W.; Guo, Q.; Geng, J. Cholecystectomy Damages Aging-Associated Intestinal Microbiota Construction. *Front. Microbiol.* **2018**, *9*, 1402. [CrossRef]
44. Yoon, W.J.; Kim, H.N.; Park, E.; Ryu, S.; Chang, Y.; Shin, H.; Kim, H.L.; Yi, S.Y. The Impact of Cholecystectomy on the Gut Microbiota: A Case-Control Study. *J. Clin. Med.* **2019**, *8*, 79. [CrossRef]
45. Nahata, M.C.; Barson, W.J. Ceftriaxone: A third-generation cephalosporin. *Drug Intell. Clin. Pharm.* **1985**, *19*, 900–906.
46. Zhao, Z.; Wang, B.; Mu, L.; Wang, H.; Luo, J.; Yang, Y.; Yang, H.; Li, M.; Zhou, L.; Tao, C. Long-Term Exposure to Ceftriaxone Sodium Induces Alteration of Gut Microbiota Accompanied by Abnormal Behaviors in Mice. *Front. Cell Infect. Microbiol.* **2020**, *10*, 258. [CrossRef]
47. Giuffrè, M.; Campigotto, M.; Campisciano, G.; Comar, M.; Crocè, L.S. A story of liver and gut microbes: How does the intestinal flora affect liver disease? A review of the literature. *Am. J. Physiol. Gastrointest. Liver Physiol.* **2020**, *318*, G889–G906. [CrossRef]

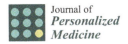

Journal of Personalized Medicine

Article

'Statistical Irreproducibility' Does Not Improve with Larger Sample Size: How to Quantify and Address Disease Data Multimodality in Human and Animal Research

Abigail R. Basson [1,2], Fabio Cominelli [1,2,3,4] and Alexander Rodriguez-Palacios [1,2,3,4,*]

1. Division of Gastroenterology and Liver Diseases, Case Western Reserve University School of Medicine, Cleveland, OH 44106, USA; axb860@case.edu (A.R.B.); Fabio.Cominelli@uhhospitals.org (F.C.)
2. Digestive Health Research Institute, University Hospitals Cleveland Medical Center, Cleveland, OH 44106, USA
3. Mouse Models, Silvio O'Conte Cleveland Digestive Diseases Research Core Center, Cleveland, OH 44106, USA
4. Germ-Free and Gut Microbiome Core, Digestive Health Research Institute, Case Western Reserve University, Cleveland, OH 44106, USA
* Correspondence: axr503@case.edu; Tel.: +216-368-8545; Fax: +216-844-7371

Citation: Basson, A.R.; Cominelli, F.; Rodriguez-Palacios, A. 'Statistical Irreproducibility' Does Not Improve with Larger Sample Size: How to Quantify and Address Disease Data Multimodality in Human and Animal Research. *J. Pers. Med.* **2021**, *11*, 234. https://doi.org/10.3390/jpm11030234

Academic Editor: Lucrezia Laterza

Received: 20 February 2021
Accepted: 18 March 2021
Published: 23 March 2021

Publisher's Note: MDPI stays neutral with regard to jurisdictional claims in published maps and institutional affiliations.

Copyright: © 2021 by the authors. Licensee MDPI, Basel, Switzerland. This article is an open access article distributed under the terms and conditions of the Creative Commons Attribution (CC BY) license (https://creativecommons.org/licenses/by/4.0/).

Abstract: Poor study reproducibility is a concern in translational research. As a solution, it is recommended to increase sample size (N), i.e., add more subjects to experiments. The goal of this study was to examine/visualize data multimodality (data with >1 data peak/mode) as cause of study irreproducibility. To emulate the repetition of studies and random sampling of study subjects, we first used various simulation methods of random number generation based on preclinical published disease outcome data from human gut microbiota-transplantation rodent studies (e.g., intestinal inflammation and univariate/continuous). We first used unimodal distributions (one-mode, Gaussian, and binomial) to generate random numbers. We showed that increasing N does not reproducibly identify statistical differences when group comparisons are repeatedly simulated. We then used multimodal distributions (>1-modes and Markov chain Monte Carlo methods of random sampling) to simulate similar multimodal datasets A and B (*t*-test-*p* = 0.95; N = 100,000), and confirmed that increasing N does not improve the 'reproducibility of statistical results or direction of the effects'. Data visualization with violin plots of categorical random data simulations with five-integer categories/five-groups illustrated how multimodality leads to irreproducibility. Re-analysis of data from a human clinical trial that used maltodextrin as dietary placebo illustrated multimodal responses between human groups, and after placebo consumption. In conclusion, increasing N does not necessarily ensure reproducible statistical findings across repeated simulations due to randomness and multimodality. Herein, we clarify how to quantify, visualize and address disease data multimodality in research. Data visualization could facilitate study designs focused on disease subtypes/modes to help understand person–person differences and personalized medicine.

Keywords: violin plots; random sampling; analytical reproducibility; microbiome; fecal matter transplantation; data disease subtypes; personalized medicine; maltodextrin; dip test

1. Introduction

Multimodal diseases are those in which affected subjects can be divided into subtypes; for instance, "mild" vs. "severe" disease, based on (known/unknown) modifiers of disease severity. Data subtypes, also known as "data modes", can be visualized as "peaks" and "valleys" within a violin or Kernel plot. There is emerging interest in understanding dataset multimodality and identifying strategies to address such source of variability in disease and medical research (brain [1,2], biobanking [3], genomics [4,5], and orthopedics [6]). In animals, for example those that receive human gut/fecal microbiota transplantations (hGM-FMT) or animals administered special diets or treatments may also exhibit "high", "middle", or "low reactivity" (e.g., gut inflammation) in response to the intervention. Although high/low ranging responses often appear in study datasets (biological and nonbiological) as multimodal distributions, little is known about how these could affect rodent research reproducibility or how to address such multimodal and random variance. Herein, we illustrate how multimodality via random sampling affects study reproducibility in research using, as an example, fecal microbiota transplantation studies in rodents as a way to exemplify variability and randomness resulting from data multimodality

To establish the causal connection between human diseases and the microbiome, animal models, primarily germ-free models transplanted with hGM, have been widely used as tools in translational research. Unfortunately, despite efforts to help scientists improve their studies (e.g., ARRIVE guidelines), there are still concerns on poor study reproducibility, in part owing to microbiome variability [7,8]. Novel sources of artificial microbiome heterogeneity that could explain variable hGM study results have been described [8–12]. Recently, we also illustrated how scientists often lack appropriate methods for the analysis of cage-clustered data, and with examples, we showed how to use study power ($p = 1 - \beta$) to help investigators monitor their study validity and sample size (N) [8].

With respect to N, published recommendations often include to increase N, i.e., adding more subjects (e.g., human, mice, cells) to improve research reproducibility. The objective of our study was to illustrate via simulations (using as an example hGM rodent disease data dispersion/variability) the impact of repeated random sampling from a population of subjects (at various N) on (i) the data distribution, (ii) the shape of said data distribution, and (iii) the cumulative probability of generating a statistically significant result for simulated repeated hGM-transplanted group comparisons for a hypothetical disease outcome. By using various methods of random number generation, encompassing unimodal and multimodal distributions, we illustrate that randomness alone introduces large-scale 'random analytical–statistical irreproducibility' patterns, regardless of number type (continuous or integer/categorical), especially for multimodal data distributions.

After examining the statistical content of 38 high-quality studies [13–50] assessed in a recent systematic review [51], herein, we found that scientists who increased N, concurrently reduced the number of mice/donor (MxD), indicating that statistically, scientists replace the disease variance in mice by the disease variance in humans in their hGM-FMT studies. Furthermore, supporting our previous report [8,52], studies lacked proper statistics methods to control for animal density, and most importantly with respect to data modality, we found that none of the studies considered data multimodality/violin plots. Herein, we clarify how to visualize, quantify and address disease data multimodality in human and animal research.

2. Materials and Methods

2.1. Overall Approach

To verify our hypothesis using, as an example, the context of hGM rodent studies and N, we used published (observed) preclinical rodent univariate data (e.g., intestinal inflammation) to make simulations with randomly generated numbers to then conduct repeated standard statistical and visualization analyses. Simulations were conducted using (i) integer data that could represent, for instance, categories of disease severity varying on scoring scale systems made of positive whole numbers categories (categorical), names (nominal), or orders (ordinal data), and (ii) continuous data that could represent, for instance, body weight or inflammation severity outcomes given in positive decimal numbers, or transmembrane electric resistance which oscillate around zero between negative and positive decimal numbers. Across multiple scenarios (details below), we used various number generator software and methods encompassing at least three major statistical probability distribution classes. The first, having no data modes with equal probability of sampling numbers across a min and max range bounds (uniform, rectangle shape); the second, having one data mode where the probability of sampling a number is higher when it is closer to the center of the data set (mean) and decreases away from the center (Gaussian unimodal and bell shape); and the third, having at least two data modes where the probability of sampling a number resulted from the combined joint probabilities of at least two Gaussian probability distributions interconnected using Markov chain principles of sampling dependency (mixed Gaussian Markov chain, multimodal, and partly overlapping bell shapes). In doing so, we generated a wide array of dataset possibilities, with varying N (from 3 to 100,000/group), which we then compared statistically as treatment/subject groups using standard tests (*t*-test, or ANOVA; see Methods and sections below for justification and nonparametric alternatives). Therein, we monitored and quantified the extent to which data analysis reproducibility was influenced by randomness alone during the sampling of subjects from hypothetical populations within varying N, as well as dataset shapes numerically restricted nonarbitrarily around published means $\pm$ SD, or upper and lower values. Lastly, we used random arbitrary range parameters for additional validation.

2.2. Published Preclinical hGM-FMT Rodent Data Used for Simulations

To facilitate the visualization of how random sampling and disease variability influence study conclusions (significant vs. nonsignificant *p*-values) in the context of N, we conducted a series of simulations based on existing statistical methods (see simulations described below), using, as an example, preclinical hGM-FMT disease phenotyping data estimates from our own IBD studies (Basson et al.) [52] and that of Baxter et al. [21] (a study listed in a recent systematic review [7]). In brief, by transplanting feces from inflammatory bowel disease (IBD), namely Crohn's disease ("Dis1") and ulcerative colitis ("Dis2"), and "Healthy" donors (n = 3 donors for each "disease/healthy" state) into a germ-free spontaneous mouse model of cobblestone/ileal Crohn's disease (SAMP1/YitFc) [52,53], Basson et al. [52] observed with ~90% engraftment of human microbial taxa after 60 days, that the hGM-FMT effect on mouse IBD-phenotype was independent of the disease state of the donor. Specifically, samples from some IBD patients and some healthy donors did not affect the severity of intestinal inflammation in mice, while the remaining donors exacerbated inflammation, indicating the presence of disease data multimodality in animal models. Comparably, Baxter et al. [17] found that differences in the number of tumors resulting in a hGM-FMT mouse model of chemically induced colorectal cancer (CRC) were independent of the cancer status of the human donors (n = 3 colorectal cancer, n = 3 healthy individuals).

In addition to published parameters, actual data points inferred from published plots, or the dataset itself were used to define the data distribution using histograms and normality density plots using Wessa.net [54]. Inspection of the distribution of observed experimental data was performed using Excel or R software, as described in [55], which uses R code, as described in [56]. To further assist in the examination of which distribution fit the data best, the R-interface implementation of the Tukey Lambda PPCC plot was used to distinguish normal, u shape, uniform, Cauchy, and logistic distributions, as described in [54,57], using R code based on [58]. To identify the best fitting distribution function that the observed data has, we used the Excel functions (TRENDLINE and Equation) and examined the R^2 for the linear, exponential, and logarithm function (unimodal distributions) or used polynomial functions with two or more terms to describe the shape of the data distribution. Each term approximately corresponds to a mode/peak in the dataset. Model fitting used the same interface as that used for model fitting of a normal distribution to observed data, as described by [59], which used R code as described in [56].

For clarity, the purpose of this study was to illustrate the effect of randomness as an analytical component in preclinical research datasets and not to examine the validity of rodents as models of human diseases. As such, we used simulated data generated within the data distribution parameters of published data or used completely random number sets drawn from various distributions within arbitrary number ranges, e.g., common to gut inflammation scores in rodents. Factors such as batch effect, gender, and cage density, among others, were not considered in the simulations, because the main objective was to examine 'random sampling' and because such factors are not often reported in rodent publications or are inherently part of the data distribution of the published datasets [8].

2.3. Simulation of Hypothetical Disease Outcome Sets Using Random Numbers

Iteration of random number generation [60] was conducted to illustrate the effect of random sampling on the reproducibility of analysis of mouse preclinical datasets generated using established software. In sequence, we first defined and used the published (observed) rodent disease outcome parameters when available (e.g., mean and SD, or the min and max data ranges, for at least two "subject/treatment groups"). We then used such parameters as input for random generation software (Excel, GraphPad, R software, wessa.net, and random.org), which for each iteration, generated sets of "randomly sampled treatment groups" of random numbers, which were then statistically compared using standard methods and software to determine (i) to what extent the differences were significant, (ii) the difference in magnitude between the compared groups (treatment effect difference), and (iii) which group was higher mean (direction of the effect). Each set of random numbers (a subject/treatment group) used for statistical analysis was generated at various sample sizes N to examine the effect of N on statistical reproducibility for the simulated published datasets. Results were monitored manually for each iteration and plotted to illustrate effects in manuscript figures, recorded using Excel functions by creating an analysis template simulator for readers use, or used Monte Carlo simulations in statistical software (GraphPad, or R) to compute thousands of iterations and summarize the statistical results for cumulative reproducibility and compute Monte Carlo adjusted p-values.

2.4. Group Simulations Using Pseudorandom Integer and Continuous Numbers

To enable the visualization of the simulation strategy and analytical comparisons across integers and continuous data over various Ns, and to visualize the impact of adding three subjects to each group for each statistical simulation, we used Excel with the embedded formulas and functions (see Supplementary File 1). The supplementary file contains two spreadsheets. One sheet shows the layout for the generation of random integer numbers in increments of 3, as well as the cumulative statistics using t-test functions to compare pairs of data with N ranging from 3 to 63, expandable to ~1 million rows, and for uniform and Gaussian (based on inverse Gaussian functions as described below). The other sheet follows the same format, based on the same distributions, but it generates continuous random numbers, instead of integers. Pre-set bar plots with standard deviations and line plots with the cumulative summary of statistical results illustrate there is no difference between uniform or Gaussian distribution-based simulations. To allow for reproducibility, statistical analyses were completed with a suited two-group parametric (t test) statistical functions available in Excel, because corresponding nonparametric tests are not available in the software, and their performance is similar to parametric in numerous scenarios, especially with large N. Nonparametric statistical functions are available for Excel using third-party open-access macros and extensions that vary in implementation across platforms (e.g., Real Statistics Using Excel [61]).

As laid out in Supplementary File 1, random numbers were generated using uniform distributions, which is the standard function for Excel RAND (continuous) and RANDBE-TWEEN (integer) functions. However, for the generation of numbers, based on a Gaussian distribution (not readily available in Excel), we nested the RAND formula inside of the NORMINV formula for the probability input, which, in turn, returns the inverse of the normal cumulative distribution for the specified mean and standard deviation. Additional options available in Excel were not used in this study. To constrain the data range within positive numbers, since inflammation scores are not negative, we used the formula = MIN (MAX(NORM.INV(RAND(), C$16, C$17), 0),80) to limit numbers between 0 and 80, which is beyond the absolute probability of 1 of having the maximum possible inflammatory score within the expectations of the published parameters (i.e., maximum inflammation is unlikely to be 80) [62,63].

2.5. Visualization of Randomly Generated Numbers

In all depicted illustrations, the randomly generated numbers used computer-software/automated-pseudorandom (seeded and unseeded) methods [64,65]. Unless described otherwise, the numbers generated (generated using uniform and Gaussian distributions) were restricted to be confined within biologically meaningful data boundaries based on published data (for example, 0 as minimum for normal histological score or intestinal inflammation and 80 as arbitrary ~3-fold the maximum possible histological score) as described. For illustration purposes, the x- or y-axes in plots were generically labeled as outcome disease severity. Simulating a situation where a scientist would recruit a trio of donors (three donors) per group at a time and was interested in conducting interim statistical analysis following the addition of every trio of donors to the study, we summarized the pairwise group analysis for the simulated disease comparisons, for various N, and for consecutively added donors as an aggregate "cumulative probability of being a significant simulation" statistic. Comparisons were deemed significant if at least one p-value was <0.05 across simulations.

2.6. Parametric vs. Nonparametric Group Statistics and Monte Carlo p-Value Estimates

Because parametric and nonparametric statistical methods often produce interchangeably/similar p-values, especially when data have normal distribution, and also as the group sample size N increases, as previously described, herein, for illustrative purposes, we used, unless otherwise described, primarily parametric tests to conduct the statistical analysis because in most cases N was larger than 3–6, with simulations conducted with N = 6, 9, 18, 21, and additional increments of 3 up to 63, or with N = 100, 200, 600, 1000, 10,000, or 100,000. When applicable for further validation of the data generation and specific simulations datasets in Excel, the data was exported to GraphPad, a statistical software widely used in the literature, to conduct Student's unpaired t-test and/or one-way ANOVA with Tukey statistical comparisons (or the nonparametric in some scenarios with low N < 6, or as needed see below) to calculate adjusted p-values using Monte Carlo simulations for decimal numbers with Gaussian distribution, and to determine the % of simulations that were significant or not. For post hoc analysis, nonseeded Monte Carlo simulation function was used.

2.7. Markov Chain Monte Carlo Multimodal Simulations of Continuous Data

To illustrate the major role of random sampling across multiple N from multimodal data distributions, we used Markov chain Monte Carlo multimodal simulation functions and R software to obtain groups of numbers from such distributions for statistical comparisons using two-group statistics. The scripts are available in Supplementary Figure S5. Specifically, to illustrate the effect of random sampling from data simulations from multimodal distribution functions, unconstrained-parameter simulations of two mixed, yet separate, normal distributions were performed using the random walk Metropolis–Hastings algorithm [66,67], a form of dependent sampling from a proposed posterior distribution, as a well-established method of Markov chain Monte Carlo (MCMC) simulations [68], using R and STATA (v15.1). In the latter, the MCMC sampling of a new individual is dependent on the prior probability of being part of a mode within a multimodal distribution, instead of being completely random from a unimodal distribution, using a log-likelihood correction to prevent negative sigma values and also allow for asymmetrical distributions. This method is beneficial as it asymptotically converges to the true proposal distribution and so represents a more robust method of data simulation compared to other alternatives of simulating sampling from multimodal distributions (i.e., binomial and mixed normal distributions).

2.8. Multimodality Tests and Variability of Statistical Results

The test of multimodality was conducted using the dip test (which measures the departure of a sample from unimodality, using the uniform distribution as the worst case as a reference) and STATA [69], with packages available in R [70]. The tabulation of modes from a variable in a dataset was computed using the *modes* and *hsmode* function in STATA [71,72]. Statistical and simulation analyses were conducted or plotted with Excel, R, Stata, and GraphPad.

To determine the sources of statistical methods variability in hGM-FMT rodent studies, we reviewed the content of 38 studies listed in ref [51]. For computation purposes, we searched each article for the following keywords: "cage," "stat*", "housed", "multiple", "multivariable", "cluster", "mixed", "individual*", and "random*", and appropriately extracted details to additional inserted columns of an excel file. Detailed statistical tests and software used, focused on assessing the effect of the hGM in the rodent phenotypes, were extracted to determine if studies used proper cluster statistical analysis and/or controlled for random effects introduced by caging, when needed, that is, if more than one mouse was housed per cage. Data including descriptions of animal density (numbers, e.g., 1–5) were assigned to the sourced keywords to allow for statistical analysis. If a range was provided for N or animal density, estimations were computed using the median value within the range, as well as the minimum and maximum values. The average of estimated center values was used for analysis and graphical summaries

3. Results

3.1. ". Disease Data Subtypes" (Modes) Occur with Uniform and Gaussian Random Sampling

In microbiome rodent studies, the selection of a sufficient number of human donors, as well as the number of mice/group which required the testing of each human donor (MxD), is critical to account for the effects of random sampling, which exist when the hGM induces variable disease severity in humans and rodents. Thus, to visualize the variability of disease severity (data subtypes/modes) in hGM-FMT rodents and the effect of N on the reproducibility of said pairwise statistical comparisons from, hypothetically, randomly selected human donors, we first conducted a series of simulations using as input, the mean $\pm$ SD (disease outcome, continuous data) from hGM-FMT mice in Basson et al. [52] to generate random numbers (Figure 1a; note dispersed overlapping data). We also generated separate random datasets of integer and decimal numbers using functions designed to draw numbers from a uniform and Gaussian distribution (see details in Methods, and formulas and visualization strategy in Supplementary File 1 and Supplementary Figure S1). We showed that under the conditions simulated, the integer-uniform dataset is statistically similar to the one generated using decimal-Gaussian methods (Figure 1b), and we demonstrated how the random selection of N (sampled as groups for each of three iterative datasets) influences the direction and significance in pairwise comparative statistics.

Simulations showed that the number of MxD is important because mice have various response patterns to the hGM (i.e., disease severity and disease data subtypes/modes), which can be consistently detected depending on the MxD and thus the variability introduced by random sampling. Simulations showed that for the three hGM-FMT group datasets (plotted as Dis1, Dis2, and Healthy), it was possible to reproducibly identify from two to three unique donor disease severity subtypes (data modes) in mice induced by the hGM ("high", "middle", and "low" disease severity).

Simulation plots made it visually evident that testing <4–5 MxD yielded mean values more likely to be affected by intrinsic variability of random sampling, thus making studies with >6 MxD more stable and preferable. Conversely, studies with 1–2 MxD are at risk of being strongly dependent on randomness. Iterative simulations showed that the mean effect (e.g., ileal histology) in transplanted mice varies minimally (i.e., stabilizes) after 7 ± 2 MxD, depending on the random dataset iterated. Beyond that, increasing MxD becomes less cost-effective/unnecessary if the focus is the human donors (Figure 1c).

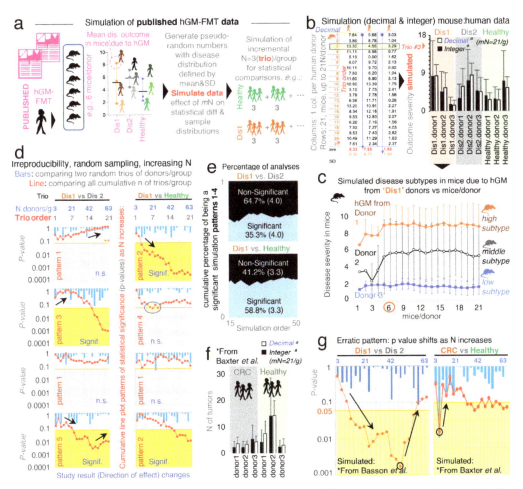

Figure 1. Random sampling from overlapping datasets yield unexpected "linear patterns of cumulative statistical irreproducibility". Simulations on observed data from Basson et al. [52] to visualize disease vs. healthy datasets. (**a**) Method overview to generate pseudorandom numbers and simulations from published (observed) data (see details/formulas in Supplementary File 1 and Supplementary Figure S1). (**b**) Visualization of simulated outcomes using random decimal and integer numbers datasets generated based on 3 donors/group for Disease 1 ("Dis1"), Disease 2 ("Dis2"), and "Healthy" groups. Bar plot of N = 21 mice/donor, notice no differences between integer and decimal datasets group pattern, or absolute differences, superscript letter "a", paired-t $p > 0.05$. (**c**) Simulation of human gut/fecal microbiota transplantations (hGM-FMT) mice data yields reproducible simulated "disease data subtypes" from 6 mice/group. (**d**) Cumulative line plots depicting patterns of statistical irreproducibility and pairwise statistical directions of effect estimates (n.s.:signif., signif.:signif., signif.:n.s., and n.s:n.s.). Representative simulations comparing two groups of donors, with N ranging from three (trio) donors/group to 63, in multiples of three (cumulative addition of new trios per group). Note Y-axis, p-value of differences using two-group Student's t-test. Notice as N increases, the cumulative significance (red line) exhibit different linear patterns due to variance introduced by random sampling. (**e**) Percentage of simulated analysis with significant or nonsignificant pairwise difference (blue; significant, black; non-significant; and parentheses, SD). Comparison deemed significant, if at least one p-value < 0.05 across simulations with N between 3 and 63 donors/group. (**f**) Visualization of simulated outcome using observed data from Baxter et al. [21]. No differences between integer and decimal datasets, superscript letter "a", paired-t $p > 0.05$. (**g**) Random simulations illustrate "erratic" statistical patterns. Notice as N increases, group differences become more significant, until an inflection point, where adding more donors makes the significance disappear. See Supplementary Figure S2 for additional examples and computed R^2 value to illustrate the linearity of the correlation between N and statistical significance.

3.2. Random Sampling from Overlapping Datasets Yield "Linear Patterns of Statistical Irreproducibility"

Often, published literature contains figures and statistical analysis conducted with three donors per disease group. Thus, to mimic this scenario and to examine the role of random sampling of subjects on the reproducibility of pairwise statistical results (significant vs. nonsignificant) in the context of hGM-FMT rodent studies, we compared two groups of donors, each having three donors/group (donor "trio"), with N increasing in multiples of three (ranging from 3 to 62 donors/group). We conducted (i) multiple donor/group ("trio–trio") pairwise comparisons and (ii) a simultaneous overall analysis for the cumulative sum of all the donor trios (i.e., the cumulative addition of new trios per group) simulated for each disease group. That is, we monitored and quantified whether results for each random iteration (simulation event) were significant (using univariate Student's t-statistics $p < 0.05$) or nonsignificant ($p > 0.05$) for groups of simulated donor datasets (Dis1, Dis2, or Healthy). Assessing the effect of random sampling at various N and also as N accumulated, we were able to illustrate that pairwise "trio–trio" comparisons between the simulated rodent disease outcome datasets almost always produced nonsignificant results when iterative trios were compared (due to large SD overlapping; see bars in Figure 1d representing 21 sets of pairwise trio–trio p-values). However, as N increases by the cumulative addition of all (mostly nonsignificant) donor trios (i.e., N increases in multiples of three, for a range of N between 3 and 63 donors/group; (3, 6, 9, 12, ... ,63)), pairwise statistical comparisons between the simulated datasets did not produce consistent results (see line plots in Figure 1d representing p-value for cumulative addition of donors when sampling iterations were simulated).

Results are clinically relevant because the simulated N, being much larger (63 donors/group) than the largest N tested by one of the hGM-FMT studies examined in a recent systematic review [51] (21 donors/group) [45] demonstrates that the analysis of randomly selected subjects would not always yield reproducible results due to the chance of sampling aleatory sets of individuals with varying degrees of disease severity, regardless of how many donors are recruited in an study. To provide a specific example, using Dis1 as a referent, cumulative pairwise comparisons (vs. Dis2 and vs. Healthy) revealed at least five different patterns of irreproducible statistical results (rodent disease outcome) as N increased between 3 and 63 per group. Figure 1d illustrates four of these variable cumulative linear patterns of statistical irreproducibility in which, remarkably, (i) Dis1 becomes significantly different vs. Dis2, and vs. Healthy, as N increases, (ii) Dis1 becomes significantly different from Dis2 but not vs. Healthy, (iii) Dis1 was significantly different from healthy but not vs. Dis2, and (iv) Dis1 never becomes significantly different despite sampling up to 63 donors/group. See Supplementary Figure S2 for complementary plots illustrating linearity of patterns (R^2, mean 0.51 ± 0.23, 21 simulations).

Hence, the results clearly illustrate that seeking funds to recruit more donors as recently suggested is not a prudent statistical solution to the problem of understanding disease causality of widely variable conditions in both humans and animals. By statistical irreproducibility, herein, we refer to the inability to reproduce the direction and statistical significance of a test effect when analyses are conducted between groups created by the random selection of subjects from distributions defined using observed data.

To investigate the cumulative probability of generating a statistically significant simulation that collectively would lead to the inconsistent patterns (statistical irreproducibility) observed via random sampling, we computed an aggregate "cumulative probability of being a significant simulation" for 50 pairwise statistical simulation sets fulfilling the four linear patterns described above. Emphasizing the concept that increasing N is not a reproducible solution, Figure 1e shows that only $35.3 \pm 4.0\%$ of comparisons between Dis1 and Dis2, and $58.8 \pm 3.3\%$ for Dis1 and Healthy, were significant.

3.3. "Erratic Patterns" of Statistical Irreproducibility as N Increases

To increase the external validity of our observations, we next simulated the data published from a hGM-FMT study on colorectal cancer conducted by Baxter et al. [21]. In agreement with Basson et al. [52], Baxter et al. revealed comparably bimodal colorectal cancer phenotypes in mice resulting from both the diseased (colorectal cancer) patients and healthy human donors (Figure 1f).

Unexpectedly, we observed for both Basson et al. [52] and Baxter et al. [21], as simulations were conducted, an "erratic" shift on the significance of the cumulative analysis occurred as N increased (Figure 1g). In some cases, the increasing addition of donor trios/group (as simulations proceeded for increasing values of N) made it possible to identify simulations where erratic changes in the statistical significance for group comparisons switched randomly, yet gradually, from being significant to nonsignificant as more donor trios were "recruited" into the simulations (Figure 1g). Clinically relevant simulations indicated that adding extra subjects could at times actually invert the overall cumulative effect of the p-value, possibly due to the variable distribution and multimodal nature of the host responses to experimental interventions. As such, simulations indicate that it is advisable to conduct several a priori determined interim data analysis in clinical trials to ensure that significance is numerically stable ($p < 0.05$), as well as the relevance of personalized analysis to examine disease variance in populations. Unfortunately, there are no guidelines or examples available to assist in determining how many donors would be sufficient, and to visualize the effect of random sampling of individuals from a vastly heterogeneous population of healthy and diseased subjects.

3.4. Monte Carlo Simulations and Probability of Statistical Reproducibility

Expanding the reproducibility of these uniform and Gaussian distributions, we then made simulations using solely Gaussian distributions for N = 63 donors/group and conducted (i) Monte Carlo adjusted Student's unpaired t-tests and (ii) Monte Carlo adjusted one-way ANOVA with Tukey correction for family errors and multiple comparisons. Monte Carlo simulations were used to indicate how many tests will yield a significant result and the direction of effect. Monte Carlo simulations with normal Gaussian distribution around the group means and a pooled SD of ± 4 were also computed. See Supplementary Figure S3 and Supplementary File 2 for methods employed in GraphPad for this Monte Carlo simulation and the corresponding dataset. Supporting the observations above, Monte Carlo Gaussian simulations showed that, using pairwise comparison, Dis1 would be significantly different from Dis 2 (adjusted t-test $p < 0.05$) only 57.7% of the time (95% CI = 58–57.4), with 1540 simulations producing negative (contradictory) mean differences between the groups. Compared to Healthy, Dis1, and Dis2 were significant only 9.1% (95% CI = 9.2–8.9) and 78.3% (95% CI = 78.6–78.1) of the time, respectively. Statistical analyses were compared, for p-values computed by parametric t-tests and nonparametric Mann–Whitney statistics, findings were comparable, yet distinct, with borderline significant p-values.

Under the "Weak Law of Large Numbers" [73–75] and randomization principles, it is almost always possible to detect some level of statistical significance(s) and mean group differences when asymptotic mathematical methods based on numerous simulations are used. For example, when simulations are used as a surrogate for multiple experiments which are not possible in real research settings. However, in this case, the mean simulated differences yielding from 100,000 simulations were minuscule (Dis1-Dis2 = 1.6; Healthy-Dis2 = -1.97; and Healthy-Dis1 = 0.42). Compared to the range of disease variance for each disease, such minuscule differences may not be clinically relevant to explain disease variance at the individual level. Note that the SD was 4; therefore, it is intuitive to visualize in a numerical context such small differences across greatly overlapping unimodal simulations.

Correcting for family errors, one-way ANOVA corrected with 10,000 Monte Carlo simulations with N = 63/group showed that at least one of the three groups would be statistically different in approximately only 67.2% of the simulations (95% CI = 64.2–

70.0), whereas in 32.8% (95% CI = 64.2–70.0) of simulations, the groups would appear as statistically similar (see Supplementary Table S1 for estimations after 100,000 Monte Carlo simulations (R software); note narrower CI as simulations increase, Supplementary Figure S4). The comparison of Dis1 vs. Dis2 in supplementary Table S1 demonstrates that the percentage of cases in which a simulation could be significant, depending on the degree of data dispersion. For example, simulations with SD of 4, compared to SD of 10, produce significant results less often, illustrating how data with larger dispersions contribute to poor statistical reproducibility, which cannot necessarily be corrected by increasing N.

3.5. Violin Plots to Visualize, and Tests to Quantify, Multimodal "Disease Data Subtypes"

To visualize and to illustrate how to address the underlying mechanisms that could explain the "linear and erratic patterns of statistical irreproducibility" that is introduced by random sampling, we first used dot plots based on observed and simulated data, followed by kernel-based statistics and plots (violin, box, bar). Plot appearance and one-way ANOVA statistics showed that when N is increased, significant results, when present for largely overlapping phenotypes, are primarily due to small differences between sample means (Figure 2a,b).

Simulations that compared three groups of 65 donors/group almost always yielded a significantly different group; however, dot plots show that the significant differences between means are just a small fraction of the total disease variability as verified with Monte Carlo simulations. That is, as N increases, comparisons can become significant (see plot with 65 donors in Figure 2c). In this context, a significant difference of such a narrow magnitude may not be clinically relevant, or generalizable, to explain the presence of a disease phenotype in a population, especially for subjects at the extreme ranges of the disease distribution.

Mechanistically, the detection of significant comparisons can be attributed to the effect that increasing N has on the data mean and variance, which increases at a higher rate for the variance as shown in Figure 2d. Instead of increasing N as a general solution, we suggest that scientists use violin plots over other plots commonly encouraged by publishers [76] (e.g., bar, boxplot, and dot plots), because violin plots provide an informative approach to make inferences about "disease data subtypes" in the population (see subtypes shown with arrows in Figure 2e,f).

Violin plots are similar to a box plot, as they show a marker for the data median, interquartile ranges, and the individual data points [77]. However, as a unique feature, violin plots show the probability density of the data at different values, usually smoothed by a kernel density estimator. The idea of a kernel average smoother is that within a range of aligned data points, for each data point to be smoothed (X0), there is a constant distance size (λ) of choice for the kernel window (radius or width), around which a weighted average for nearby data points are estimated. Weighted analysis gives data points that are closer to X0 higher weights within the kernel window, thus identifying areas with higher data densities (which correspond to the disease data modes). As an example of the benefits of using violin plots, Figure 2g shows that as N increases, as does the ability of scientists to subjectively infer the presence of disease subtypes.

To strengthen the reproducibility of "subtype" mode identification, herein, we also suggest the use of statistical methods to identify disease data modes (e.g., see the statistical function *modes* in Methods and Discussion), because as N increases, the visual detection of modes becomes increasingly more subjective as shown in Figure 2g.

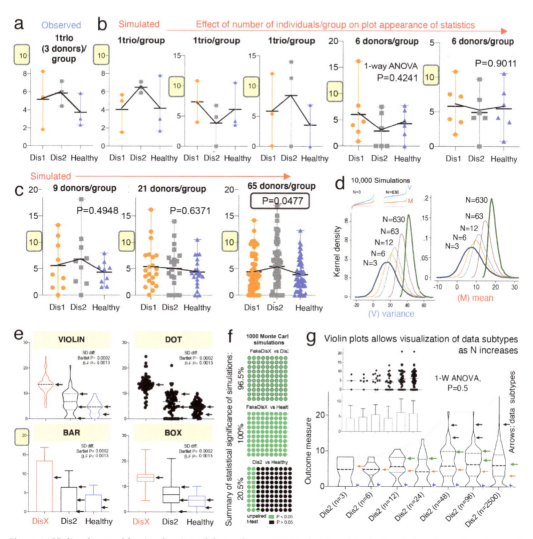

Figure 2. Violin plots enable visualization of data subtypes in simulations of random sampling for various N sample size. Observed raw data derived from Basson et al. (**a**,**b**) Dot plots (mean, range) of observed (1 "trio"; 3 donors/group), and simulated data (3 and 6 donors/group; panel B). Note that differences are not significant because of the variability between diseases. (**c**) Dot plots (mean, range) of simulated data for 9, 21, and 65 donors per group. Note that simulated mean effects became significant with 65 donors/group. However, the mean difference is small compared to the variance of the groups and the difference is not biologically different because it is a function of the total variance (23%). (**d**) Kernel density simulations (10,000) based on observed (n = 3) and simulated data. Note that as N increases the mean becomes narrower while the variance widens. See 100,000 Monte Carlo simulations in Supplementary Table S1. (**e**) Comparison of visual appearance and data display for violin, dot, bar, and box plots of simulated data to illustrate "disease data subtypes" (arrows). (**f**) Plot illustrates cumulative proportion of simulation runs that generated a significant (green, $p < 0.05$) or nonsignificant value (black, $p > 0.05$). Analysis illustrates how Monte Carlo adjusted analysis could be reported with observed findings. See Supplementary Figure S4 for 100,000 Monte Carlo simulations of random numbers generated in R. (**g**) Violin plots allow visualization of data subtypes as N increases (arrows, subtypes).

3.6. Violin Plots Guide Subtype Analysis to Identify Biologically Significant Results

Violin plots and kernel density distribution curves in Figure 3 illustrate why comparing groups of randomly sampled individuals may not yield biologically relevant information, even though statistical analysis identifies that the mean values differ between compared groups. Figure 3a illustrates the different patterns of potential donor subtypes (i.e., data modes visualized in violin plots as disease data/curve "peaks") that would yield significant results in a single experiment depending on the donors sampled.

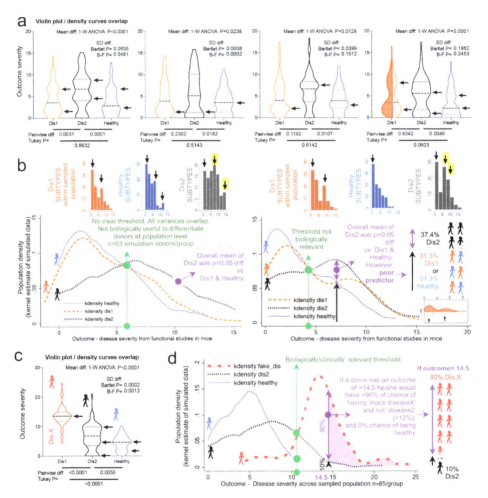

Figure 3. Violin plots illustrate that statistical differences with large N may not have clinical predictive value at individual level. Violin and kernel plots illustrate statistical vs. biologically relevant differences and thresholds. (**a**) Violin plots of four simulated random number sets illustrate that each set of donors may have unique subtypes of disease illustrated with arrowheads (disease severity scores with higher number of simulated donors). Arrows indicate "disease data subtypes" vary with every simulation of 63 donors/group. (**b**) Kernel density curves illustrate large overlap of sample population from simulated data (see panel 3a). Significant differences are highlighted by shaded area. Note the threshold does not have distinctive separation for the plots indicating that it is not biologically useful as a predictor of outcome. (**c**) Violin plots illustrate meaningful statistical difference for population (compared to panel 3b). "Fake disease X" ("DisX") was generated as a "mock" disease following Gaussian distribution around the mean. Monte Carlo simulations were significant 96.5% (upper limit 97.6, lower limit 95.4%). (**d**) Kernel density curves of panel 3c illustrate example of distribution separation with both statistical difference and biological relevance.

However, the kernel density plots in Figure 3b show that significant findings do not necessarily indicate/yield clinically relevant thresholds or parameters to differentiate between the populations (due to the overlapping and inflation of data "peaks" in some subjects within the samples). To contrast the data simulated from Basson et al., we replaced data from Dis1 dataset with a Gaussian distributed (R software) sample of random numbers (within 13.5 ± 3.5, labeled as "fake disease X"; vs. 6.4 ± 4.3, and 4.5 ± 2.5 for Dis2 and Healthy, respectively) to illustrate how a kernel plot would appear when significant differences have a clinically relevant impact in differentiating subtypes (Figure 3c,d).

Collectively, simulations indicate that the uneven random sampling of subtypes across a disease group would be an important factor in determining the direction of significance if studies were repeated, owing primarily to the probability of sampling data "modes" or "peaks/valleys" in both healthy and diseased populations.

3.7. Multimodal Datasets Illustrate How Statistical Irreproducibility Occurs

Thus far, we have used unimodal distributions to show how random sampling affects statistical results. However, there has been an increased interest in understanding data multimodality in various biological processes [78,79] for which new statistical approaches have been proposed. Methods to simulate multimodal distributions are however not trivial, in part due to the unknown nature of multimodality in biological processes.

To facilitate the understanding of the conceptual mechanisms that influence the effect of data multimodality and random sampling on statistical significance, Figure 4a–e schematically contextualizes the statistical and data distribution principles that can interfere with reproducibility of statistical results when simulations are repeated.

Random simulations from unimodal distributions work on the assumption that numbers (e.g., donors' disease severity) are drawn from a population, independently from one another. That is, the probability of sampling or drawing a number from a population is not influenced by the number that was selected prior. While this form of random sampling is very useful in deterministic mathematics, it does not capture the dependence of events that occur in multimodal biology. That is, in biology, the probability of an event to occur depends on the nature of the preceding events. To increase the external validity of our report, we thus conducted simulations based on three strategies to draw density curves resembling multimodal distributions.

To simulate the statistical comparison of two hypothetical multimodal data distribution, we (i) ran Markov chain Monte Carlo (MCMC) simulations for two datasets ("drug A" vs. "drug B") each with two data modes (Figure 5a,b), (ii) used the statistical *dip test* (STATA) to determine if the simulated data were statistically multimodal, and (iii) used the Student's *t*-test to determine the statistical significance, the mean differences, and directions for the simulated distributions ("drug A" vs. "drug B"), using various N (Figure 5c). The MCMC simulations clearly illustrate how random sampling of two multimodal hypothetical datasets lead to inconsistent patterns of statistical results when compared, indicating that biological data are multimodal, have multiple peaks/modes, and that two groups intended for comparison may have different or mismatching shapes and thus real data may not have Gaussian distribution. Notice that the data dispersion increases as N increases; see summary statistics in Figure 5c.

Collectively, Figure 5 underscores the notion that randomness alone elicits effect on irreproducible results, and that mean-SD are imperfect to visualize data shape. See Supplementary Figure S5 for wider range of N and the scripts for the *dip test* and *modes* analysis using STATA and R commands.

Figure 5d,e depicts distributions derived from both "truncated beta", and the combination of two "mixed unimodal" distribution functions (e.g., two independent Gaussian curves in one plot), which are illustrative of multimodality, but not necessarily reliable methods to examine the effects from dependent random sampling in multimodality. Thus, we used "Random walk Markov chain Metropolis–Hastings algorithms" using R software to simulate random sampling, accounting for the hypothetical dependence between two different disease subtypes.

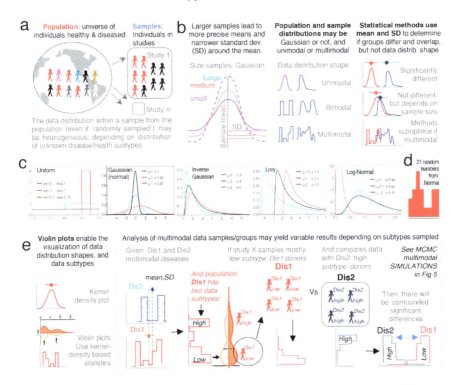

Figure 4. Conceptual overview of the effect of random sampling and analysis of multimodal data. (**a**) Schematic conceptualization of random sampling from a population of heterogeneous individuals. (**b**) Representation of various unidimensional data distributions. Notice that mean and SD do not represent the shape of the distribution. (**c**). Examples of probability density functions of unimodal distributions. Wolfram language [80]. (**d**) Example of a random sampling of numbers generated in this study using decimal Gaussian distribution generates a non-Gaussian distribution (bimodal; two peaks/modes, as in disease distribution subtypes). This illustrates that even under seemingly unbiased circumstances (randomness), a set of random subjects from a population may be of two subtypes and not represent the population in its "universe" of disease possibilities. (**e**) Multimodal distributions. Use of violin and kernel plots to visualize subtypes.

Conclusively, MCMC illustrations emphasize that increasing N in the study of multimodal diseases in a single study should not be assumed to provide results that can be directly extrapolated to the population, but rather, MCMC emphasizes that the target study of data subtypes could lead to the identification of mechanisms which could explain why diseases vary within biological systems (e.g., humans and mice).

3.8. Categorical Data Exhibit Multimodality

Until this point, the majority of data simulations reported herein were based on continuous data, using various methods computer pseudorandom number algorithms. Statistical comparisons were then made between two and three groups per simulation using *t*-tests or one-way ANOVAs, or their nonparametric equivalent, as it is common in rodent literature. To further understand the effect of randomness on preclinical datasets, we further simulated categorical outcomes [81,82]. We simulated five categories of gut inflammation, with changing severity in steps of 1, between 1-(category "normal") to 6-(category "most inflamed"). To illustrate how randomness affects the reproducibility of statistical analysis in studies with >3 treatments, we simulated five treatment groups (untreated, placebo, and treatments X, Y and Z).

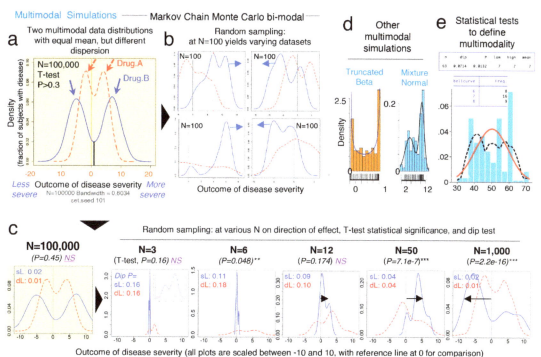

Figure 5. Comparison of two statistically similar multimodal datasets yields highly irreproducible results due to random sampling at various N. Markov chain Monte Carlo (MCMC) simulations emphasize the need to identify disease subtypes for the study of multimodal diseases. MCMC are random-number-generating strategies to simulate two multimodal distributions, wherein a random walk MCMC Metropolis–Hastings' algorithm simulates random sampling accounting for inter-/within-mode dependence of two "data disease subtypes". (**a**) MCMC simulations of two statistically similar multimodal datasets (hypothetical effect of "drug A"; red dash line vs. "drug B"; blue solid line), "real" distributions set at N = 100,000; grey reference line at x = 0, downward arrows; data modes. (**b**) Random sampling of multimodal dataset (from panel 5a) at N = 100 yields varying dataset distributions and a different mean, SD. (**c**) Effect of random sampling dataset (from panel 5a) on increasing N on *t*-test significance and direction of effect for "drug A" vs. "drug B" (arrow), including dip test for MCMC simulations (*set.seed* 101). See Supplementary Figure S5 for wider range of N and the STATA and R command scripts for the *dip test* and *modes* analyses. (**d**) Example of other multimodal distributions derived from "truncated beta" and the combination of two "mixed unimodal" distribution functions. (**e**) Example of a Hartigan–Hartigan (Hartigans') unimodality *dip test* and a *modes* test [69,83,84] showing a multimodal data distribution (black dotted line) compared to normal univariate density plot (red line). To identify data subtypes (modes), the dip test [69] computes a *p*-value to help determine unimodal or multimodal; does not require a priori knowledge of potential multimodality; it is interpreted from test statistics (if *p* < 0.05 data is not unimodal, if *p* > 0.05–1.0 at least one data mode in dataset). Asterisks indicate significance *p* < 0.05.

Using an integer generator which draws true random numbers from atmospheric noise (random.org), we set the algorithm to draw random numbers between 1 and 6 (representing the six categories), creating equal group sets of N = 6, 12, 100, and 1000 integers/group, with no differences between the five groups.

One-way ANOVA (and Kruskal–Wallis) statistics with post hoc pairwise comparisons across groups for >250 study dataset simulations, illustrated that increasing N from 6 to

1000/group do not prevent the occurrence of expected false significant findings (i.e., *Ho* = at least one group is different) with *p*-value < 0.05. Random groups with N = 1000 expected to be similar, showed statistical significances in 3 of 50 iterations, which is expectedly similar to the expected five false discoveries for 100 if *p* = 0.05 (3/50 vs. 5/100; Fisher exact *p* = 1); however, the directions of the effects changed drastically within treatment groups, across the significantly different simulations.

Supporting our hypothesis, increasing N does not necessarily prevent false discoveries, as we did not see more false discoveries than linearly expected [51] when N decreased from "optimal" 1000 to "less optimal" 100, 12 and 6 (3/50 vs. 2/40, 4/40 and 1/40, respectively; Fisher exact *p* < 0.6261; Figure 6a–c).

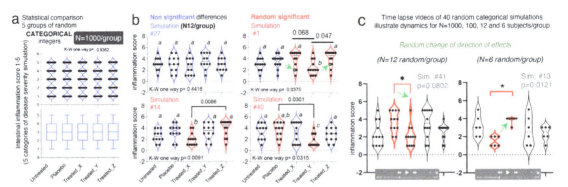

Figure 6. Categorical data simulations and violin plots illustrate that integer data exhibit multimodality and affect statistical reproducibility as simulations are performed randomly with various N. (**a**) N = 1000/group, simulation #1, violin plot and correspondent box plot for nonsignificant expected similarity across five groups (one-way K-W *p* > 0.05). See *p*-values and violin plots for >40 consecutive simulations in Supplementary Figure S7. (**a**,**b**) N = 12/group, violin plots for simulations #27 (non-significant), and #1, #14, and #40 (significant) illustrate comparisons due to randomness, result in irreproducible "treatment effects" and "direction of effects". Arrows, data points with statistical influence (see boxplots in Supplementary Figure S7). (**c**) Screenshots of time-lapse videos to show dynamically how statistical irreproducibility occurs at random for various N. Arrows indicate direction of effect. See Supplementary Video S1 doi:10.6084/m9.figshare.13377407. Asterisks indicate significance *p* < 0.05.

Visualization of these integer datasets with violin plots, illustrates that in all cases, categorical data follow multimodal distribution principles that accentuate the random irreproducibility of statistical analysis, and more importantly, the irreproducibility of the direction of effect as simulations are repeated. Violin plots illustrate how with lower N, there is the risk that investigators misperceive a data point as an outlier, when it is not, and proceed to exclude such points, consciously or unconsciously favoring the appearance of significant findings, especially when using small N for categorical data. As an alternative to categorical data, we have proposed the use of decimal scoring systems, instead of univariate integers, where decimals further carry information relevant to disease severity, making the system intrinsically more multivariable (see validated examples from Rodriguez-Palacios et al. for colonoscopy scores, and pathological scores for intestinal pathologies in [53,85]). To appreciate the advantages of violin plots in understanding integer multimodality for integers, simulations at various N are available as time-lapse videos at doi:10.6084/m9.figshare.13377407 (https://figshare.com/s/dcf154ce73c5bc086e80).

3.9. "Data Disease Subtyping" and "Cage-Cluster" Statistics

One important caveat to consider across animal studies is that increasing N alone is unhelpful if clustered-data statistics are not used to control for animal cage-density (>1 mouse/cage), which our group showed contributes to "artificial heterogeneity", "cyclical microbiome bias", and false-positive/false-negative conclusions [8,86].

To infer the role of scientific decision on the need for particular statistical methods, we examined the published studies [51] for "animal density" and "statistical" content (see Methods). Supporting the need for "modernizing" data analysis, we found that only one of the 38 studies (2.6%, 95% CI = 0.1–13.8%) used proper statistical methods (mixed models) to control for cage-clustering [23].

Although on average, studies tested 6.6 patients and 6.4 controls/group (range = 1–21), most studies were below the average (65.7%, 25/38, 95% CI = 48.6–80.4%), with 14 having <4 donors/group (Figure 7a). However, of interest, the number of human donors included in a study was inversely correlated with the number of mice/per donor used in the FMT experiments Figure 7b.

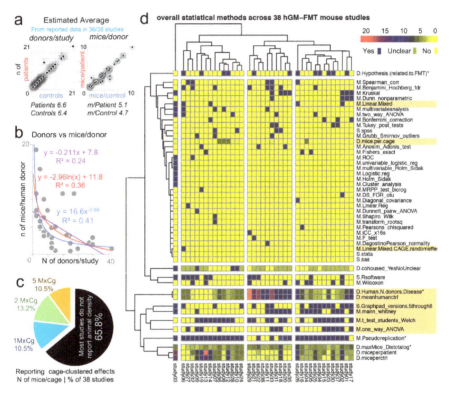

Figure 7. Study design and statistical methods among 38 hGM-FMT studies reveal lack of cage-clustered analysis and dominance of univariate analysis. Analysis of 38 studies reviewed in ref [51]. (a) Average and correlation of human donors with disease vs. healthy controls hN (left) and number of mice mN per human donor across studies (right plot). (b) Correlation plot with exponential, logarithmic and linear fits shows that scientists tend to use less mice when more donors are tested, creating a "trade-off" between data uncertainty due to variance in human disease with that of variance in animal models for disease of interest. (c) Pie chart, distribution of studies reporting mice/cage (MxCg), which indicates cage-clustered effects (search within study text keywords cage/cluster*, individual/house*, mice per*, density*, mixed/random/fix/methods/stat*, $p = *$). Most studies do not report MxCg (animal density). (d) Heatmap, overall statistical methods (M), statistical software (S), and study design (D) used across 38 studies. Only "study 6" [23] used linear mixed methods to control for the random effects of cage clustering. *Asterisk indicate variables examined in ref. [51]. Most statistical software reported in studies appear to be used for univariate statistics.

Unfortunately, the majority of studies (25/38, 65.8%, 95% CI = 48.6–80.4%) did not report animal density, consistent with previous analyses [8]; while 10.5% of the studies (4/38, 95% CI = 2.9–24.8%) housed their mice individually, which is advantageous because study designs are free of intraclass correlation coefficient, eliminating the need for cage-cluster statistics (Figure 7c).

Our review of the statistical methods used across the 38 studies also revealed that most scientists used GraphPad chiefly for graphics and univariate analysis of mouse phenotype data. This finding suggests an underutilization of the available functions in statistical software, for example, Monte Carlo simulations, to help understand the effect of random sampling on the reproducibility and significance of observed study results, and the likelihood of repeatability by others (Monte Carlo adjusted 95% confidence intervals) (Figure 7d). Of note, none of the studies considered multimodality or used violin plots (0%, 0/38, 95% CI = 6.9e−18, 9.1).

3.10. Multimodality in Human Outcome Data

To expand our analysis from that of microbiome hGM-FMT studies to that of other multifactorial diseases, we then examined published data from a double-blind, randomized, placebo-controlled, crossover design study in which the efficacy of a prebiotic dietary fiber (polydextrose) in improving cognitive performance an acute stress response in healthy individuals was investigated [87]. Using pre- and post-intervention data extrapolated from a figure in the publication, herein, we show that multimodality is present in human-derived outcomes. (Figure 8a–e). In the context of the simulations herein presented, this analysis represents the complexity of biomedical research and illustrate means to visualize disease subtypes. In this example, we show the "high", "middle", or "low" responders to cold stress regardless of the treatment (placebo vs. prebiotic fiber). Note that at baseline, two samples of individuals have two different distributions (normality tests and multimodality). In the figure, panels 8B and D illustrate that two different groups of individuals sampled for the study have different degrees of susceptibility. It is also important to note that at baseline, the two samples of individuals have two different distributions (normality tests and multimodality; Figure 8b,d). In conclusion, re-analysis of data from this human clinical trial that used maltodextrin as dietary placebo illustrates multimodal variability/differences in the stress responses between the two human groups and after the placebo consumption.

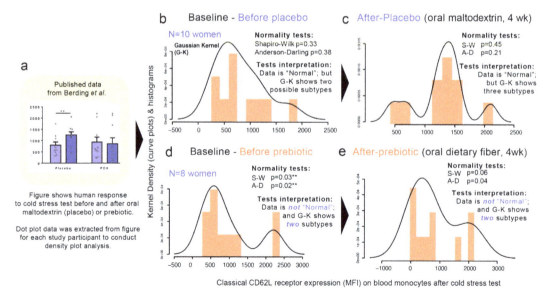

Figure 8. Example of multimodality in human outcome data. (a) Data was extrapolated from dot plot in study published by Berding et al. [87] (b,c) Outcome data for "placebo" maltodextrin group before and after cold stress test. (d,e) Outcome data for "prebiotic" fiber group before and after cold stress test. Panels B and D illustrate that two different groups of individuals sampled for the study have different degrees of susceptibility. Asterisks indicate significance $p < 0.05$.

4. Discussion

Understanding dataset multimodality and identifying strategies to address such source of variability in statistics is an emerging field in applied statistics to help address the complexity of multipeak data sets to improve study inferences and reproducibility in various fields of science, including biomedical research. Despite the inclusion of large numbers of human subjects in microbiome studies, the causal role of the human microbiome in disease remains uncertain. Exemplifying that a large N is not necessarily informative with complex human diseases, a large metanalysis [88] of raw hGM data from obese and IBD patients showed that human disease phenotypes do not always yield reproducible interlaboratory predictive biological signatures. Even when hundreds of individuals are studied, especially, if the "effect size for the disease of interest" is narrow (i.e., in obesity; larger in IBD) relative to the variability of the disease. For the human IBD subtypes (i.e., ulcerative colitis and Crohn's disease), the metanalysis [88] concluded that only the ileal form of Crohn's disease showed consistent hGM signatures compared to both healthy control donors and patients with either colonic Crohn's disease or ulcerative colitis [89], but no consistent signatures were observed for obesity.

Using a simple strategy of assuming random numbers drawn from an observed sample distribution, we have analytically illustrated that increasing N yields aberrant and/or conflicting statistical predictions, which depend on the patterns of disease variability and presence of disease subtypes (data modes). Specifically, our simulations revealed that the number of discernable data subtypes may wax and wane as N increases, and that increasing N does not uniformly enable the identification of statistical differences between groups. Furthermore, subjects randomly selected from a multimodal diseased population may create groups with statistical differences that do not always have the same direction. Especially, (i) if the human disease of interest exhibits variable phenotypes (e.g., cancer, obesity, or asthma) and (ii) if multivariable cage-clustered data analyses are not used to account for intraclass correlation coefficient of phenotypes within/between animal cages.

Under the "weak law of large numbers" principle in mathematics (Bernoulli's theorem [73–75]; see references for further illustration [90]), as N increases, the distribution of the study/sample means approximates the mean of the actual population, which facilitates the identification of statistically significant (but not biologically meaningful) differences between otherwise overlapping sample datasets. Commonly used statistical methods (e.g., t-tests; parametric vs. nonparametric) are designed to quantify differences around the sample centers (mean, median) and range of dispersion (standard errors or deviation) of two groups. However, these methods do not account for the distribution shape (unimodal vs. bi/multimodal) of the compared datasets. With arbitrary increases in N, what is insignificant becomes significant, thus increasing the tendency for the null hypothesis to be rejected despite clinically subtle differences [91,92].

To guide the selection of sufficient N (cases) or disease data subtype, herein we highlight the use of two simple statistical steps: (i) to first determine if the shape of the dataset is unimodal (e.g., dip test), and if not unimodal, then (ii) to use statistical simulations and tests to determine the number of modes/data values of interest, and finally, to (iii) perform Monte Carlo simulations using the statistical analysis conducted by scientists on their experimental data to quantify the frequency by which random sampling could interfere with the p-value computed. Such forms of Monte Carlo adjusted p-values can easily be performed using GraphPad or similar software (R, STATA), which are widely used in the literature. Doing so facilitates the objective design of personalized/disease subtyping experiments. Although comparisons between group means is important because some diseases are truly different, findings from our own hGM-FMT study [52] and others [21,23] highlight the relevance of studying disease subtypes and the sources of variability by personalizing the functional analysis of the hGM in mice (i.e., that both "pathological" and "beneficial" effects can be seen in hGM-FMT mice independent of donor disease status). For example, in our own work, the functional characterization of "beneficial" or "nonbeneficial" disease microbiome subtypes in IBD patients at times of remission could lead to the identification of an ideal patient fecal sample for future autologous transplantation during times of active disease. Therefore, personalized research has the potential to identify different functional microbiome subtypes (on a given outcome, e.g., assay or hGM-FMT mice) for one individual.

One pitfall of traditional statistics that are based either on mean and SD, or on non-parametric median and ranking methods, is that only central and dispersion parameters are used for analysis, which does not represent the data distribution shape. With mean and SD consistent with the observed data, there is no guarantee that the simulated data would match the whole distribution of the observed data.

With respect to determining unimodality, easily implementable tests to quantify data modality are available in STATA (statistical functions *diptest* and *mode*; proprietary and community contributed) and R (Package *multimode*, community contributed) [93]. The dip test [69] quantifies departures from unimodality and does not require a priori knowledge of potential multimodality, and thus, information can be easily interpreted from the test statistics and the *p*-value [83,94]. Although reports and comparative analysis of statistical performance have been described for various multimodality tests (e.g., dip test, bimodality test, Silverman's test, and likelihood ratio test [95], and kernel methods), including simpler alternatives that use benchmarks to determine the influence of data outliers [78,79,83,96], it is important to emphasize that every method depends on its intended application and data set/shape [84], and thus must be accompanied by the inspection of the data distributions modes.

5. Conclusions

In conclusion, by conducting a series of simulations and a review of statistical methods in current hGM-FMT literature, we extensively illustrate the constraints of increasing N as a main solution to identify causal links between the hGM and disease. We also highlight the integral role of multivariable cage-clustered data analyses, as previously described by our group [8]. Herein, we provided a conceptual framework that integrates the dynamics of sample center means and range of dispersion from the compared datasets with kernel and violin plots to identify "data disease subtypes" to address sample size and data multimodality. Biological insights from well-controlled, analyzed, and personalized analyses will lead to precise "person-specific" principles of disease, or identification of anti-inflammatory hGM, that could explain clinical/treatment outcomes in patients with certain disease subtypes and self-correct, guide, and promote the personalized investigation of disease subtype mechanisms.

Supplementary Materials: The following are available online at https://www.mdpi.com/2075-442 6/11/3/234/s1, Figure S1: Generation of random datasets of integer and decimal numbers using functions designed to draw numbers from a uniform and gaussian distribution, Figure S2: Further examples for data simulations with R2 value illustrate linearity as illustrated in Figure 1D, Figure S3: GraphPad Methods for Monte Carlo simulation, Figure S4: Monte Carlo Gaussian 100,000 simulations, Figure S5: Markov chain Monte Carlo (MCMC) simulations and examples of dip test, Figure S6: 16S microbiome profiles of hGM-SAMP fed an AD or AD-modified diet for 24 weeks, S7: Categorical data simulations and violin plots illustrate that categorical data exhibit multimodality and affects statistical reproducibility of random data. Table S1: Comparative percentages of simulations that yielded significant results for two statistical approaches, Video S1: Time-Lapse Examples doi:10.6084/m9.figshare.13377407 (https://figshare.com/s/dcf154ce73c5bc086e80).

Author Contributions: A.R.-P. conceptualized the study and proposed analytical arguments, conducted statistical analysis and simulations. A.R.B. and A.R.-P. conducted the survey, interpreted/analyzed data, and wrote the manuscript. F.C. contributed scientific suggestions. All authors have read and agreed to the published version of the manuscript.

Funding: A.R.-P. receives support from NIH grant R21 DK118373 entitled "Identification of pathogenic bacteria in Crohn's disease." We acknowledge the Biorepository Core of the NIH Silvio O. Conte Cleveland Digestive Disease Research Core Center (P30DK097948). Partial support also originates for A.R.-P. from the NIH grant P01DK091222 (Germ-Free and Gut Microbiome Core to A.R.-P. and to

F.C., Case Western Reserve University). A.B. received support from NIH grant T32DK083251 and F32DK117585.

Institutional Review Board Statement: Not Applicable.

Informed Consent Statement: Not Applicable.

Data Availability Statement: All datasets analyzed for this report are included in the following published articles [21,51,52] and/or their supplementary information files.

Acknowledgments: AB would like to thank the Raffners for their unwavering support.

Conflicts of Interest: The authors declare no conflict of interest.

References

1. Yalcin, A.; Rekik, I. A Diagnostic Unified Classification Model for Classifying Multi-Sized and Multi-Modal Brain Graphs Using Graph Alignment. *J. Neurosci. Methods* **2020**, 109014. [CrossRef]
2. Li, S.; Jamadar, S.D.; Ward, P.G.D.; Egan, G.F.; Chen, Z. Estimation of simultaneous BOLD and dynamic FDG metabolic brain activations using a multimodality concatenated ICA (mcICA) method. *Neuroimage* **2020**, 117603. [CrossRef]
3. Medina-Martinez, J.S.; Arango-Ossa, J.E.; Levine, M.F.; Zhou, Y.; Gundem, G.; Kung, A.L.; Papaemmanuil, E. Isabl Platform, a digital biobank for processing multimodal patient data. *BMC Bioinform.* **2020**, *21*, 549. [CrossRef] [PubMed]
4. Zeng, P.; Wangwu, J.; Lin, Z. Coupled co-clustering-based unsupervised transfer learning for the integrative analysis of single-cell genomic data. *Brief. Bioinform.* **2020**. [CrossRef] [PubMed]
5. Stelzer, C.; Benenson, Y. Precise determination of input-output mapping for multimodal gene circuits using data from transient transfection. *PLoS Comput. Biol.* **2020**, *16*, e1008389. [CrossRef]
6. Visell, Y. Fast Physically Accurate Rendering of Multimodal Signatures of Distributed Fracture in Heterogeneous Materials. *IEEE Trans. Vis. Comput. Graph.* **2015**, *21*, 443–451. [CrossRef]
7. Kilkenny, C.; Browne, W.J.; Cuthill, I.C.; Emerson, M.; Altman, D.G. Improving bioscience research reporting: The ARRIVE guidelines for reporting animal research. *PLoS Biol.* **2010**, *8*, e1000412. [CrossRef] [PubMed]
8. Basson, A.; LaSalla, A.; Lam, G.; Kulpins, D.; Moen, E.; Sundrud, M.; Miyoshi, J.; Ilic, S.; Theriault, B.; Cominelli, F.; et al. Artificial microbiome heterogeneity spurs six practical action themes and examples to increase study power-driven reproducibility. *Sci. Rep.* **2019**, *10*, 5039. [CrossRef] [PubMed]
9. Franklin, C.L.; Ericsson, A.C. Microbiota and reproducibility of rodent models. *Lab Anim.* **2017**, *46*, 114–122. [CrossRef]
10. Ericsson, A.C.; Gagliardi, J.; Bouhan, D.; Spollen, W.G.; Givan, S.A.; Franklin, C.L. The influence of caging, bedding, and diet on the composition of the microbiota in different regions of the mouse gut. *Sci. Rep.* **2018**, *8*. [CrossRef]
11. Stappenbeck, T.S.; Virgin, H.W. Accounting for reciprocal host-microbiome interactions in experimental science. *Nature* **2016**, *534*, 191–199. [CrossRef]
12. Arrieta, M.C.; Walter, J.; Finlay, B.B. Human Microbiota-Associated Mice: A Model with Challenges. *Cell Host Microbe* **2016**, *19*, 575–578. [CrossRef] [PubMed]
13. Soderborg, T.K.; Clark, S.E.; Mulligan, C.E.; Janssen, R.C.; Babcock, L.; Ir, D.; Young, B.; Krebs, N.; Lemas, D.J.; Johnson, L.K.; et al. The gut microbiota in infants of obese mothers increases inflammation and susceptibility to NAFLD. *Nat. Commun.* **2018**, *9*, 4462. [CrossRef]
14. Liu, R.; Kang, J.D.; Sartor, R.B.; Sikaroodi, M.; Fagan, A.; Gavis, E.A.; Zhou, H.; Hylemon, P.B.; Herzog, J.W.; Li, X.; et al. Neuroinflammation in Murine Cirrhosis Is Dependent on the Gut Microbiome and Is Attenuated by Fecal Transplant. *Hepatology* **2020**, *71*, 611–626. [CrossRef] [PubMed]
15. Fielding, R.A.; Reeves, A.R.; Jasuja, R.; Liu, C.; Barrett, B.B.; Lustgarten, M.S. Muscle strength is increased in mice that are colonized with microbiota from high-functioning older adults. *Exp. Gerontol.* **2019**, *127*, 110722. [CrossRef]
16. Maeda, Y.; Kurakawa, T.; Umemoto, E.; Motooka, D.; Ito, Y.; Gotoh, K.; Hirota, K.; Matsushita, M.; Furuta, Y.; Narazaki, M.; et al. Dysbiosis Contributes to Arthritis Development via Activation of Autoreactive T Cells in the Intestine. *Arthritis Rheumatol.* **2016**, *68*, 2646–2661. [CrossRef] [PubMed]
17. Stoll, M.L.; Pierce, M.K.; Watkins, J.A.; Zhang, M.; Weiss, P.F.; Weiss, J.E.; Elson, C.O.; Cron, R.Q.; Kumar, R.; Morrow, C.D.; et al. Akkermansia muciniphila is permissive to arthritis in the K/BxN mouse model of arthritis. *Genes Immun.* **2019**, *20*, 158–166. [CrossRef]
18. Petursdottir, D.H.; Nordlander, S.; Qazi, K.R.; Carvalho-Queiroz, C.; Ahmed Osman, O.; Hell, E.; Bjorkander, S.; Haileselassie, Y.; Navis, M.; Kokkinou, E.; et al. Early-Life Human Microbiota Associated With Childhood Allergy Promotes the T Helper 17 Axis in Mice. *Front. Immunol.* **2017**, *8*, 1699. [CrossRef]
19. Feehley, T.; Plunkett, C.H.; Bao, R.; Choi Hong, S.M.; Culleen, E.; Belda-Ferre, P.; Campbell, E.; Aitoro, R.; Nocerino, R.; Paparo, L.; et al. Healthy infants harbor intestinal bacteria that protect against food allergy. *Nat. Med.* **2019**, *25*, 448–453. [CrossRef] [PubMed]
20. Battaglioli, E.J.; Hale, V.L.; Chen, J.; Jeraldo, P.; Ruiz-Mojica, C.; Schmidt, B.A.; Rekdal, V.M.; Till, L.M.; Huq, L.; Smits, S.A.; et al. Clostridioides difficile uses amino acids associated with gut microbial dysbiosis in a subset of patients with diarrhea. *Sci. Transl. Med.* **2018**, *10*. [CrossRef] [PubMed]

21. Baxter, N.T.; Zackular, J.P.; Chen, G.Y.; Schloss, P.D. Structure of the gut microbiome following colonization with human feces determines colonic tumor burden. *Microbiome* **2014**, *2*, 20. [CrossRef]
22. Wong, S.H.; Zhao, L.; Zhang, X.; Nakatsu, G.; Han, J.; Xu, W.; Xiao, X.; Kwong, T.N.Y.; Tsoi, H.; Wu, W.K.K.; et al. Gavage of Fecal Samples From Patients With Colorectal Cancer Promotes Intestinal Carcinogenesis in Germ-Free and Conventional Mice. *Gastroenterology* **2017**, *153*, 1621–1633.e1626. [CrossRef]
23. Tomkovich, S.; Dejea, C.M.; Winglee, K.; Drewes, J.L.; Chung, L.; Housseau, F.; Pope, J.L.; Gauthier, J.; Sun, X.; Muhlbauer, M.; et al. Human colon mucosal biofilms from healthy or colon cancer hosts are carcinogenic. *J. Clin. Investig.* **2019**, *130*, 1699–1712. [CrossRef]
24. Kelly, J.R.; Borre, Y.; Brien, C.O.; Patterson, E.; El Aidy, S.; Deane, J.; Kennedy, P.J.; Beers, S.; Scott, K.; Moloney, G.; et al. Transferring the blues: Depression-associated gut microbiota induces neurobehavioural changes in the rat. *J. Psychiatr. Res.* **2016**, *82*, 109–118. [CrossRef]
25. Zheng, P.; Zeng, B.; Zhou, C.; Liu, M.; Fang, Z.; Xu, X.; Zeng, L.; Chen, J.; Fan, S.; Du, X.; et al. Gut microbiome remodeling induces depressive-like behaviors through a pathway mediated by the host's metabolism. *Mol. Psychiatry* **2016**, *21*, 786–796. [CrossRef]
26. Fujii, Y.; Nguyen, T.T.T.; Fujimura, Y.; Kameya, N.; Nakamura, S.; Arakawa, K.; Morita, H. Fecal metabolite of a gnotobiotic mouse transplanted with gut microbiota from a patient with Alzheimer's disease. *Biosci. Biotechnol. Biochem.* **2019**, *83*, 2144–2152. [CrossRef]
27. Zheng, P.; Zeng, B.; Liu, M.; Chen, J.; Pan, J.; Han, Y.; Liu, Y.; Cheng, K.; Zhou, C.; Wang, H.; et al. The gut microbiome from patients with schizophrenia modulates the glutamate-glutamine-GABA cycle and schizophrenia-relevant behaviors in mice. *Sci. Adv.* **2019**, *5*, eaau8317. [CrossRef]
28. Li, S.X.; Sen, S.; Schneider, J.M.; Xiong, K.N.; Nusbacher, N.M.; Moreno-Huizar, N.; Shaffer, M.; Armstrong, A.J.S.; Severs, E.; Kuhn, K.; et al. Gut microbiota from high-risk men who have sex with men drive immune activation in gnotobiotic mice and in vitro HIV infection. *PLoS Pathog.* **2019**, *15*, e1007611. [CrossRef] [PubMed]
29. Smith, M.I.; Yatsunenko, T.; Manary, M.J.; Trehan, I.; Mkakosya, R.; Cheng, J.; Kau, A.L.; Rich, S.S.; Concannon, P.; Mychaleckyj, J.C.; et al. Gut microbiomes of Malawian twin pairs discordant for kwashiorkor. *Science* **2013**, *339*, 548–554. [CrossRef]
30. Kau, A.L.; Planer, J.D.; Liu, J.; Rao, S.; Yatsunenko, T.; Trehan, I.; Manary, M.J.; Liu, T.C.; Stappenbeck, T.S.; Maleta, K.M.; et al. Functional characterization of IgA-targeted bacterial taxa from undernourished Malawian children that produce diet-dependent enteropathy. *Sci. Transl. Med.* **2015**, *7*. [CrossRef]
31. Wagner, V.E.; Dey, N.; Guruge, J.; Hsiao, A.; Ahern, P.P.; Semenkovich, N.P.; Blanton, L.V.; Cheng, J.; Griffin, N.; Stappenbeck, T.S.; et al. Effects of a gut pathobiont in a gnotobiotic mouse model of childhood undernutrition. *Sci. Transl. Med.* **2016**, *8*, 366ra164. [CrossRef]
32. Natividad, J.M.; Pinto-Sanchez, M.I.; Galipeau, H.J.; Jury, J.; Jordana, M.; Reinisch, W.; Collins, S.M.; Bercik, P.; Surette, M.G.; Allen-Vercoe, E.; et al. Ecobiotherapy Rich in Firmicutes Decreases Susceptibility to Colitis in a Humanized Gnotobiotic Mouse Model. *Inflamm. Bowel Dis.* **2015**, *21*, 1883–1893. [CrossRef] [PubMed]
33. Nagao-Kitamoto, H.; Shreiner, A.B.; Gillilland, M.G., 3rd; Kitamoto, S.; Ishii, C.; Hirayama, A.; Kuffa, P.; El-Zaatari, M.; Grasberger, H.; Seekatz, A.M.; et al. Functional Characterization of Inflammatory Bowel Disease-Associated Gut Dysbiosis in Gnotobiotic Mice. *Cell. Mol. Gastroenterol. Hepatol.* **2016**, *2*, 468–481. [CrossRef]
34. De Palma, G.; Lynch, M.D.J.; Lu, J.; Dang, V.T.; Deng, Y.K.; Jury, J.; Umeh, G.; Miranda, P.M.; Pastor, M.P.; Sidani, S.; et al. Transplantation of fecal microbiota from patients with irritable bowel syndrome alters gut function and behavior in recipient mice. *Sci. Transl. Med.* **2017**, *9*. [CrossRef] [PubMed]
35. Touw, K.; Ringus, D.L.; Hubert, N.; Wang, Y.; Leone, V.A.; Nadimpalli, A.; Theriault, B.R.; Huang, Y.E.; Tune, J.D.; Herring, P.B.; et al. Mutual reinforcement of pathophysiological host-microbe interactions in intestinal stasis models. *Physiol. Rep.* **2017**, *5*. [CrossRef] [PubMed]
36. Chen, Y.J.; Wu, H.; Wu, S.D.; Lu, N.; Wang, Y.T.; Liu, H.N.; Dong, L.; Liu, T.T.; Shen, X.Z. Parasutterella, in association with irritable bowel syndrome and intestinal chronic inflammation. *J. Gastroenterol. Hepatol.* **2018**, *33*, 1844–1852. [CrossRef]
37. Britton, G.J.; Contijoch, E.J.; Mogno, I.; Vennaro, O.H.; Llewellyn, S.R.; Ng, R.; Li, Z.; Mortha, A.; Merad, M.; Das, A.; et al. Microbiotas from Humans with Inflammatory Bowel Disease Alter the Balance of Gut Th17 and RORgammat (+) Regulatory T Cells and Exacerbate Colitis in Mice. *Immunity* **2019**, *50*, 212–224.e214. [CrossRef]
38. Torres, J.; Hu, J.; Seki, A.; Eisele, C.; Nair, N.; Huang, R.; Tarassishin, L.; Jharap, B.; Cote-Daigneault, J.; Mao, Q.; et al. Infants born to mothers with IBD present with altered gut microbiome that transfers abnormalities of the adaptive immune system to germ-free mice. *Gut* **2020**, *69*, 42–51. [CrossRef]
39. Sampson, T.R.; Debelius, J.W.; Thron, T.; Janssen, S.; Shastri, G.G.; Ilhan, Z.E.; Challis, C.; Schretter, C.E.; Rocha, S.; Gradinaru, V.; et al. Gut Microbiota Regulate Motor Deficits and Neuroinflammation in a Model of Parkinson's Disease. *Cell* **2016**, *167*, 1469–1480.e1412. [CrossRef]
40. Berer, K.; Gerdes, L.A.; Cekanaviciute, E.; Jia, X.; Xiao, L.; Xia, Z.; Liu, C.; Klotz, L.; Stauffer, U.; Baranzini, S.E.; et al. Gut microbiota from multiple sclerosis patients enables spontaneous autoimmune encephalomyelitis in mice. *Proc. Natl. Acad. Sci. USA* **2017**, *114*, 10719–10724. [CrossRef]

41. Cekanaviciute, E.; Yoo, B.B.; Runia, T.F.; Debelius, J.W.; Singh, S.; Nelson, C.A.; Kanner, R.; Bencosme, Y.; Lee, Y.K.; Hauser, S.L.; et al. Gut bacteria from multiple sclerosis patients modulate human T cells and exacerbate symptoms in mouse models. *Proc. Natl. Acad. Sci. USA* **2017**, *114*, 10713–10718. [CrossRef]

42. Sharon, G.; Cruz, N.J.; Kang, D.W.; Gandal, M.J.; Wang, B.; Kim, Y.M.; Zink, E.M.; Casey, C.P.; Taylor, B.C.; Lane, C.J.; et al. Human Gut Microbiota from Autism Spectrum Disorder Promote Behavioral Symptoms in Mice. *Cell* **2019**, *177*, 1600–1618.e1617. [CrossRef]

43. Koren, O.; Goodrich, J.K.; Cullender, T.C.; Spor, A.; Laitinen, K.; Backhed, H.K.; Gonzalez, A.; Werner, J.J.; Angenent, L.T.; Knight, R.; et al. Host Remoding of the Gut Microbiome and Metabolic Changes during Pregnancy. *Cell* **2012**, *150*, 470–480. [CrossRef]

44. Ridaura, V.K.; Faith, J.J.; Rey, F.E.; Cheng, J.Y.; Duncan, A.E.; Kau, A.L.; Griffin, N.W.; Lombard, V.; Henrissat, B.; Bain, J.R.; et al. Gut Microbiota from Twins Discordant for Obesity Modulate Metabolism in Mice. *Science* **2013**, *341*, 1241214. [CrossRef]

45. Goodrich, J.K.; Waters, J.L.; Poole, A.C.; Sutter, J.L.; Koren, O.; Blekhman, R.; Beaumont, M.; Van Treuren, W.; Knight, R.; Bell, J.T.; et al. Human genetics shape the gut microbiome. *Cell* **2014**, *159*, 789–799. [CrossRef] [PubMed]

46. Kovatcheva-Datchary, P.; Nilsson, A.; Akrami, R.; Lee, Y.S.; De Vadder, F.; Arora, T.; Hallen, A.; Martens, E.; Bjorck, I.; Backhed, F. Dietary Fiber-Induced Improvement in Glucose Metabolism Is Associated with Increased Abundance of Prevotella. *Cell Metab.* **2015**, *22*, 971–982. [CrossRef]

47. Chiu, C.C.; Ching, Y.H.; Li, Y.P.; Liu, J.Y.; Huang, Y.T.; Huang, Y.W.; Yang, S.S.; Huang, W.C.; Chuang, H.L. Nonalcoholic Fatty Liver Disease Is Exacerbated in High-Fat Diet-Fed Gnotobiotic Mice by Colonization with the Gut Microbiota from Patients with Nonalcoholic Steatohepatitis. *Nutrients* **2017**, *9*, 1220. [CrossRef] [PubMed]

48. Li, J.; Zhao, F.; Wang, Y.; Chen, J.; Tao, J.; Tian, G.; Wu, S.; Liu, W.; Cui, Q.; Geng, B.; et al. Gut microbiota dysbiosis contributes to the development of hypertension. *Microbiome* **2017**, *5*, 14. [CrossRef] [PubMed]

49. Zhang, L.; Bahl, M.I.; Roager, H.M.; Fonvig, C.E.; Hellgren, L.I.; Frandsen, H.L.; Pedersen, O.; Holm, J.-C.; Hansen, T.; Licht, T.R. Environmental spread of microbes impacts the development of metabolic phenotypes in mice transplanted with microbial communities from humans. *ISME J.* **2017**, *11*, 14. [CrossRef] [PubMed]

50. Ge, X.; Zhao, W.; Ding, C.; Tian, H.; Xu, L.; Wang, H.; Ni, L.; Jiang, J.; Gong, J.; Zhu, W.; et al. Potential role of fecal microbiota from patients with slow transit constipation in the regulation of gastrointestinal motility. *Sci. Rep.* **2017**, *7*, 441. [CrossRef]

51. Walter, J.; Armet, A.M.; Finlay, B.B.; Shanahan, F. Establishing or exaggerating causality for the gut microbiome: Lessons from human microbiota-associated rodents. *Cell* **2020**, *180*, 221–232. [CrossRef] [PubMed]

52. Basson, A.; Gomez-Nguyen, A.; Menghini, P.; Butto, L.; Di Martino, L.; Aladyshkina, N.; Osme, A.; LaSalla, A.; Fischer, D.; Ezeji, J.C.; et al. Human gut microbiome transplantation in ileitis prone mice: A tool for the functional characterization of the microbiota in inflammatory bowel disease patients. *Inflamm. Bowel Dis.* **2019**, *26*, 347–359. [CrossRef]

53. Rodriguez-Palacios, A.; Kodani, T.; Kaydo, L.; Pietropaoli, D.; Corridoni, D.; Howell, S.; Katz, J.; Xin, W.; Pizarro, T.T.; Cominelli, F. Stereomicroscopic 3D-pattern profiling of murine and human intestinal inflammation reveals unique structural phenotypes. *Nat. Commun.* **2015**, *6*, 7577. [CrossRef]

54. Wessa, P. *Free Statistics Software*; Version 1.2.1; Office for Research Development and Education: Denver, CO, USA, 2020; Available online: https://www.wessa.net/ (accessed on 5 October 2020).

55. Wessa, P. Histogram (v1.0.21). In *Free Statistics Software (v1.2.1)*; Office for Research Development and Education: Denver, CO, USA, 2020; Available online: http://www.wessa.net/rwasp_histogram.wasp/ (accessed on 5 October 2020).

56. Venables, W.N.; Ripley, B.D. *Modern Applied Statistics with S*, 4th ed.; Springer: New York, NY, USA, 2002. [CrossRef]

57. Wessa, P. Tukey Lambda PPCC Plot (v1.0.3). In *Free Statistics Software (v1.2.1)*; Office for Research Development and Education: Denver, CO, USA, 2013; Available online: http://www.wessa.net/rwasp_tukeylambda.wasp/ (accessed on 5 October 2020).

58. NIST. *NIST/SEMATECH e-Handbook of Statistical Methods*; NIST: Gaithersburg, MD, USA, 2003. Available online: http://www.itl.nist.gov/div898/handbook/ (accessed on 5 October 2020). [CrossRef]

59. Wessa, P. Maximum-Likelihood Normal Distribution Fitting and QQ Plot (v1.0.8). In *Free Statistics Software (v1.2.1)*; Office for Research Development and Education: Denver, CO, USA, 2021; Available online: https://www.wessa.net/rwasp_fitdistrnorm.wasp/ (accessed on 5 October 2020).

60. DiCarlo, D.; David, F. Random Number Generation: Types and Techniques. Senior Honors Theses, Liberty University, Lynchburg, VA, USA, 2012; p. 308. Available online: https://digitalcommons.liberty.edu/honors/308 (accessed on 6 October 2020).

61. Real Statistics Using Excel. Available online: https://www.real-statistics.com (accessed on 4 October 2020).

62. Devroye, L. *Non-Uniform Random Variate Generation*; Springer: New York, NY, USA, 1986.

63. R.Documentation. Available online: https://stat.ethz.ch/R-manual/R-devel/library/base/html/Random.html (accessed on 10 October 2020).

64. Haahr, M. Introduction to Randomness and Random Numbers. Available online: www.random.org/randomness/ (accessed on 15 December 2020).

65. Ehrhardt, J.C. Generation of pseudorandom numbers. *Med. Phys.* **1986**, *13*, 240–241. [CrossRef]

66. van Ravenzwaaij, D.; Cassey, P.; Brown, S.D. A simple introduction to Markov Chain Monte-Carlo sampling. *Psychon. Bull. Rev.* **2018**, *25*, 143–154. [CrossRef] [PubMed]

67. Peng, R.D. Advanced Statistical Computing. 2020. Available online: https://bookdown.org/rdpeng/advstatcomp/metropolis-hastings.html (accessed on 10 October 2020).

68. Gilks, W.R. *Markov Chain Monte Carlo in Practice*; Chapman &Amp; Hall/CRC: Boca Raton, FL, USA, 1996.

69. Hartigan, J.A.; Hartigan, P.M. The Dip Test of Unimodality. *Ann. Stat.* **1985**, *13*, 70–84. [CrossRef]
70. Maechler, M. *Hartigan's Dip Test Statistic for Unimodality—Corrected, 0.75–7*; R Foundation for Statistical Computing: Vienna, Austria, 2016.
71. Cox, N.J. sg113_2: Tabulation of modes. *Stata Tech. Bull.* **1999**, *50*, 26–27.
72. Bickel, D.R.; Fruhwirth, R. On a fast, robust estimator of the mode: Comparisons to other robust estimators with applications. *Comput. Stat. Data Anal.* **2006**, *50*, 3500–3530. [CrossRef]
73. Papoulis, A. *Probability, Random Variables, and Stochastic Processes*, 2nd ed.; McGraw-Hill: New York, NY, USA, 1984.
74. Feller, W. Law of Large Numbers for Identically Distributed Variables. In *An Introduction to Probability Theory and Its Applications*; Wiley: New York, NY, USA, 1971; Volume 3, pp. 69–71.
75. Weisstein, E.W. Weak Law of Large Numbers. from MathWorld—A Wolfram Web Resource. Available online: http://mathworld.wolfram.com/WeakLawofLargeNumbers.html (accessed on 4 March 2020).
76. Krzywinski, M.; Altman, N. Visualizing samples with box plots. *Nat. Methods* **2014**, *11*, 119–120. [CrossRef]
77. Hintze, J.; Nelson, R. Violin Plots: A Box Plot-Density Trace Synergism. *Am. Stat.* **1998**, *52*, 181–184. [CrossRef]
78. Johnsson, K.; Linderoth, M.; Fontes, M. What is a "unimodal" cell population? Using statistical tests as criteria for unimodality in automated gating and quality control. *Cytom. A* **2017**, *91*, 908–916. [CrossRef]
79. Testroet, E.D.; Sherman, P.; Yoder, C.; Testroet, A.; Reynolds, C.; O'Neil, M.; Lei, S.M.; Beitz, D.C.; Baas, T.J. A novel and robust method for testing bimodality and characterizing porcine adipocytes of adipose tissue of 5 purebred lines of pig. *Adipocyte* **2017**, *6*, 102–111. [CrossRef]
80. Wolfram Alpha LLC. Wolfram|Alpha. 2009. Available online: https://www.wolframalpha.com/ (accessed on 15 December 2020).
81. Weber, S.; Eye, A. Simulation Methods for Categorical Variables. In *Wiley StatsRef: Statistics Reference Online*; John Wiley & Sons, Ltd.: Hoboken, NJ, USA, 2014.
82. Goovaerts, P. Stochastic simulation of categorical variables using a classification algorithm and simulated annealing. *Math. Geol.* **1996**, *28*, 909–9821. [CrossRef]
83. Freeman, J.B.; Dale, R. Assessing bimodality to detect the presence of a dual cognitive process. *Behav. Res. Methods* **2013**, *45*, 83–97. [CrossRef]
84. Kang, Y.-J.; Noh, Y. Development of Hartigan's Dip Statistic with Bimodality Coefficient to Assess Multimodality of Distributions. In *Mathematical Problems in Engineering*; Hindawi: London, UK, 2019; Volume 4819475, p. 17.
85. Kodani, T.; Rodriguez-Palacios, A.; Corridoni, D.; Lopetuso, L.; Di Martino, L.; Marks, B.; Pizarro, J.; Pizarro, T.; Chak, A.; Cominelli, F. Flexible Colonoscopy in Mice to Evaluate the Severity of Colitis and Colorectal Tumors Using a Validated Endoscopic Scoring System. *J. Vis. Exp.* **2013**. [CrossRef]
86. Rodriguez-Palacios, A.; Aladyshkina, N.; Ezeji, J.C.; Erkkila, H.L.; Conger, M.; Ward, J.; Webster, J.; Cominelli, F. 'Cyclical Bias' in Microbiome Research Revealed by A Portable Germ-Free Housing System Using Nested Isolation. *Sci. Rep.* **2018**, *8*, 18. [CrossRef]
87. Berding, K.; Long-Smith, C.M.; Carbia, C.; Bastiaanssen, T.F.S.; van de Wouw, M.; Wiley, N.; Strain, C.R.; Fouhy, F.; Stanton, C.; Cryan, J.F.; et al. A specific dietary fibre supplementation improves cognitive performance-an exploratory randomised, placebo-controlled, crossover study. *Psychopharmacology* **2021**, *238*, 149–163. [CrossRef]
88. Walters, W.A.; Xu, Z.; Knight, R. Meta-analyses of human gut microbes associated with obesity and IBD. *FEBS Lett.* **2014**, *588*, 4223–4233. [CrossRef]
89. Gevers, D.; Kugathasan, S.; Denson, L.A.; Vazquez-Baeza, Y.; Van Treuren, W.; Ren, B.; Schwager, E.; Knights, D.; Song, S.J.; Yassour, M.; et al. The treatment-naive microbiome in new-onset Crohn's disease. *Cell Host Microbe* **2014**, *15*, 382–392. [CrossRef] [PubMed]
90. Hanck, C.; Arnold, M.; Gerber, A.; Schmelzer, M. Convergence in Probability, Consistency and the Law of Large Numbers. In *Introduction to Econometrics with R*; University of Duisburg-Essen: Essen, Germany, 2019.
91. Biau, D.J.; Kerneis, S.; Porcher, R. Statistics in brief: The importance of sample size in the planning and interpretation of medical research. *Clin. Orthop. Relat. Res.* **2008**, *466*, 2282–2288. [CrossRef]
92. Faber, J.; Fonseca, L.M. How sample size influences research outcomes. *Dent. Press J. Orthod.* **2014**, *19*, 27–29. [CrossRef] [PubMed]
93. Ameijeiras-Alonso, J.; Crujeiras, R.M.; The R Core Team; The R Foundation. *Package 'Multimode'*. 1.4. 2018. Available online: https://cran.r-project.org/web/packages/multimode/multimode.pdf (accessed on 22 March 2021).
94. Stanbro, M. *Hartigan's Dip Test of Unimodality Applied on Terrestrial Gamma—Ray Flashes*. Honors Thesis, University of Alabama, Tuscaloosa, AL, USA. Available online: https://www.uah.edu/images/administrative/Honors/Papers/v03n2-Stanbro.pdf. (accessed on 6 October 2020).
95. Wolfe, J.H. Pattern clustering by multivariate mixture analysis. *Multivar. Behav. Res.* **1970**, *5*, 329–350. [CrossRef] [PubMed]
96. Xu, L.; Bedrick, E.J.; Hanson, T.; Restrepo, C. A Comparison of Statistical Tools for Identifying Modality in Body Mass Distributions. *J. Data Sci.* **2014**, *12*, 175–196. [CrossRef]

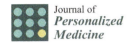

Article

Differences in the Microbial Composition of Hemodialysis Patients Treated with and without β-Blockers

Yi-Ting Lin [1,2,3], Ting-Yun Lin [4,5], Szu-Chun Hung [4,5], Po-Yu Liu [6], Wei-Chun Hung [7], Wei-Chung Tsai [8], Yi-Chun Tsai [2,9,10], Rachel Ann Delicano [11], Yun-Shiuan Chuang [1], Mei-Chuan Kuo [2,10,12], Yi-Wen Chiu [2,10,12] and Ping-Hsun Wu [2,3,12,*]

1. Department of Family Medicine, Kaohsiung Medical University Hospital, Kaohsiung 80708, Taiwan; 960254@kmuh.org.tw (Y.-T.L.); kinkipag@gmail.com (Y.-S.C.)
2. Faculty of Medicine, College of Medicine, Kaohsiung Medical University, Kaohsiung 80708, Taiwan; lidam65@yahoo.com.tw (Y.-C.T.); mechku@kmu.edu.tw (M.-C.K.); chiuyiwen@kmu.edu.tw (Y.-W.C.)
3. Graduate Institute of Clinical Medicine, College of Medicine, Kaohsiung Medical University, Kaohsiung 80708, Taiwan
4. Division of Nephrology, Taipei Tzu Chi Hospital, Buddhist Tzu Chi Medical Foundation, New Taipei City 23142, Taiwan; water_h2o_6@hotmail.com (T.-Y.L.); szuchun.hung@gmail.com (S.-C.H.)
5. School of Medicine, Tzu Chi University, Hualien 97071, Taiwan
6. Department of Internal Medicine, College of Medicine, National Taiwan University, Taipei 100225, Taiwan; poyu.liu@gmail.com
7. Department of Microbiology and Immunology, Kaohsiung Medical University, Kaohsiung 80708, Taiwan; wchung@kmu.edu.tw
8. Division of Cardiology, Department of Internal Medicine, Kaohsiung Medical University Hospital, Kaohsiung Medical University, Kaohsiung 80708, Taiwan; k920265@gap.kmu.edu.tw
9. Division of General Medicine, Department of Internal Medicine, Kaohsiung Medical University, Kaohsiung 80708, Taiwan
10. Faculty of Renal Care, College of Medicine, Kaohsiung Medical University, Kaohsiung 80708, Taiwan
11. Institute of Surgical Sciences, Uppsala University, 752 36 Uppsala, Sweden; rachel.delicano@surgsci.uu.se
12. Division of Nephrology, Department of Internal Medicine, Kaohsiung Medical University Hospital, Kaohsiung Medical University, Kaohsiung 80708, Taiwan
* Correspondence: 970392@kmuh.org.tw; Tel.: +886-7-3121101

Abstract: β-blockers are commonly prescribed to treat cardiovascular disease in hemodialysis patients. Beyond the pharmacological effects, β-blockers have potential impacts on gut microbiota, but no study has investigated the effect in hemodialysis patients. Hence, we aim to investigate the gut microbiota composition difference between β-blocker users and nonusers in hemodialysis patients. Fecal samples collected from hemodialysis patients (83 β-blocker users and 110 nonusers) were determined by 16S ribosomal RNA amplification sequencing. Propensity score (PS) matching was performed to control confounders. The microbial composition differences were analyzed by the linear discriminant analysis effect size, random forest, and zero-inflated Gaussian fit model. The α-diversity (Simpson index) was greater in β-blocker users with a distinct β-diversity (Bray–Curtis Index) compared to nonusers in both full and PS-matched cohorts. There was a significant enrichment in the genus *Flavonifractor* in β-blocker users compared to nonusers in full and PS-matched cohorts. A similar finding was demonstrated in random forest analysis. In conclusion, hemodialysis patients using β-blockers had a different gut microbiota composition compared to nonusers. In particular, the *Flavonifractor* genus was increased with β-blocker treatment. Our findings highlight the impact of β-blockers on the gut microbiota in hemodialysis patients.

Keywords: microbiome; beta-blocker; hemodialysis; next-generation sequencing; propensity score matching methods

1. Introduction

The gut microbiota has a crucial role in metabolic, nutritional, physiological, defensive, and immunological processes in the human body, with its composition linked to human health and the development of diseases [1,2]. Human-microbiome association can be considered as integration in evolution. The microbiome can modulate and restore human health [3]. Changes in this microbial equilibrium, that is, dysbiosis, promotes and influences the course of many intestinal and extra-intestinal diseases [4–6]. In addition to genetic and environmental factors, several common medications (e.g., proton pump inhibitors, nonsteroidal anti-inflammatory drugs, atypical antipsychotics, selective serotonin reuptake inhibitors, antibiotics, statins, and antidiabetic drugs) are associated with the specific gut microbiota composition [7–13]. Indeed, drug-microbiome-host interactions are complex and multifactorial, impacting host metabolism [14,15]. Hence, they should be part of the core phenotype set for human gut microbiota research [16].

Patients with chronic kidney disease (CKD) have altered gut microbiota, with a bidirectional causal effect relationship [17,18]. Among the cardiovascular preventive drugs for patients with end-stage renal disease (ESRD), β-blockers are commonly prescribed in higher cardiovascular risk patients to prevent sudden cardiac death [19,20]. Beyond the clinical effect of β-blockers in ESRD patients, they also have a potential impact on gut microbiota [7,16]. Besides, the benefit of beta-blockers may be attributed to preventing the activity of the gut microbe-generated metabolite, such as phenylacetylglutamine [21]. However, limited study has investigated the impact on ESRD patients. Herein, we evaluate the gut microbiota composition of β-blocker users and nonusers in Taiwanese hemodialysis patients.

2. Materials and Methods

2.1. Study Participants

The Ethics Committee approved the study protocols of Kaohsiung Medical University Hospital (KMUHIRB-E(I)-20160095 and KMUHIRB-E(I)-20180118) and Taipei Tzu Chi Hospital (07-X01-002). All participants provided written informed consent. Hemodialysis patients were recruited from the dialysis unit of Taipei Tzu Chi Hospital and Kaohsiung Medical University Hospital in Taiwan from August 2017 to February 2018. The inclusion criteria were patients with age more than 18 years old and received regular hemodialysis three times per week, 3.5–4 h with high-flux dialyzers. The exclusion criteria included patients with partial or total colectomy, inflammatory bowel diseases, active malignancies, or patients who were prescribed antibiotics within three months before enrollment. Fecal samples were collected from 193 stable hemodialysis patients and analyzed by high-throughput 16S ribosomal RNA gene sequencing to compared participants with and without β-blocker treatment. All β-blocker users were prescribed for at least one month.

2.2. Comorbidity, Laboratory, and Clinical Variables

All baseline characteristics of sociodemographic data, age, sex, body mass index, dialysis vintage, arteriovenous shunt type, comorbidities, medications, and biochemical data were collected in the built-in electronic health care system. Blood samples were collected after overnight fasting through the arteriovenous fistula or graft before scheduled hemodialysis sessions. The biochemical data included serum values for hemoglobin, albumin, high sensitivity C reactive protein, total cholesterol, low-density lipoprotein, triglycerides, ion calcium, and phosphate from routine blood samples obtained within 30 days before stool sample collection. Diet was evaluated by a licensed dietitian using a modified short-form food frequency questionnaire. No specific antioxidant supplements (i.e., tea, cocoa products, or wine) were recorded because of strict dietary restrictions in hemodialysis patients. Participants have followed the nutrition guideline of the National Kidney Foundation's Kidney Disease Outcomes Quality Initiative (KDOQI™) [22], which recommends a high-protein intake (1.1–1.4 g/kg/day) and reduced consumption of fruits, vegetables, and dietary fiber to avoid potassium overload. Diabetes was defined as HbA1C

6.5% or higher or use of oral antidiabetic agents or insulin. Hypertension was defined as 140/90 mmHg or higher or taking blood pressure-lowering drugs. A history of myocardial infarction or documented by coronary angiography, class III or IV congestive heart failure, or a cerebrovascular accident were defined as cardiovascular disease.

2.3. Fecal Sample Collection and Bacterial 16S rRNA Amplicon Sequencing and Processing

All stool samples were frozen immediately after collection by each participant, then delivered in cooler bags to the laboratory (Germark Biotechnology, Taichung, Taiwan) within 24 h. A QIAamp DNA Stool Mini Kit (Qiagen, MD, USA) was used to extract DNA from fecal samples. Barcode-indexed PCR primers (341F and 805R) were used to create an amplicon library by amplifying the variable regions 3 and 4 (V3–V4) of the 16S rRNA gene [23]. The amplicons were sequenced (300 bp paired-end) using an Illumina MiSeq sequencer at the same time in the same laboratory to avoid batch effects (Germark Biotechnology, Taichung, Taiwan). The 16S-amplicon pipeline was adapted from 16S Bacteria/Archaea SOP v1 of Microbiome Helper workflows [24]. Paired-End reAd mergeR (PEAR; version 0.9.8) [25] was used to merge paired-end reads to raw reads, then filtered low-quality reads by thresholds of sequence length $\geq$400 bp and quality score of 90% bases of reads $\geq$20. Quantitative Insight Into Microbial Ecology (QIIME; version 1.9.1) software was used to select operational taxonomic units (OTU) [26]. The SILVA (version 123) 16S database [27,28] was applied to cluster OTUs and assign taxonomy using the UCLUST algorithm (version v1.2.22q) [29] with a 97% sequence identity threshold. Reads were dereplicated, and singletons were discarded. The final OTU table was rarefied into minimum sequencing depth in the data set.

2.4. Propensity Score Matching

Propensity score (PS) matching [30,31] was performed to balance confounders between the comparisons of interest (i.e., β-blocker users versus nonusers) and minimize the confounding by indication resulting from nonrandom treatment study. Using a logistic regression model, β-blocker use was accessed to estimate the propensity to receive a β-blocker for each participant based on potential confounders, including age, sex, body mass index, dialysis vintage, smoking history, vascular access type, Bristol stool scale, dietary intake, comorbidities (diabetes mellitus, hypertension, dyslipidemia, coronary artery disease, heart failure, cerebrovascular disease, and parathyroidectomy history), concomitant drugs used (including ACEI (angiotensin converting enzyme inhibitors)/ARB (angiotensin-receptor blockers), glucose-lowering drugs (such as sulfonylurea, dipeptidyl peptidase-4 inhibitors, insulin), statin, calcium carbonate, and proton pump inhibitors), and clinical laboratory data (hemoglobin, albumin, total cholesterol, triglyceride, high sensitivity C reactive protein (hsCRP), sodium, potassium, total calcium, phosphate, parathyroid hormone, serum iron, ferritin, normalized protein catabolic rate (nPCR), and single pool Kt/V). In this study, 193 hemodialysis patients were enrolled, including 83 β-blocker users and 110 nonusers (full cohort). PS-matched (1:1) analysis was used to match participants with β-blocker treatment ($N = 62$) to participants without β-blocker treatment ($N = 62$) (PS-matched cohort, Figure 1).

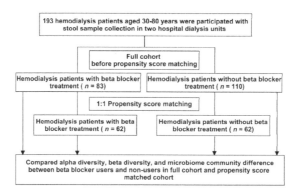

Figure 1. Study design.

2.5. Statistical and Bioinformatics Analyses of Microbiota

The study design is presented in Figure 1. Demographic characteristics are shown as the mean, median, or frequency, with differences between β-blocker users and nonusers determined using an independent T-test or chi-squared test, as appropriate. A rarefaction curve was built to prevent methodological artifacts originating from variations in sequencing depth. The α-diversity indices (Shannon and Simpson's indices) estimated the evenness of taxa within each sample and were generated using the R "vegan" package and calculated the *p*-value by the Kruskal–Wallis test. The β-diversity provides a comparison of the taxonomic profiles' differences between pairs of individual samples. The β-diversity was calculated based on the Bray–Curtis distance matrices and was visualized using principal coordinates analysis (PCoA) and calculated using homogeneity of group dispersions by Permutational Analysis of Multivariate Dispersions (PERMDISP) [32].

Co-occurrence analysis was used to determine the relationships within communities, with core microbiome analysis performed at the genus level using MicrobiomeAnalyst [33], in which sample prevalence and relative abundance cut-off values were set at 20 and 0.2%, respectively. For visualization of the internal interactions and further measurement of the microbial community, Sparse Correlations for Compositional data (SparCC) was used to calculate the Spearman correlation coefficient with the corresponding *p*-value between every two taxa. Microbiota community structure was assessed by co-occurrence networks built by the SparCC algorithm [34]. The *p*-values were estimated by 100 random permutations and iterations for each SparCC calculation, and correlation matrices were computed from the resampled data matrices. Only OTUs with correlation scores greater than 0.4 and *p*-value less than 0.05 were categorized into co-abundance groups (CAGs); these coefficients were also used to assess the length of edges on the network. An undirected network, weighted by SparCC correlation magnitude, was generated using bioinformatics tools in MicrobiomeAnalyst [33].

The bacterial OTU difference between β-blocker users and nonusers was analyzed by the linear discriminant analysis (LDA) of effect size (LEfSe) analysis with samples presenting more than 0.1% relative abundance and found >30% of all samples. The LEfSe analysis employed the nonparametric factorial Kruskal–Wallis test or Wilcoxon rank-sum test and LDA to identify differentially abundant taxa between the groups. Only taxa with LDA score greater than two or less than two at a *p*-value < 0.05 were considered significantly enriched. All statistical tests are two-tailed, and a *p*-value < 0.05 was considered statistically significant. The random forest method [35] was performed to determine a ranked list of all bacterial taxa to identify the most predictive bacterial community to classify β-blocker users and nonusers. The random forest is a supervised learning algorithm ranking OTUs based on their ability to discriminate among the groups, while accounting for the complex interrelationships in high dimensional data. The MetagenomeSeq method was also used to evaluate differential abundance in sparse marker-gene survey data using a zero-inflated

Gaussian (ZIG) fit model to account for undersampling and sparsity in OTU count data after normalizing the data through cumulative sum scaling (CSS) [36]. Finally, the log-transformed read counts difference of the top selected genera from the ZIG fit model between β-blocker users and nonusers was analyzed in the full and PS-matched cohorts.

Co-occurrence and random forest analyses were performed by MicrobiomeAnalyst [33]. The other statistical analyses were performed using R statistical software (version 3.5.1) and STATA statistical software (version 14; StataCorp LLC, College Station, TX, USA).

2.6. Functional Prediction Analysis

Phylogenetic Investigation of Communities by Reconstruction of Unobserved States (PICRUSt2) [37] was used to predict the metagenome, which was based on Integrated Microbial Genomes (IMG) database [38] to evaluate the functions of gut microbiota among β blocker users and nonusers in the full cohort and PS-matched cohort. An OTU table was used for predicting metagenome based on Kyoto Encyclopedia of Genes and Genomes (KEGG) Orthology (KO) annotations. Metabolic module enrichment analysis was done with functional sets enrichment analysis (FSEA) described by Liu et al. [39]. The 'FSEA' function in the MARco R package based on the Liu et al. paper was applied in this study [39]. The 'FSEA' was embedded with the 'gage' R-package [40]. Enrichment scores were scored based on the GSEA algorithm of the Database for Annotation, Visualization, and Integrated Discovery (DAVID) bioinformatics resources [41,42].

3. Results

3.1. Patient Characteristics

Patient characteristics are shown in Table 1, with those receiving β-blockers having a higher proportion of diabetes, hypertension, dyslipidemia, coronary artery disease, heart failure, cerebrovascular disease, and more commonly used ACEI/ARB, glucose-lowering drugs (such as dipeptidyl peptidase-4 inhibitors or insulin) and statin. PS matching resulted in 62 matched pairs with balanced baseline characteristics (Table 1).

3.2. Gut Microbiota Profile Differs in Hemodialysis Patients with and without β Blocker Treatment

The rarefaction curves were close to asymptotic based on the number of OTUs observed. To represent the microbiome community with enough coverage, the rarefaction curves reached saturation at a cutoff point of 45,000 sequences per sample (Supplementary Figure S1). Compared to the gut microbiota composition and structure between β-blocker users and nonusers, no substantial differences were observed in the relative abundance proportion in the full and PS-matched cohorts (Supplementary Figure S2). Hemodialysis patients taking β-blockers had a higher α-diversity and a distinct β-diversity compared to nonusers in the full and PS-matched cohorts (Figure 2). The core microbiome was Bacteroides in hemodialysis patients (Supplementary Figure S3A), with a similar core microbiome in β-blocker users and nonusers (Supplementary Figure S3B).

Table 1. Baseline characteristics of hemodialysis patients with and without β blocker treatment.

Baseline Characteristics	Before Propensity Score Matching			After Propensity Score Matching		
	β-Blocker Users (N = 83)	β-Blocker Nonusers (N = 110)	*p*-Value	β-Blocker Users (N = 62)	β-Blocker Nonusers (N = 62)	*p*-Value
Age (years)	64.3 ± 11.4	65.4 ± 11.2	0.511	64.7 ± 11.6	66.3 ± 11.8	0.446
Male	49 (59.0%)	57 (51.8%)	0.318	37 (59.7%)	28 (45.2%)	0.106
Body mass index	23.4 ± 3.25	23.6 ± 3.91	0.708	23.5 ± 3.34	23.5 ± 3.93	0.988
Dialysis vintage (months)	86.24 ± 56.53	96.54 ± 63.21	0.243	93.22 ± 57.61	85.4 ± 55.67	0.444
Smoking history	15 (18.1%)	12 (10.9%)	0.156	9 (14.5%)	6 (9.7%)	0.409
Arteriovenous fistula	75 (90.4%)	99 (90.0%)	0.934	57 (91.9%)	57 (91.9%)	>0.999
Comorbidities						
Diabetes mellitus	45 (54.2%)	34 (30.9%)	0.001	24 (38.7%)	30 (48.4%)	0.277
Hypertension	80 (96.4%)	87 (79.1%)	<0.001	59 (95.2%)	59 (95.2%)	>0.999
Dyslipidemia	31 (37.3%)	24 (21.8%)	0.018	16 (25.8%)	15 (24.2%)	0.836
Coronary artery disease	34 (41.0%)	22 (20.0%)	0.001	21 (33.9%)	18 (29.0%)	0.562
Heart failure	22 (26.5%)	15 (13.6%)	0.025	14 (22.6%)	11 (17.7%)	0.502
Cerebrovascular disease	31 (37.3%)	24 (21.8%)	0.018	5 (8.1%)	8 (12.9%)	0.379
Parathyroidectomy history	7 (8.4%)	18 (16.4%)	0.104	6 (9.7%)	6 (9.7%)	>0.999
Medications						
ACEI/ARB	29 (34.9%)	24 (21.8%)	0.043	23 (37.1%)	15 (24.2%)	0.119
Glucose lowering drugs	34 (41.0%)	23 (20.9%)	0.003	20 (32.3%)	19 (30.6%)	0.847
Sulfonylurea	14 (16.9%)	13 (11.8%)	0.317	6 (9.7%)	11 (17.7%)	0.192
Dipeptidyl peptidase 4 inhibitors	28 (33.7%)	13 (11.8%)	<0.001	17 (27.4%)	11 (17.7%)	0.198
Insulin	17 (20.5%)	10 (9.1%)	0.024	9 (14.5%)	8 (12.9%)	0.794
Statin	29 (34.9%)	17 (15.5%)	0.002	17 (27.4%)	12 (19.4%)	0.289
Calcium carbonate	67 (80.7%)	94 (85.5%)	0.382	51 (82.3%)	50 (80.6%)	0.817
Proton pump inhibitors	13 (15.7%)	10 (9.1%)	0.163	9 (14.5%)	7 (11.3%)	0.592
Clinical laboratory data						
Hemoglobin (g/dL)	10.62 ± 1.14	10.71 ± 1.41	0.650	10.6 ± 1.05	10.74 ± 1.49	0.555
Albumin (g/dL)	3.52 ± 0.51	3.56 ± 0.46	0.538	3.53 ± 0.46	3.54 ± 0.47	0.902

Table 1. *Cont.*

Baseline Characteristics	Before Propensity Score Matching			After Propensity Score Matching		
	β-Blocker Users (*N* = 83)	β-Blocker Nonusers (*N* = 110)	*p*-Value	β-Blocker Users (*N* = 62)	β-Blocker Nonusers (*N* = 62)	*p*-Value
Total cholesterol (mg/dL)	154.01 ± 33.75	161.89 ± 33.62	0.109	151.94 ± 33.57	163.51 ± 35.30	0.064
Triglyceride (mg/dL)	140.52 ± 103.77	129.61 ± 90.35	0.437	136.21 ± 105.99	131.14 ± 95.51	0.780
High sensitivity CRP (mg/dL)	2.15 ± 4.65	2.5 ± 4.21	0.589	2.45 ± 5.23	2.21 ± 3.95	0.779
Sodium (mmol/L)	136.92 ± 2.68	137.07 ± 2.62	0.700	137.19 ± 2.80	136.64 ± 2.44	0.241
Potassium (mmol/L)	4.73 ± 0.68	4.61 ± 0.62	0.195	4.77 ± 0.66	4.65 ± 0.65	0.294
Total calcium (mg/dL)	9.15 ± 0.86	9.29 ± 0.94	0.277	9.19 ± 0.92	9.25 ± 0.86	0.683
Phosphate (mg/dL)	5.08 ± 1.21	4.95 ± 1.24	0.453	5.16 ± 1.15	5.09 ± 1.35	0.768
Parathyroid hormone (pg/mL)	376.53 ± 338.79	383.5 ± 278.13	0.876	394.16 ± 370.62	357.29 ± 245.84	0.515
Serum iron (μg/dL)	63.57 ± 26.73	65.85 ± 21.16	0.508	63.94 ± 26.61	67.52 ± 22.93	0.424
Ferritin (ng/mL)	567.53 ± 549.64	496.67 ± 377.33	0.291	534.93 ± 330.67	538.54 ± 413.54	0.957
nPCR (g/kg/day)	1.12 ± 0.21	1.16 ± 0.27	0.326	1.12 ± 0.20	1.18 ± 0.28	0.180
Single pool Kt/V	1.67 ± 0.27	1.65 ± 0.27	0.591	1.67 ± 0.28	1.68 ± 0.27	0.817
Dietary intake (serving/day)						
Meat	0.86 ± 0.57	0.82 ± 0.53	0.652	0.86 ± 0.57	0.74 ± 0.52	0.241
Vegetable	2.01 ± 1.09	1.86 ± 1.11	0.265	2.05 ± 1.06	1.91 ± 1.18	0.499
Fruit	0.93 ± 0.72	0.95 ± 0.72	0.583	0.86 ± 0.63	0.89 ± 0.75	0.837
Bristol stool scale	3.94 ± 1.86	3.74 ± 1.76	0.448	4 ± 1.78	3.71 ± 1.67	0.352

Abbreviation: ACEI/ARB, angiotensin-converting enzyme inhibitors/angiotensin-receptor blockers; CRP, C reactive protein; nPCR, normalized protein catabolic rate.

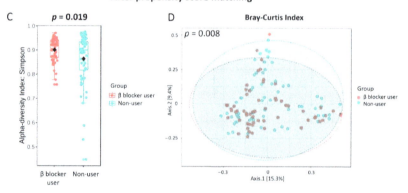

Figure 2. The α-diversity and β-diversity in hemodialysis patients with and without β blocker used in full cohort (**A,B**) and propensity score matching cohort (**C,D**). β blocker users had a higher α-diversity than β blocker nonusers in full cohort (**A**) and propensity score matching cohort (**C**) β blocker users had a different β-diversity (Bray–Curtis index) compared to β blocker nonusers in full cohort (**B**) and propensity score matching cohort (**D**). The β-diversity *p*-value was calculated using the homogeneity of group dispersions by the Permutational Analysis of Multivariate Dispersions (PERMDISP) test.

3.3. Specific Microbial Taxa Differences between β-Blocker Users and Nonusers

Discriminant analysis using LEfSe identified the significant differentiating taxa between study groups. In the full cohort, the genera *Ruminococcus 2*, *Collinsella*, *Ruminococcaceae UCG-004*, *Ruminiclostridium 5*, *Anaerotruncus*, *Eisenbergiella*, and *Flavonifractor* were enriched in β-blocker users compared to nonusers (Figure 3A). In the PS-matched cohort, the enriched genera were *Faecalibacterium*, *Subdoligranulum*, *Tyzzerella*, *Pantoea*, *Lachnospiraceae UCG-004*, and *Flavonifractor* were found (Figure 3B). Using random forest models for taxonomy prediction, the top three ranked genera to discriminate between β-blocker users and nonusers were *Parabacteroides*, *Flavonifractor*, and *Ruminococcaceae UCG-004* in the full cohort (Figure 4A), *Prevotella 9*, *Flavonifractor*, and *Tyzzerella* in the PS-matched cohort (Figure 4B).

To reduce the effect of zero-inflation in the microbiome data, we performed the MetagenomeSeq algorithm integrating the CSS method and a statistical model based on the ZIG distribution. Evaluating the significant difference in genus taxonomy between β-blocker users and nonusers, we found eight genera differences in the full cohort and PS-matched cohort (Supplementary Table S1). There were three different genera (*Flavonifractor*, *Tyzzerella*, and *Prevotellaceae NK3B31 group*) in both the full and PS-matched cohorts

(Figure 5A). Focusing on the ZIG fit model to predict specific genera, there was an increased *Flavonifractor* genus in β-blocker users compared to nonusers using a classical univariate test (Kruskal–Wallis test) in the full ($p = 0.023$) and PS-matched cohorts ($p = 0.01$) (Figure 5B). However, no differences were found in *Tyzzerella* or *Prevotellaceae NK3B31 group* (Figure 5B).

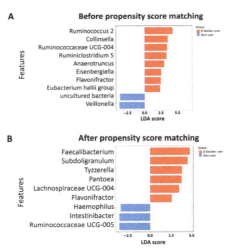

Figure 3. Taxonomic differences were detected between β blocker users and nonusers in the full cohort (**A**) and propensity score matching cohort (**B**). Linear discriminative analysis (LDA) effect size (LEfSe) analysis between β blocker users (red) and nonusers (blue) with an LDA score > 2.0 or < −2 with *p*-value > 0.1 among β blocker users and nonusers.

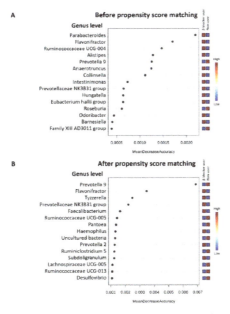

Figure 4. Determination of specific bacteria for discriminatory across hemodialysis patients with and without β blocker treatment in full cohort (**A**) and propensity score matching cohort (**B**). The discriminatory taxa were determined by applying Random Forest analysis using the genus-level abundance.

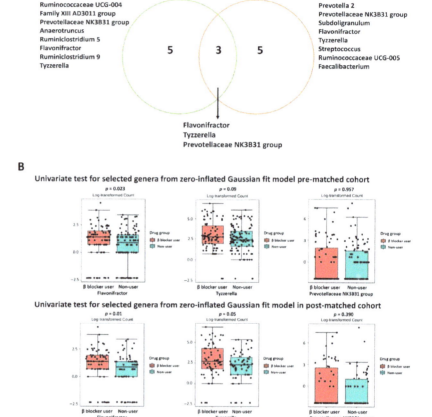

Figure 5. The genera difference between β blocker users and nonusers in the full cohort and propensity score matching cohort using zero-inflated Gaussian fit model. (**A**) The Venn diagram showed the different significant genera in the full cohort and propensity score-matched cohort. (**B**) Univariate test between selected genera from zero-inflated Gaussian fit model. Significance was considered for $p < 0.05$.

Using PICRUSt2 as a metagenome predictive exploratory tool, genes were categorized into KEGG Orthology metabolic pathways. All predicted KEGG Orthology (KOs) were mapped to KEGG metabolic pathways. Each pathway was tested with gene-set enrichment by comparing expected gene abundance between β blocker users and nonusers in full and PS-matched cohorts. However, no significant KEGG enriched pathways were observed (Figures S4 and S5).

4. Discussion

In the present study, hemodialysis patients treated with β-blockers had a higher α-diversity and a distinct β-diversity compared to nonusers. The microbial communities contained higher levels of *Bacteroidetes* and lower levels of *Firmicutes* in all hemodialysis patients, which is similar to CKD rat microbial communities [43] and in a human CKD microbiota study [44]. Co-occurrence analysis revealed no difference in keystone taxa

Bacteroides between β-blocker users and nonusers. Overall, there was an enriched genus *Flavonifractor* in β-blocker users in the full and PS-matched cohorts. Furthermore, LEfSe analysis, random forest algorithm, ZIG fit model, and univariate test all confirmed this difference between groups. However, we did not determine KEGG metabolic pathways between β blocker users and nonusers using PICRUSt2 functional prediction analysis.

β-blocker use was associated with a higher α-diversity than nonusers in hemodialysis patients, which was linked to a favorable healthy state [45]. Increased α-diversity has been associated with foods generally considered healthy, such as plant consumption or red wine [46–48]. Furthermore, commonly used medications such as antibiotics or proton pump inhibitors can decrease gut α-diversity [49]. Regarding the specific taxonomy of the gut microbiome, the genus *Flavonifractor* was enriched in β-blocker users in both the full and PS-matched cohorts. *Flavonifractor* is associated with several diseases, such as obesity [50], atrial fibrillation [51], coronary artery disease [52], and medications (antidiabetic drugs, such as Metformin and Glucagon-like peptide 1 Receptor agonist [53]). It can convert quercetin or other flavonoids into acetic acid and butyric acid [54] and is also correlated with oxidative stress and inflammation [55]. The presence of *Flavonifractor* was found in association with circulating inflammatory markers (i.e., interleukin-6, interleukin-8, interleukin-1β) [56], which were linked to cardiovascular disease. Besides, oral administration of *Flavonifractor plautii* was involved in the inhibition of tumor necrosis factor-α expression in obese adipose tissue inflammatory environments [57]. Thus, the increased abundance of *Flavonifractor* by β-blocker treatment may have a potential benefit in cardiovascular disease via gut microbiota regulation.

We also identified a potential link between β-blocker use and the genus *Tyzzerella* in the PS-matched cohort. Importantly, *Tyzzerella* was enriched in those with a high cardiovascular risk profile [58]. However, the small sample size limited the potential association between β-blocker use and *Tyzzerella* in univariate analysis, so more extensive studies are needed to confirm this association. Regarding the link between β-blocker and microbiota changes; a chimera mouse model suggested bone marrow beta1/2 adrenergic receptor signaling can regulate host-microbiota interactions, leading to the generation of novel anti-inflammatory treatments for gut dysbiosis [59]. Therefore, depletion of this sympathetic regulation in bone marrow promotes beneficial shifts in gut microbiota associated with gut immune suppression [59]. It is proposed that beta-blockers may provide a beneficial microbiome in such conditions.

We compared the microbiota differences between β-blocker users and nonusers using PS matching analysis in the present study. Since β-blocker intake is highly correlated with age, cardiovascular risk, comorbidities, and concurrent medication, each factor represents a relevant confounder for microbiome analyses [16,60]. Most observational studies have controlled for possible confounding variables, but even rigorous data adjustment cannot eliminate the risk of bias. PS matching is an alternative to reduce the effect of influencing factors on gut microbiota analysis [30,31]; thus, we selected variables of interest as potential confounders and then performed PS matching to reduce these effects deviations and confounding variables to conduct a reasonable comparison between groups. The intestinal microbiota was affected by various factors, including demographic data, comorbidities, concomitant medications, and clinical laboratory data, and the application of PS matching eliminated confounding factors. Using PS analysis, there was still a higher α-diversity and different β-diversity in β-blocker users compared to nonusers. We also identified six genera associated explicitly with the β-blocker user in the LEfSe analysis, four top-ranked genera in random forest analysis, and eight genera in ZIG fit model analysis. Although there were some differences in bacterial associations with β-blocker use in our full (before PS matching) and PS-matched cohorts, we investigated the taxa represented in both the full and PS-matched cohorts. Importantly, three genera (*Flavonifractor*, *Tyzzerella*, and *Prevotellaceae NK3B31 group*) were both significant differences in ZIG fit model among the full and PS-matched cohorts. The genera abundance differences between β-blocker users and nonusers were changed in the PS matching procedure. The genera abundance significant differences in *Ruminiclostridium 9*, *Ruminococcaceae UCG-004*, *Anaerotruncus*, and *Ruminiclostridium 5* were attenuated after PS matching, suggesting that these genera abundances may be more strongly associated with other confounding variables, such as comorbidities or concomitant medications, which was accounted for in the PS models. In specific, genus *Anaerotruncus* was reported related to hypertension [61–63], diabetes mellitus [64], and dipeptidyl peptidase 4 inhibitors used [65], which were unbalance in the pre-matched cohort. The genus *Ruminiclostridium* and *Ruminococcaceae* were correlated to hypertension in the previous study [66–68]. Thus, the change of gut microbiome difference in β-blockers users and nonusers before and after PS matching reflected confounders' influence. Since many factors influencing gut microbiota, we performed PS matching as an alternative technique to account for multiple confounders in this study.

In addition, there were more zeros than expected under the assumption of Poisson or negative binomial distributions for microbiome OTU counts, known as zero-inflation. One popular strategy to circumvent the zero-inflation problem is to add a pseudo-count [69]; however, this assumption may not be appropriate due to the large extent of structural zeros due to physical absence. Moreover, the pseudo-count choice is arbitrary, and the clustering results can be highly dependent upon the choice [70]. Thus, CSS was developed for microbiome sequencing data, and a zero-inflated model was used to model read counts that have an excess of zeros [36,71,72]. In CSS, raw counts are divided by the cumulative sum of counts up to a percentile determined using a data-driven approach to capture the relatively invariant count distribution for a dataset. To solve the zero-inflation issue, we applied the ZIG fit model and calculated the CSS. Interestingly, the four genera in the full (*Ruminococcaceae UCG-004*, *Ruminiclostridium 5*, *Anaerotruncus*, and *Flavonifractor*) and PS-matched cohorts (*Flavonifractor*, *Tyzzerella*, *Faecalibacterium*, *Subdoligranulum*) overlapped in the LEfSe analysis and ZIG fit model analysis.

Several limitations should be mentioned. First, cross-sectional studies only provide an impression of the relative abundance of bacterial taxa at a single time point, so causal inference cannot be addressed. Besides, the observational study only demonstrates the association rather than the causality. Second, the microbiota was assessed with a fecal sample, which may differ from microbiota from other parts of the intestine. Besides, 16S rRNA sequencing is limited as it cannot differentiate viable from non-viable bacteria. A significant portion of the taxa identified by sequencing may not be metabolically active. Thus, further study is needed to investigate various samples, such as small intestine or colon mucosal bacteria. Third, PS matching might not fully balance the overall effects of medications or disease severity, such as the dose of medications or the status between controlled and uncontrolled DM. Finally, the study was performed in Asia hemodialysis patients whose diet is different from other populations, so dietary effects on the gut microbiome should be interpreted with caution.

5. Conclusions

This study demonstrated that the composition of the gut microbiota was different in hemodialysis patients treated with β-blockers, with a higher level of α-diversity and genus *Flavonifractor*. These findings support the additional benefits of β-blocker treatment, which may mediate the microbiota in hemodialysis patients. However, the functional relevance of the β-blocker induced microbial differences is unclear. Hence, larger prospective treatment naïve studies are warranted to understand the impact of β-blockers on the gut microbiome of CKD patients and their implications for health and disease.

Supplementary Materials: The following are available online at https://www.mdpi.com/2075-4426/11/3/198/s1, Figure S1: Rarefaction curves of the number of OTUs versus the sequencing effort per sample in the full cohort. Figure S2: The relative abundance percentage of intestinal microbiota between β-blocker users and nonusers in the full cohort and propensity score matching cohort. (**A**) Phylum level (**B**) Class level (**C**) Order level. Figure S3: Core microbiome analysis in hemodialysis patients with and without β-blocker used. (**A**) SparCC correlation analysis (genus level using 100 SparCC permutations, 0.35 correlation threshold, and 0.05 *p*-value threshold) in all hemodialysis patients with and without β-blocker used (**B**) Relative abundance and sample prevalence of bacterial genus in β-blocker users and nonusers. Figure S4: Enrichment analysis for predictive Kyoto Encyclopedia of Genes and Genomes (KEGG) metabolic modules between β-blocker users and nonusers in full (before propensity score matching) cohort. No significant KEGG enriched pathways were observed (all p-value > 0.05). Figure S5: Enrichment analysis for predictive Kyoto Encyclopedia of Genes and Genomes (KEGG) metabolic modules between β-blocker users and nonusers in propensity score-matched cohort. No significant KEGG enriched pathways were observed (all p-value > 0.05). Table S1: Summary table of significant genus difference in hemodialysis patients with and without β-blocker treatment in zero-inflated Gaussian fit model.

Author Contributions: Conceptualization, P.-H.W., Y.-T.L., Y.-W.C., and M.-C.K.; methodology, P.-H.W., Y.-T.L., P.-Y.L., Y.-W.C., and M.-C.K.; formal analysis, P.-H.W., Y.-T.L., and P.-Y.L.; investigation, P.-H.W., Y.-T.L., P.-Y.L.; data curation, P.-H.W., Y.-T.L., and P.-Y.L.; writing—original draft preparation, P.-H.W., Y.-T.L., and P.-Y.L.; writing—review and editing, W.-C.H., W.-C.T., Y.-C.T., Y.-W.C., M.-C.K., T.-Y.L., S.-C.H., R.A.D., and Y.-S.C.; funding acquisition, P.-H.W. and Y.-T.L. All authors have read and agreed to the published version of the manuscript.

Funding: This research was funded by grants from the Ministry of Science and Technology, Taiwan (MOST 107-2314-B-037-104, MOST 107-2314-B-037-098-MY3, and MOST 109-2314-B-037-088), Kaohsiung Medical University Hospital, Taiwan (KMUH108-8M11, KMUH108-8R70, KMUH109-9R16, KMUH109-9R81, KMUH-DK(B)110003-1, and KMUH-DK(B)110003-4), Kaohsiung Medical University, Taiwan (KMU-Q108024, KMU-Q108027, KMU-DK(B)110003, and KMU-DK(B)110003-2), and NSYSU-KMU JOINT RESEARCH PROJECT (NSYSUKMU 105-I005 and NSYSUKMU 106-I005).

Institutional Review Board Statement: The study was conducted according to the guidelines of the Declaration of Helsinki and approved by the Ethics Committee of Kaohsiung Medical University Hospital (KMUHIRB-E(I)-20160095 and KMUHIRB-E(I)-20180118) and Taipei Tzu Chi Hospital (07-X01-002).

Informed Consent Statement: Informed consent was obtained from all subjects involved in the study.

Data Availability Statement: Raw FASTQ data files of samples from hemodialysis patients have been deposited in the NCBI Sequence Read Archive database under BioProject accession number PRJNA648014.

Acknowledgments: We acknowledge Germark Biotechnology Lab for the stool sample analysis of gut microbiota.

Conflicts of Interest: The authors declare no conflict of interest.

References

1. Lynch, S.V.; Pedersen, O. The Human Intestinal Microbiome in Health and Disease. *N. Engl. J. Med.* **2016**, *375*, 2369–2379. [CrossRef] [PubMed]
2. Jandhyala, S.M.; Talukdar, R.; Subramanyam, C.; Vuyyuru, H.; Sasikala, M.; Nageshwar Reddy, D. Role of the normal gut microbiota. *World J. Gastroenterol.* **2015**, *21*, 8787–8803. [CrossRef]
3. Salvucci, E. The human-microbiome superorganism and its modulation to restore health. *Int. J. Food Sci. Nutr.* **2019**, *70*, 781–795. [CrossRef]
4. Belizario, J.E.; Faintuch, J.; Garay-Malpartida, M. Gut Microbiome Dysbiosis and Immunometabolism: New Frontiers for Treatment of Metabolic Diseases. *Mediators Inflamm.* **2018**, *2018*, 2037838. [CrossRef] [PubMed]
5. DeGruttola, A.K.; Low, D.; Mizoguchi, A.; Mizoguchi, E. Current Understanding of Dysbiosis in Disease in Human and Animal Models. *Inflamm. Bowel. Dis.* **2016**, *22*, 1137–1150. [CrossRef]
6. Carding, S.; Verbeke, K.; Vipond, D.T.; Corfe, B.M.; Owen, L.J. Dysbiosis of the gut microbiota in disease. *Microb. Ecol. Health Dis.* **2015**, *26*, 26191. [CrossRef]
7. Jackson, M.A.; Verdi, S.; Maxan, M.E.; Shin, C.M.; Zierer, J.; Bowyer, R.C.E.; Martin, T.; Williams, F.M.K.; Menni, C.; Bell, J.T.; et al. Gut microbiota associations with common diseases and prescription medications in a population-based cohort. *Nat. Commun.* **2018**, *9*, 2655. [CrossRef]
8. Imhann, F.; Bonder, M.J.; Vich Vila, A.; Fu, J.; Mujagic, Z.; Vork, L.; Tigchelaar, E.F.; Jankipersadsing, S.A.; Cenit, M.C.; Harmsen, H.J.; et al. Proton pump inhibitors affect the gut microbiome. *Gut* **2016**, *65*, 740–748. [CrossRef] [PubMed]
9. Makivuokko, H.; Tiihonen, K.; Tynkkynen, S.; Paulin, L.; Rautonen, N. The effect of age and non-steroidal anti-inflammatory drugs on human intestinal microbiota composition. *Br. J. Nutr.* **2010**, *103*, 227–234. [CrossRef] [PubMed]

10. Bahr, S.M.; Tyler, B.C.; Wooldridge, N.; Butcher, B.D.; Burns, T.L.; Teesch, L.M.; Oltman, C.L.; Azcarate-Peril, M.A.; Kirby, J.R.; Calarge, C.A. Use of the second-generation antipsychotic, risperidone, and secondary weight gain are associated with an altered gut microbiota in children. *Transl. Psychiatry* **2015**, *5*, e652. [CrossRef]
11. Forslund, K.; Hildebrand, F.; Nielsen, T.; Falony, G.; Le Chatelier, E.; Sunagawa, S.; Prifti, E.; Vieira-Silva, S.; Gudmundsdottir, V.; Pedersen, H.K.; et al. Disentangling type 2 diabetes and metformin treatment signatures in the human gut microbiota. *Nature* **2015**, *528*, 262–266. [CrossRef]
12. Freedberg, D.E.; Toussaint, N.C.; Chen, S.P.; Ratner, A.J.; Whittier, S.; Wang, T.C.; Wang, H.H.; Abrams, J.A. Proton Pump Inhibitors Alter Specific Taxa in the Human Gastrointestinal Microbiome: A Crossover Trial. *Gastroenterology* **2015**, *149*, 883–885.e9. [CrossRef] [PubMed]
13. Jackson, M.A.; Goodrich, J.K.; Maxan, M.E.; Freedberg, D.E.; Abrams, J.A.; Poole, A.C.; Sutter, J.L.; Welter, D.; Ley, R.E.; Bell, J.T.; et al. Proton pump inhibitors alter the composition of the gut microbiota. *Gut* **2016**, *65*, 749–756. [CrossRef] [PubMed]
14. Fu, J.; Bonder, M.J.; Cenit, M.C.; Tigchelaar, E.F.; Maatman, A.; Dekens, J.A.; Brandsma, E.; Marczynska, J.; Imhann, F.; Weersma, R.K.; et al. The Gut Microbiome Contributes to a Substantial Proportion of the Variation in Blood Lipids. *Circ. Res.* **2015**, *117*, 817–824. [CrossRef] [PubMed]
15. Buffie, C.G.; Pamer, E.G. Microbiota-mediated colonization resistance against intestinal pathogens. *Nat. Rev. Immunol.* **2013**, *13*, 790–801. [CrossRef]
16. Zhernakova, A.; Kurilshikov, A.; Bonder, M.J.; Tigchelaar, E.F.; Schirmer, M.; Vatanen, T.; Mujagic, Z.; Vila, A.V.; Falony, G.; Vieira-Silva, S.; et al. Population-based metagenomics analysis reveals markers for gut microbiome composition and diversity. *Science* **2016**, *352*, 565–569. [CrossRef]
17. Evenepoel, P.; Poesen, R.; Meijers, B. The gut-kidney axis. *Pediatr. Nephrol.* **2017**, *32*, 2005–2014. [CrossRef] [PubMed]
18. Vaziri, N.D.; Wong, J.; Pahl, M.; Piceno, Y.M.; Yuan, J.; DeSantis, T.Z.; Ni, Z.; Nguyen, T.H.; Andersen, G.L. Chronic kidney disease alters intestinal microbial flora. *Kidney Int.* **2013**, *83*, 308–315. [CrossRef]
19. Weir, M.A.; Herzog, C.A. Beta blockers in patients with end-stage renal disease-Evidence-based recommendations. *Semin. Dial.* **2018**, *31*, 219–225. [CrossRef]
20. Bakris, G.L.; Hart, P.; Ritz, E. Beta blockers in the management of chronic kidney disease. *Kidney Int.* **2006**, *70*, 1905–1913. [CrossRef]
21. Nemet, I.; Saha, P.P.; Gupta, N.; Zhu, W.; Romano, K.A.; Skye, S.M.; Cajka, T.; Mohan, M.L.; Li, L.; Wu, Y.; et al. A Cardiovascular Disease-Linked Gut Microbial Metabolite Acts via Adrenergic Receptors. *Cell* **2020**, *180*, 862–877.e22. [CrossRef]
22. Ikizler, T.A.; Burrowes, J.D.; Byham-Gray, L.D.; Campbell, K.L.; Carrero, J.J.; Chan, W.; Fouque, D.; Friedman, A.N.; Ghaddar, S.; Goldstein-Fuchs, D.J.; et al. KDOQI Clinical Practice Guideline for Nutrition in CKD: 2020 Update. *Am. J. Kidney Dis.* **2020**, *76*, S1–S107. [CrossRef] [PubMed]
23. Herlemann, D.P.; Labrenz, M.; Jurgens, K.; Bertilsson, S.; Waniek, J.J.; Andersson, A.F. Transitions in bacterial communities along the 2000 km salinity gradient of the Baltic Sea. *ISME J.* **2011**, *5*, 1571–1579. [CrossRef]
24. Comeau, A.M.; Douglas, G.M.; Langille, M.G. Microbiome Helper: A Custom and Streamlined Workflow for Microbiome Research. *mSystems* **2017**, *2*, e00127-16. [CrossRef] [PubMed]
25. Zhang, J.; Kobert, K.; Flouri, T.; Stamatakis, A. PEAR: A fast and accurate Illumina Paired-End reAd mergeR. *Bioinformatics* **2014**, *30*, 614–620. [CrossRef]
26. Caporaso, J.G.; Kuczynski, J.; Stombaugh, J.; Bittinger, K.; Bushman, F.D.; Costello, E.K.; Fierer, N.; Pena, A.G.; Goodrich, J.K.; Gordon, J.I.; et al. QIIME allows analysis of high-throughput community sequencing data. *Nat. Methods* **2010**, *7*, 335–336. [CrossRef]
27. Quast, C.; Pruesse, E.; Yilmaz, P.; Gerken, J.; Schweer, T.; Yarza, P.; Peplies, J.; Glockner, F.O. The SILVA ribosomal RNA gene database project: Improved data processing and web-based tools. *Nucleic. Acids. Res.* **2013**, *41*, D590–D596. [CrossRef]
28. Yilmaz, P.; Parfrey, L.W.; Yarza, P.; Gerken, J.; Pruesse, E.; Quast, C.; Schweer, T.; Peplies, J.; Ludwig, W.; Glockner, F.O. The SILVA and "All-species Living Tree Project (LTP)" taxonomic frameworks. *Nucleic. Acids. Res.* **2014**, *42*, D643–D648. [CrossRef] [PubMed]
29. Edgar, R.C. Search and clustering orders of magnitude faster than BLAST. *Bioinformatics* **2010**, *26*, 2460–2461. [CrossRef]
30. Sturmer, T.; Wyss, R.; Glynn, R.J.; Brookhart, M.A. Propensity scores for confounder adjustment when assessing the effects of medical interventions using nonexperimental study designs. *J. Intern. Med.* **2014**, *275*, 570–580. [CrossRef] [PubMed]
31. Ali, M.S.; Groenwold, R.H.; Belitser, S.V.; Pestman, W.R.; Hoes, A.W.; Roes, K.C.; Boer, A.; Klungel, O.H. Reporting of covariate selection and balance assessment in propensity score analysis is suboptimal: A systematic review. *J. Clin. Epidemiol.* **2015**, *68*, 112–121. [CrossRef]
32. Lozupone, C.A.; Hamady, M.; Kelley, S.T.; Knight, R. Quantitative and qualitative beta diversity measures lead to different insights into factors that structure microbial communities. *Appl. Environ. Microbiol.* **2007**, *73*, 1576–1585. [CrossRef]
33. Chong, J.; Liu, P.; Zhou, G.; Xia, J. Using MicrobiomeAnalyst for comprehensive statistical, functional, and meta-analysis of microbiome data. *Nat. Protoc.* **2020**, *15*, 799–821. [CrossRef] [PubMed]
34. Friedman, J.; Alm, E.J. Inferring correlation networks from genomic survey data. *PLoS Comput. Biol.* **2012**, *8*, e1002687. [CrossRef]
35. Svetnik, V.; Liaw, A.; Tong, C.; Culberson, J.C.; Sheridan, R.P.; Feuston, B.P. Random forest: A classification and regression tool for compound classification and QSAR modeling. *J. Chem. Inf. Comput. Sci.* **2003**, *43*, 1947–1958. [CrossRef] [PubMed]
36. Paulson, J.N.; Stine, O.C.; Bravo, H.C.; Pop, M. Differential abundance analysis for microbial marker-gene surveys. *Nat. Methods* **2013**, *10*, 1200–1202. [CrossRef]

37. Douglas, G.M.; Maffei, V.J.; Zaneveld, J.R.; Yurgel, S.N.; Brown, J.R.; Taylor, C.M.; Huttenhower, C.; Langille, M.G.I. PICRUSt2 for prediction of metagenome functions. *Nat. Biotechnol.* **2020**, *38*, 685–688. [CrossRef]
38. Markowitz, V.M.; Chen, I.M.; Palaniappan, K.; Chu, K.; Szeto, E.; Grechkin, Y.; Ratner, A.; Jacob, B.; Huang, J.; Williams, P.; et al. IMG: The Integrated Microbial Genomes database and comparative analysis system. *Nucleic. Acids. Res.* **2012**, *40*, D115–D122. [CrossRef]
39. Liu, P.-Y. poyuliu/MARco: MARco: Microbiome Analysis RcodeDB (Version v1.0). Zenodo. Available online: http://doi.org/10.5281/zenodo.4589898 (accessed on 1 February 2021).
40. Luo, W.; Brouwer, C. Pathview: An R/Bioconductor package for pathway-based data integration and visualization. *Bioinformatics* **2013**, *29*, 1830–1831. [CrossRef]
41. Huang da, W.; Sherman, B.T.; Lempicki, R.A. Systematic and integrative analysis of large gene lists using DAVID bioinformatics resources. *Nat. Protoc.* **2009**, *4*, 44–57. [CrossRef]
42. Huang, D.W.; Sherman, B.T.; Tan, Q.; Collins, J.R.; Alvord, W.G.; Roayaei, J.; Stephens, R.; Baseler, M.W.; Lane, H.C.; Lempicki, R.A. The DAVID Gene Functional Classification Tool: A novel biological module-centric algorithm to functionally analyze large gene lists. *Genome Biol.* **2007**, *8*, R183. [CrossRef]
43. Lau, W.L.; Vaziri, N.D.; Nunes, A.C.F.; Comeau, A.M.; Langille, M.G.I.; England, W.; Khazaeli, M.; Suematsu, Y.; Phan, J.; Whiteson, K. The Phosphate Binder Ferric Citrate Alters the Gut Microbiome in Rats with Chronic Kidney Disease. *J. Pharmacol. Exp. Ther.* **2018**, *367*, 452–460. [CrossRef]
44. Lun, H.; Yang, W.; Zhao, S.; Jiang, M.; Xu, M.; Liu, F.; Wang, Y. Altered gut microbiota and microbial biomarkers associated with chronic kidney disease. *Microbiologyopen* **2019**, *8*, e00678. [CrossRef]
45. Le Chatelier, E.; Nielsen, T.; Qin, J.; Prifti, E.; Hildebrand, F.; Falony, G.; Almeida, M.; Arumugam, M.; Batto, J.M.; Kennedy, S.; et al. Richness of human gut microbiome correlates with metabolic markers. *Nature* **2013**, *500*, 541–546. [CrossRef]
46. McDonald, D.; Hyde, E.; Debelius, J.W.; Morton, J.T.; Gonzalez, A.; Ackermann, G.; Aksenov, A.A.; Behsaz, B.; Brennan, C.; Chen, Y.; et al. American Gut: An Open Platform for Citizen Science Microbiome Research. *mSystems* **2018**, *3*, e00031-18. [CrossRef] [PubMed]
47. Le Roy, C.I.; Wells, P.M.; Si, J.; Raes, J.; Bell, J.T.; Spector, T.D. Red Wine Consumption Associated With Increased Gut Microbiota alpha-Diversity in 3 Independent Cohorts. *Gastroenterology* **2020**, *158*, 270–272. [CrossRef]
48. Leeming, E.R.; Johnson, A.J.; Spector, T.D.; Le Roy, C.I. Effect of Diet on the Gut Microbiota: Rethinking Intervention Duration. *Nutrients* **2019**, *11*, 2862. [CrossRef]
49. Le Bastard, Q.; Al-Ghalith, G.A.; Gregoire, M.; Chapelet, G.; Javaudin, F.; Dailly, E.; Batard, E.; Knights, D.; Montassier, E. Systematic review: Human gut dysbiosis induced by non-antibiotic prescription medications. *Aliment. Pharmacol. Ther.* **2018**, *47*, 332–345. [CrossRef] [PubMed]
50. Kasai, C.; Sugimoto, K.; Moritani, I.; Tanaka, J.; Oya, Y.; Inoue, H.; Tameda, M.; Shiraki, K.; Ito, M.; Takei, Y.; et al. Comparison of the gut microbiota composition between obese and non-obese individuals in a Japanese population, as analyzed by terminal restriction fragment length polymorphism and next-generation sequencing. *BMC Gastroenterol.* **2015**, *15*, 100. [CrossRef]
51. Zuo, K.; Li, J.; Li, K.; Hu, C.; Gao, Y.; Chen, M.; Hu, R.; Liu, Y.; Chi, H.; Wang, H.; et al. Disordered gut microbiota and alterations in metabolic patterns are associated with atrial fibrillation. *Gigascience* **2019**, *8*, giz058. [CrossRef] [PubMed]
52. Zhu, Q.; Gao, R.; Zhang, Y.; Pan, D.; Zhu, Y.; Zhang, X.; Yang, R.; Jiang, R.; Xu, Y.; Qin, H. Dysbiosis signatures of gut microbiota in coronary artery disease. *Physiol. Genom.* **2018**, *50*, 893–903. [CrossRef] [PubMed]
53. Gurung, M.; Li, Z.; You, H.; Rodrigues, R.; Jump, D.B.; Morgun, A.; Shulzhenko, N. Role of gut microbiota in type 2 diabetes pathophysiology. *EBioMedicine* **2020**, *51*, 102590. [CrossRef]
54. Carlier, J.P.; Bedora-Faure, M.; K'Ouas, G.; Alauzet, C.; Mory, F. Proposal to unify Clostridium orbiscindens Winter et al. 1991 and Eubacterium plautii (Seguin 1928) Hofstad and Aasjord 1982, with description of Flavonifractor plautii gen. nov., comb. nov., and reassignment of Bacteroides capillosus to Pseudoflavonifractor capillosus gen. nov., comb. nov. *Int. J. Syst. Evol. Microbiol.* **2010**, *60*, 585–590. [CrossRef]
55. Coello, K.; Hansen, T.H.; Sorensen, N.; Munkholm, K.; Kessing, L.V.; Pedersen, O.; Vinberg, M. Gut microbiota composition in patients with newly diagnosed bipolar disorder and their unaffected first-degree relatives. *Brain Behav. Immun.* **2019**, *75*, 112–118. [CrossRef] [PubMed]
56. Huang, S.; Mao, J.; Zhou, L.; Xiong, X.; Deng, Y. The imbalance of gut microbiota and its correlation with plasma inflammatory cytokines in pemphigus vulgaris patients. *Scand. J. Immunol.* **2019**, *90*, e12799. [CrossRef] [PubMed]
57. Mikami, A.; Ogita, T.; Namai, F.; Shigemori, S.; Sato, T.; Shimosato, T. Oral administration of Flavonifractor plautii attenuates inflammatory responses in obese adipose tissue. *Mol. Biol. Rep.* **2020**, *47*, 6717–6725. [CrossRef] [PubMed]
58. Kelly, T.N.; Bazzano, L.A.; Ajami, N.J.; He, H.; Zhao, J.; Petrosino, J.F.; Correa, A.; He, J. Gut Microbiome Associates With Lifetime Cardiovascular Disease Risk Profile Among Bogalusa Heart Study Participants. *Circ. Res.* **2016**, *119*, 956–964. [CrossRef]
59. Yang, T.; Ahmari, N.; Schmidt, J.T.; Redler, T.; Arocha, R.; Pacholec, K.; Magee, K.L.; Malphurs, W.; Owen, J.L.; Krane, G.A.; et al. Shifts in the Gut Microbiota Composition Due to Depleted Bone Marrow Beta Adrenergic Signaling Are Associated with Suppressed Inflammatory Transcriptional Networks in the Mouse Colon. *Front. Physiol.* **2017**, *8*, 220. [CrossRef]
60. Falony, G.; Joossens, M.; Vieira-Silva, S.; Wang, J.; Darzi, Y.; Faust, K.; Kurilshikov, A.; Bonder, M.J.; Valles-Colomer, M.; Vandeputte, D.; et al. Population-level analysis of gut microbiome variation. *Science* **2016**, *352*, 560–564. [CrossRef]

61. Dan, X.; Mushi, Z.; Baili, W.; Han, L.; Enqi, W.; Huanhu, Z.; Shuchun, L. Differential Analysis of Hypertension-Associated Intestinal Microbiota. *Int. J. Med. Sci.* **2019**, *16*, 872–881. [CrossRef]
62. Robles-Vera, I.; Toral, M.; Duarte, J. Microbiota and Hypertension: Role of the Sympathetic Nervous System and the Immune System. *Am. J. Hypertens.* **2020**, *33*, 890–901. [CrossRef] [PubMed]
63. Palmu, J.; Lahti, L.; Niiranen, T. Targeting Gut Microbiota to Treat Hypertension: A Systematic Review. *Int. J. Environ. Res. Public Health* **2021**, *18*, 1248. [CrossRef]
64. Liu, C.; Shao, W.; Gao, M.; Liu, J.; Guo, Q.; Jin, J.; Meng, F. Changes in intestinal flora in patients with type 2 diabetes on a low-fat diet during 6 months of follow-up. *Exp. Ther. Med.* **2020**, *20*, 40. [CrossRef] [PubMed]
65. Whang, A.; Nagpal, R.; Yadav, H. Bi-directional drug-microbiome interactions of anti-diabetics. *EBioMedicine* **2019**, *39*, 591–602. [CrossRef] [PubMed]
66. Zuo, K.; Li, J.; Xu, Q.; Hu, C.; Gao, Y.; Chen, M.; Hu, R.; Liu, Y.; Chi, H.; Yin, Q.; et al. Dysbiotic gut microbes may contribute to hypertension by limiting vitamin D production. *Clin. Cardiol.* **2019**, *42*, 710–719. [CrossRef]
67. Durgan, D.J.; Ganesh, B.P.; Cope, J.L.; Ajami, N.J.; Phillips, S.C.; Petrosino, J.F.; Hollister, E.B.; Bryan, R.M., Jr. Role of the Gut Microbiome in Obstructive Sleep Apnea-Induced Hypertension. *Hypertension* **2016**, *67*, 469–474. [CrossRef]
68. Li, J.; Zhao, F.; Wang, Y.; Chen, J.; Tao, J.; Tian, G.; Wu, S.; Liu, W.; Cui, Q.; Geng, B.; et al. Gut microbiota dysbiosis contributes to the development of hypertension. *Microbiome* **2017**, *5*, 14. [CrossRef]
69. Mandal, S.; Van Treuren, W.; White, R.A.; Eggesbo, M.; Knight, R.; Peddada, S.D. Analysis of composition of microbiomes: A novel method for studying microbial composition. *Microb. Ecol. Health Dis.* **2015**, *26*, 27663. [CrossRef]
70. Costea, P.I.; Zeller, G.; Sunagawa, S.; Bork, P. A fair comparison. *Nat. Methods* **2014**, *11*, 359. [CrossRef]
71. Jonsson, V.; Osterlund, T.; Nerman, O.; Kristiansson, E. Modelling of zero-inflation improves inference of metagenomic gene count data. *Stat. Methods Med. Res.* **2019**, *28*, 3712–3728. [CrossRef]
72. Xu, L.; Paterson, A.D.; Turpin, W.; Xu, W. Assessment and Selection of Competing Models for Zero-Inflated Microbiome Data. *PLoS ONE* **2015**, *10*, e0129606. [CrossRef] [PubMed]

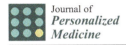

Brief Report

Intestinal Dysbiosis in Young Cystic Fibrosis Rabbits

Xiubin Liang [1], Mohamad Bouhamdan [2], Xia Hou [2], Kezhong Zhang [3], Jun Song [1], Ke Hao [4], Jian-Ping Jin [2], Zhongyang Zhang [4,*] and Jie Xu [1,*]

[1] Center for Advanced Models for Translational Sciences and Therapeutics, University of Michigan Medical Center, University of Michigan Medical School, Ann Arbor, MI 48109, USA; lixiubin@med.umich.edu (X.L.); songjun@med.umich.edu (J.S.)

[2] Department of Physiology, Wayne State University School of Medicine, Detroit, MI 48201, USA; mbouhamdan@gmail.com (M.B.); hou_xia@hotmail.com (X.H.); jjin@med.wayne.edu (J.-P.J.)

[3] Center for Molecular Medicine and Genetics, Wayne State University School of Medicine, Detroit, MI 48201, USA; kzhang@med.wayne.edu

[4] Department of Genetics and Genomic Sciences, Icahn School of Medicine at Mount Sinai, New York, NY 10029, USA; ke.hao@mssm.edu

* Correspondence: zhongyang.zhang@mssm.edu (Z.Z.); jiex@umich.edu (J.X.)

Abstract: Individuals with cystic fibrosis (CF) often experience gastrointestinal (GI) abnormalities. In recent years, the intestinal microbiome has been postulated as a contributor to the development of CF-associated GI complications, hence representing a potential therapeutic target for treatment. We recently developed a rabbit model of CF, which is shown to manifest many human patient-like pathological changes, including intestinal obstruction. Here, we investigated the feces microbiome in young CF rabbits in the absence of antibiotics treatment. Stool samples were collected from seven- to nine-week-old CF rabbits ($n = 7$) and age-matched wild-type (WT) rabbits ($n = 6$). Microbiomes were investigated by iTag sequencing of 16S rRNA genes, and functional profiles were predicted using PICRUSt. Consistent with reports of those in pediatric CF patients, the fecal microbiomes of CF rabbits are of lower richness and diversity than that of WT rabbits, with a marked taxonomic and inferred functional dysbiosis. Our work identified a new CF animal model with the manifestation of intestinal dysbiosis phenotype. This model system may facilitate the research and development of novel treatments for CF-associated gastrointestinal diseases.

Keywords: cystic fibrosis; rabbits; intestinal dysbiosis; feces microbiome

1. Introduction

Cystic fibrosis (CF) is an autosomal recessive disorder with a disease frequency of 1 in 2000 live births and a carrier rate of approximately 5% in the Caucasian population [1]. Mutations in the CF transmembrane conductance regulator (CFTR) gene lead to CF [2]. In 2019, the community celebrated the FDA's approval of Trikafta, which provides benefits to greater than 90% of CF patients [3]. However, CF is not cured yet; continuous research is needed for the development of novel therapeutics for this disease.

Clinically, CF is a progressive, chronic, and debilitating disease, affecting the lungs, sinuses, gastrointestinal (GI) tract, liver, pancreas, and others [4]. GI disease develops early and continues through adulthood in CF patients. Meconium ileus (MI) presents in up to 20% of neonates with CF, which may need surgical interventions to resolve [5]. In infancy and childhood, CF patients must be treated for pancreatic insufficiency, a condition that adversely affects intestinal nutrient absorption and subsequently weight gain and growth [6]. Constipation or distal intestinal obstruction syndrome (DIOS) often cause bloating and abdominal pain in CF patients throughout their life [7]. Furthermore, CF patients are predisposed with a 5–10 times greater risk of colorectal cancer than the general population [8].

Accumulating evidences show that the gut microbiome in CF patients is altered. In both pediatric and adult CF patients, their gut microbiome is of lower richness and diversity compared to those of healthy controls [9–11]. Such reduction of microbial diversity in CF patients is often associated with species alteration, implicating functional contributions of microbial species to CF GI diseases. However, the clinical relevance of the change in gut microorganisms is not well-established. Understanding the CF gut microbiome thus will shed light on the pathogenesis of CF GI diseases, and potentially provide hints to microbiome-based drug development.

We recently produced CF rabbits by knocking out the CFTR gene using CRISPR/Cas9 [12]. These CF rabbits manifest many typical CF pathologies, including growth retardation, airway inflammation, and metabolic disorders, among others. Comparing to other CF animal models, CF rabbits have several advantages, for example, compared to other non-rodent models (e.g., sheep and pigs), CF rabbits are relatively cost effective to house and maintain. On the other hand, compared to the mouse model, CF rabbits are large, making many experimental procedures more practical. Importantly, rabbit airway epithelial cells responded to CFTR modulator drug VX770 in a similar manner as human airway epithelial cells do, supporting the use of these animals in preclinical studies for CF [12].

Of note, almost all CF rabbits suffer from the intestinal obstruction. In this study, we investigate the composition of feces bacteria as a proxy of gut microbiome of young CF rabbits (Figure 1). We hypothesize that the composition of bacterial communities in the CF rabbit intestine is different from that in the wild-type (WT) rabbits. In support of this hypothesis, the results revealed a marked taxonomic and inferred functional dysbiosis in the CF samples when compared to WT samples. This CF rabbit model of gut dysbiosis may facilitate the research and development of novel treatments for CF GI diseases.

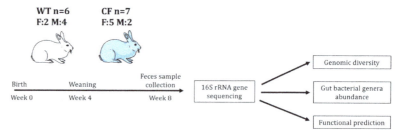

Figure 1. Illustration of experimental flow. F: female. M: male.

2. Results

2.1. CF Rabbits Exhibit Intestinal Obstruction

Intestinal obstruction is the primary cause of mortality in CF rabbits [12], as exampled in Figure 2. The proximal colon of CF rabbits is often dilated, and the distal colon presents a paucity of stool pellets (Figure 2A), which are not observed in WT animals (Figure 2B). Interestingly, unlike CF pigs and ferrets, who need immediate surgical procedures to resolve the MI condition, many CF rabbits do not develop severe obstruction until they reach four to six weeks of age. The relatively large size of the cecum may have allowed it to accumulate feces, and hence delay the onset of the obstruction in this species.

Alcian Blue-Periodic Acid Schiff (AB-PAS) stain of cross sections of CF rabbit colon illustrates the massive mucus plugging in the lumen (Figure 2C), but not in that of WT (Figure 2D). In longitudinal sections, the CF rabbit colon exhibits obvious intestinal wall thickening, inflammation accompanied by interstitial fibrosis, and visible goblet cell hyperplasia (Figure 2E) compared to the WT control (Figure 2F).

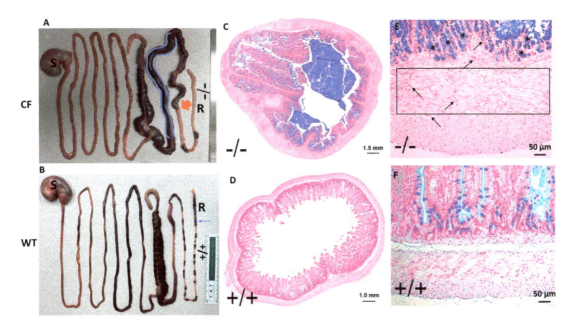

Figure 2. Intestinal obstruction is a common phenotype in CF rabbits. (**A**) Gross images of the GI tracks of a CF rabbit. The proximal colon (highlighted in blue) was dilated. Red arrow indicates the point of blockage. (**B**) Gross images of the GI tracks of a WT rabbit. Blue arrow indicates feces pellets, which are missing in the CF rabbit. (**C**) AB-PAS staining of the cross section of a CF rabbit colon. (**D**) AB-PAS staining of the cross section of a WT rabbit colon. (**E**) AB-PAS staining of the longitudinal sections of a CF rabbit colon. Region within the box is a representative area of interstitial fibrosis. Arrows indicate inflammatory infiltration; asterisks indicate goblet cell hyperplasia. (**F**) AB-PAS staining of the longitudinal sections of a WT rabbit colon. S: stomach. R: rectum. -/-: CFTR-/-. +/+: CFTR+/+.

2.2. Study Sample Characteristics

We investigated the gut microbiome, surrogated by fecal samples, of CF rabbits carrying homozygous 9 base pair (bp) deletions ($\Delta 9/\Delta 9$) on the CFTR gene ($n = 7$) and WT rabbits ($n = 6$) by iTag sequencing of the 16S rRNA gene (Figure 1). After pre-processing of the sequencing data, an average of 20.7 million base pairs (Mbp) was generated to characterize the bacteria community per sample, with an average data utilization ratio of 97.6% (Supplementary Table S1). Read pairs that passed quality control (QC) were merged into consensus sequences (i.e., tags), resulting an average of 40,889 tags of good quality per sample with a mean size of 252 bp (Supplementary Table S2). The tags were clustered and mapped to 473 operational taxonomic units (OTUs). On average, each sample had 32,885 tags assigned to 220 OTUs (Table 1). The diversity of bacteria communities in fecal samples from both CF and WT rabbits was adequately captured by the sequencing effort, which is reflected by the rarefaction curves of the observed number of OTUs and Shannon Index (Supplementary Figure S1).

Table 1. Study sample description.

Sample ID	Genotype	Age (days)	Sex	# Tags/sample	# OTUs/sample
CF01	CF	61	F	33230	217
CF02	CF	61	F	33029	144
CF03	CF	53	F	35122	176
CF04	CF	59	F	34490	139
CF05	CF	55	M	33458	160
CF06	CF	53	M	34617	118
CF07	CF	55	F	35189	299
WT01	WT	51	M	31635	269
WT02	WT	51	F	29621	281
WT03	WT	54	M	32713	275
WT04	WT	54	M	30499	306
WT05	WT	53	F	29410	313
WT06	WT	51	M	34495	170

2.3. Alpha Diversity

We first compared the alpha diversity between the CF and WT rabbits in terms of richness, measured by the observed number of OTUs and evenness measured by the Shannon index. The CF rabbits had significantly lower bacteria richness (mean difference: -90; $p = 0.017$ in a Wilcoxon one-sided test) and Shannon index (mean difference: -0.45; $p = 0.037$ in a Wilcoxon one-sided test) (Figure 3), suggesting attenuated bacteria diversity (richness and evenness) in the fecal samples of the CF rabbit model.

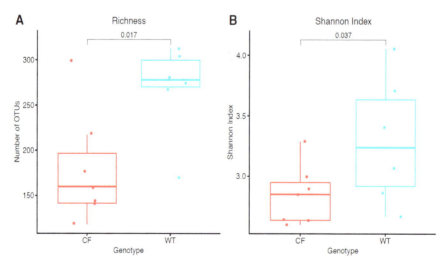

Figure 3. Sample alpha diversity in CF and WT groups. (**A**) Richness measured by the observed number of OTUs. (**B**) Evenness measured by the Shannon index. The distributions of values were summarized by boxplots. Shown from bottom to top is the minimum value, first quartile, median, third quartile, and maximum value, and the outlier value is shown as individual points. On top of the boxplots, the individual data points were super imposed; p-values were calculated by a one-sided Wilcoxon rank sum test.

2.4. Beta Diversity

Phylogeny-based beta diversity calculated by weighted and unweighted UniFrac distances [13] was visualized by non-metric multidimensional scaling (NMDS) [14] and compared between CF and WT rabbits. Figure 4 shows a clear distinction of bacteria communities in CF rabbits from those in WT rabbits. A significant difference between the CF and WT bacteria communities was also present by PERMANOVA (permutational multivariate analysis of variance) tests (weighted UniFrac distance $R2 = 0.38$, $p = 0.007$; unweighted UniFrac distance $R2 = 0.33$, $p = 0.016$), further highlighting the difference in the composition of bacteria between CF and WT rabbits (Figure 4).

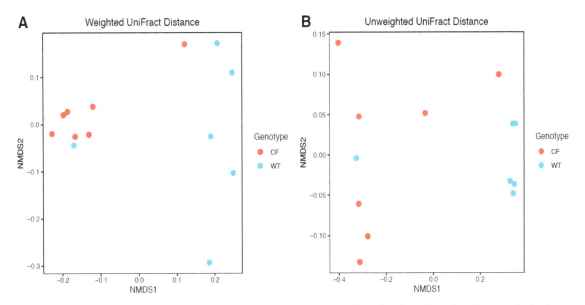

Figure 4. Beta diversity comparison between CF and WT groups based on OTU abundance. Beta diversity was calculated by phylogeny-based (**A**) weighted and (**B**) unweighted UniFrac distances based on relative abundances of identified OTUs, and visualized by non-metric multidimensional scaling (NMDS).

2.5. Relative Abundance of Bacterial Genera in CF and WT Rabbits

We further looked into the composition of bacteria communities at different taxonomical ranks, and compared them between CF and WT groups. Among the top abundant genera in rabbits (Figure 5), *Bacteroides*, *Ruminococcus*, *Blautia*, and *Parabacteroides* also appeared highly abundant in humans, while other genera, such as *Akkermansia*, *Clostridium*, *Coprococcus*, and *Oscillospira*, were present uniquely in rabbits (11). Bacteria taxa at the phylum and genus level with a significantly differential abundance (at FDR <= 0.1) between CF and WT groups are reported in Table 2. More results of differentially abundant taxa at other ranks are reported in Supplementary Table S3. In the fecal samples, CF rabbits had more *Bacteroidetes* and less *Firmicutes*, *Saccharibacteria*, and *Cyanobacteria* at the rank of phylum than WT rabbits. At the genus level, *Bacteroides*, *Blautia*, and *Holdemania* were more abundant, whereas *Oscillospira*, *Roseburia*, *Ruminococcus*, and *Dehalobacterium* were less abundant in the CF rabbit model.

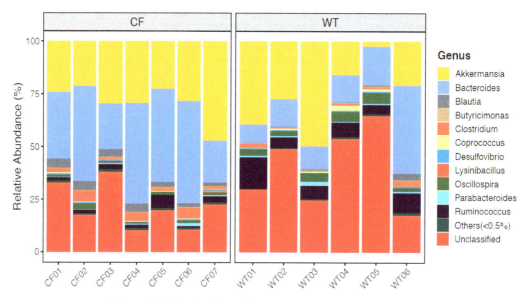

Figure 5. Relative abundance of bacterial genera in CF and WT rabbits.

Table 2. Differentially abundant phyla and genera between CF and WT groups.

Taxon	CF Relative Abundance (%) (mean ± SD)	WT Relative Abundance (%) (mean ± SD)	Mean Difference (%) (CF − WT)	p-Value	FDR
Phylum					
Firmicutes	24.234 ± 3.975	41.307 ± 11.565	−17.073	0.002	0.023
Saccharibacteria	0.001 ± 0.003	0.081 ± 0.075	−0.08	0.010	0.035
Bacteroidetes	45.023 ± 10.483	27.355 ± 11.337	17.669	0.035	0.087
Cyanobacteria	0.008 ± 0.012	0.071 ± 0.076	−0.063	0.047	0.095
Genus					
Bacteroides	37.115 ± 12.404	17.673 ± 12.282	19.442	0.008	0.060
Blautia	2.997 ± 1.147	0.67 ± 1.118	2.327	0.008	0.060
Oscillospira	1.392 ± 0.718	3.517 ± 1.347	−2.125	0.005	0.060
Roseburia	0 ± 0	0.02 ± 0.023	−0.02	0.006	0.060
Ruminococcus	2.384 ± 1.836	7.777 ± 3.881	−5.392	0.008	0.060
Holdemania	0.06 ± 0.04	0.015 ± 0.015	0.045	0.014	0.086
Dehalobacterium	0.012 ± 0.029	0.08 ± 0.063	−0.069	0.017	0.089

2.6. Predicted Functional Analysis by PICRUSt

We used PICRUSt [15] to predict the functional profiles of bacteria communities in the fecal samples of the rabbits based on 16S rRNA data, and compared the relative abundance of predicted KEGG orthology (KO) terms between the CF and WT groups (see details in Section 4.7). In total, relative abundances (in percentages) of 76 KO terms were predicted, and 18 of them had differential abundances between CF and WT rabbits at FDR <= 0.1 (Table 3). In particular, biological functions, such as short chain fatty acid (SCFAs; e.g., propanoate and butanoate) metabolism, lipid biosynthesis, bacterial motility, and chemotaxis were downregulated, while amino acid metabolism, lipopolysaccharide biosynthesis, and glycan degradation were upregulated in CF rabbits compared to WT rabbits.

Table 3. Predicted KEGG orthology terms with a significantly different abundance between CF and WT groups.

KEGG Orthology	CF Relative Abundance (%) (mean ± SD)	WT Relative Abundance (%) (mean ± SD)	Mean Difference (%) (CF − WT)	p-Value	FDR
Aminoacyl-tRNA biosynthesis	1.065 ± 0.032	1.117 ± 0.029	−0.053	0.002	0.056
Arginine and proline metabolism	1.361 ± 0.007	1.321 ± 0.041	0.041	0.005	0.056
Bacterial chemotaxis	0.304 ± 0.053	0.427 ± 0.102	−0.123	0.008	0.056
Chaperones and folding catalysts	1.05 ± 0.015	0.989 ± 0.042	0.061	0.005	0.056
Glycine, serine and threonine metabolism	0.873 ± 0.013	0.832 ± 0.025	0.041	0.005	0.056
Lipid biosynthesis proteins	0.634 ± 0.018	0.68 ± 0.025	−0.046	0.008	0.056
Membrane and intracellular structural molecules	0.712 ± 0.051	0.573 ± 0.088	0.14	0.008	0.056
Other glycan degradation	0.487 ± 0.052	0.356 ± 0.078	0.131	0.008	0.056
Propanoate metabolism	0.495 ± 0.017	0.568 ± 0.048	−0.073	0.008	0.056
Purine metabolism	2.062 ± 0.033	1.976 ± 0.028	0.086	0.001	0.056
Sporulation	0.439 ± 0.051	0.639 ± 0.159	−0.2	0.008	0.056
Bacterial motility proteins	0.728 ± 0.148	1.016 ± 0.198	−0.287	0.014	0.071
Butanoate metabolism	0.588 ± 0.022	0.661 ± 0.067	−0.074	0.014	0.071
Lipopolysaccharide biosynthesis proteins	0.549 ± 0.036	0.43 ± 0.099	0.119	0.014	0.071
RNA degradation	0.496 ± 0.01	0.456 ± 0.032	0.041	0.014	0.071
Flagellar assembly	0.224 ± 0.083	0.374 ± 0.13	−0.15	0.022	0.093
Mismatch repair	0.748 ± 0.017	0.781 ± 0.032	−0.033	0.022	0.093
Transcription factors	1.46 ± 0.049	1.609 ± 0.144	−0.149	0.022	0.093

3. Discussion

Recent studies have demonstrated altered intestinal microbiomes in CF patients across different age groups compared to those in healthy individuals. In infant CF patients, Antosca et al. reported reduced levels of *Bacterioides*, a bacterial genus associated with immune modulation, in their fecal microbiome [10]. In juvenile and young adult CF subjects aged 10–22 years, Miragoli et al. reported a lower frequency of sulfate-reducing bacteria in their fecal samples, which may have contributed to the abdominal bloating in CF patients [9]. In another study on CF children aged between 0.8 to 18 years, CF fecal samples exhibited marked taxonomic and functional changes of the gut microbiome [11]. These findings suggest that the gut microbiome plays an important role in CF-associated GI disease development, likely in an age-dependent manner.

In the present work, we report a novel CF animal model (i.e., the CF rabbits) that manifests intestinal dysbiosis. Preclinical animal models are a prerequisite to test therapeutic strategies targeting the gut microbiomes of CF patients. To date, almost all CF animal gut microbiome studies have used mice [16–18]. Interestingly, loss of functional CFTR in CF mice is associated with significant decreases in GI bacterial community richness, evenness, and diversity, and reduced relative abundance of putative protective species in some reports [16], but not in others [17]. In the other study utilizing a nonmurine model ferrets, *Streptococcus* and *Escherichia coli* were more abundant in the CF animals than in the non-CF controls; however, it is not known whether there is a reduction of bacterial diversity due to the CF condition in these animals [19]. There are no reports from other CF animals, such as rats, pigs, and sheep. The addition of CF rabbits to the gut microbiome toolbox therefore provides a new system to the research community, and is expected to facilitate study on the pathogenesis of CF-associated GI disease and accelerate the development of novel treatments for CF gastrointestinal diseases. For example, taurine conjugate ursodeoxycholic acid (TUDCA) is being tested to treat CF-related liver disease (CFLD)

(Available online: ClinicalTrials.gov ID#: NCT00004441 (accessed on 15 February 2021)). Whether TIDCA treatment alters the CF intestinal microbiome is an intriguing question, which can be tested in the CF rabbits.

Consistent with reports of those in pediatric CF patients, the fecal microbiome of CF rabbits, in comparison to that of WT rabbits, is of lower richness and diversity, with marked taxonomic and functional alterations. At the phylum level in the fecal microbiome, *Firmicutes* (↓17%) and *Bacteroidetes* (↑17%) are the two most changed in CF conditions, albeit at different directions (Table 2). The Firmicutes/Bacteroidetes (F/B) ratio is postulated as an indicator of nutritional intake status [20]. In obese individuals, this ratio is reported to be higher than that of healthy control individuals, whereas dietary restriction led to a reduction of this ratio [20]. In the young rabbits of the current study, the F/B ratio was greatly reduced in the CF fecal microbiome in comparison to that of WT, which indicates a nutritional insufficiency due to CFTR deficiency. Future studies should test whether modulating the F/B ratio can improve the nutritional status of CF individuals.

At the genus level, *Bacteroides* were increased by 19% in the CF rabbit fecal microbiome, representing the most changed species (Table 2). At the time of sample collection, rabbits were 7–9 weeks old, comparable to ~6–7 years old in human age. This observation is similar to that observed in pediatric CF individuals (aged 0.8–18 years) [11]. However, in a study of CF infants (six weeks to 12 months), the relative abundance of *Bacteroides* was consistently higher in the fecal microbiome of healthy individuals than that of the CF [10]. Our work and these studies suggest that the relative abundance of intestinal *Bacteroides* in CF subjects is age-related.

Predicted functional analysis reveals several notable changes in biological functions (BFs) associated with the intestinal microbiome in CF rabbits (Table 3). (i) The increased abundance of microbiomes that are functionally implicated in "chaperones and folding catalysts" suggests an alteration in the endoplasmic reticulum (ER) protein folding capacity and potential activation of an ER stress response in CF rabbits. (ii) There is an upregulation of BFs of lipopolysaccharide (LPS) biosynthesis in CF rabbits compared to WT rabbits. LPS is the major component of the outer membrane of Gram-negative bacteria, and is known to induce strong innate immune responses [21]. It has been previously demonstrated that challenging the airway epithelial cells with *P. Aeruginosa* decreased the CFTR function and induced an increase in pro-inflammatory cytokines [22–24].In this regard, this alteration of gut microbiomes in CF individuals may have contributed to the inflammation phenotypes. (iii) Glycans are sequences of carbohydrates that are added to proteins or lipids to modulate their structure and function. Glycans modify proteins required for regulation of immune cells, and alterations have been associated with inflammatory conditions [25]. The altered microbiome abundance involved in glycan degradation also implicates the likeness of liver disease in CF rabbits, as the alteration of protein glycosylation has been observed in GI and liver diseases [25,26]. (iv) Furthermore, decreased microbiome abundance implicated in Butanoate metabolism may also be responsible for the metabolic phenotype in CF rabbits. Hepatic mitochondria are known to be the main target of the beneficial effect of butyrate-based compounds in reverting insulin resistance and fat accumulation in diet-induced obese animal models. Butyrate, produced by fermentation in the large intestine by gut microbiota, and its synthetic derivative have been demonstrated to be protective against insulin resistance and fatty livers [27]. (v) Short chain fatty acids (SCFAs) produced by gut bacteria widely participate in energy, lipid, glucose, and cholesterol metabolism in host various tissues. The *Bacteroidetes* mainly produce acetate and propionate, whereas butyrate is the primary metabolic end product of *Firmicutes* [28]. Notably, in CF subjects, BFs of short chain fatty acid metabolism and lipid biosynthesis were downregulated, but those of amino acid metabolism and glycan degradation were upregulated. These changes may have reflected the preference for different energy sources in CF rabbits at this age.

Lastly, we should point out several limitations of the present study. First, we used fecal samples as a proxy for the intestinal microbiome. While fecal sampling is easy and non-invasive, this method has inherit disadvantages [29]; for example, it cannot provide accurate information on the spatial distribution of the microbiota along the intestine. Second, CF rabbits in this study did not receive any antibiotics, whereas antibiotics are routinely used in human patients. This factor should be considered when CF rabbits and patients' intestinal microbiomes are compared. Third, as a routine care procedure, CF rabbits (but not the WT ones) received Golytely in the present work. A strict control using WT rabbits that also receive Golytely treatment should be included in a future study. Fourth, it should be noted that rabbits are coprophagic. While this does not affect the comparison between CF and WT rabbits, caution should be taken when comparing the rabbit data with a species that is not coprophagic.

In summary, we investigated the intestinal microbiome in young CF rabbits. In comparison to that of WT rabbits, the CF rabbit intestinal microbiome is of lower richness and diversity, with a marked taxonomic and inferred functional dysbiosis. This model system may facilitate the research and development of novel treatments for CF gastrointestinal diseases.

4. Materials and Methods

4.1. Animals and Fecal Sample Collection

The animal maintenance, care, and use procedures were reviewed and approved by the Institutional Animal Care and Use Committee (protocol #PRO00008218) of the University of Michigan, an AAALAC International accredited facility. All procedures were carried out in accordance with the approved guidelines.

Heterozygous CFTRΔ9/WT (HT CF) rabbits were produced as described previously [12]. Male and female HT CF rabbits were bred to produce homozygous CFTRΔ9/Δ9, and WT rabbits were used in the present study.

Both CF and WT rabbits were fed with Laboratory Rabbit Diet #5321 (LabDiet, St. Louis, MO, USA). At two weeks of age, the CF kits were given Golytely (an osmotic laxative, Braintree Labs, Braintree, MA, USA) by oral syringe feeding daily. The CF rabbits consumed this laxative for their entire life.

Night fecal samples were collected on a morning when animals were at the corresponding age (Table 1) using sterile forceps into a sterile test tube. The samples were immediately put into a −80 °C freezer.

Approximately 300 mg fecal samples/rabbit were submitted to BGI Americas Corporation (Cambridge, MA, USA) (BGI) for sample extraction, 16S/18S/ITS amplicon sequencing, and bioinformatics.

4.2. Histology Staining

Tissues were fixed in 10% formalin for about 24 h. Fixed specimens were embedded into paraffin blocks, cut into 5 μM sections, and stained with Alcian Blue-Periodic Acid Schiff (AB-PAS). In brief, the deparaffinized tissue sections were stained with AB solution (1 g of Alcian blue, pH = 2.5, 3 mL/L of acetic acid, and 97 mL of distilled water) for 30 min, followed by rinsing in water for 10 min, oxidizing in periodic acid (5 g/L) for 5 min, and staining with Schiff reagent as a counter stain for 10 min.

4.3. 16S rRNA Sequencing Data Processing

16S rRNA sequencing was conducted at BGI. Briefly, paired-end reads of 250 bp were generated with the Illumina HiSeq platform, and then were subject to the following pre-processing procedures [30]: (i) truncation of sequence reads with an average quality below 20 (on the Phred scale) over a 30 bp sliding window and removal of trimmed reads with less than 75% of their original size, as well as their paired reads; (ii) removal of reads contaminated by the adapter (15 bases overlapped by the adapter with maximal mismatch of 3 bp); and (iii) removal of reads with ambiguous bases (N base), as well as their paired reads; (iv) removal of reads with low complexity (reads with 10 consecutive repeated bases). The clean reads were de-multiplexed and assigned to corresponding samples (0 base mismatch in barcode sequences). Summary statistics for raw and processed reads are shown in Supplementary Table S1. An average of 42,460 read pairs were generated from each sample, amounting to 21.2 million bps. After cleaning with the above procedure, an average of 41,502 read pairs remained for each sample, with an average read utilization rate of 97.8%.

After removal of cleaned paired-end reads without overlaps, overlapped paired-end reads were merged into consensus sequences (i.e., tags) by FLASH [31] with the parameters: (i) overlapping length >= 15 bp; and (ii) mismatching ratio of overlapped region <= 0.1. Furthermore, primer sequences were removed from the generated tags, where the forward and reverse amplification primers were mapped to the two ends of tags, with four consecutive bases at the 3' end of the primers being completely matched with the tags, and the mismatch bases of the remaining primer being no more than two. On average, 40,889 tags were generated per sample after removal of primer sequences, and the average length was 252 bp (Supplementary Table S2).

The generated tags were further clustered to operational taxonomic units (OTUs) by USEARCH (v7.0.1090) [32], detailed as follows: (i) the tags were clustered into OTUs with a 97% threshold using UPARSE [33], and the representative sequence for each OTU was derived; (ii) chimeras were identified and filtered by UCHIME (v4.2.40) [34], with the 16S rRNA sequences being screened against the "Gold" database (v20110519); (iii) the tags were mapped to OTU representative sequences using USEARCH (usearch_global command), and the number of tags mapped to each OTU in each sample was quantified as the abundance of OTUs; and (iv) OTU representative sequences were taxonomically classified by the Ribosomal Database Project (RDP) Classifier (v.2.2) [35] trained on the Greengenes database (version gg_13_5) [36] using a 0.6 confidence cutoff. OTUs that were not assigned to a bacteria taxonomical term were excluded from downstream analysis. A total of 427,508 tags from the 13 samples were clustered and mapped to 473 OTUs, none of which was singleton.

4.4. Alpha Diversity Analysis

The alpha diversity indices, including the observed number of OTUs and Shannon index, were calculated by Mothur (v1.31.2) [37]. The corresponding rarefaction curves were calculated based on OTUs derived from randomly extracted tags in an incremental step of 500 (Supplementary Figure S1).

4.5. Beta Diversity Analysis

Beta diversity was evaluated by phylogeny-based weighted and unweighted UniFrac distances, which take into account the distance of evolution between species to compare the composition of the bacteria community between samples [13]. Beta diversity analysis was performed by QIIME (v1.80) [38]. In the analysis, sequences (tags) were randomly sampled according to the minimum sequence number across all samples in order to account for the differences in the sequencing depth of different samples, and the abundance of OTUs was then adjusted accordingly. Weighted and unweighted UniFrac distances between samples were visualized by non-metric multidimensional scaling (NMDS), implemented by the R function isoMDS [14]. Permutational multivariate analysis of variance (PERMANOVA) tests were used to derive the significance level of the difference in beta diversity measurements between CF and WT groups, which was implemented by the function adonis in the R package vegan (v2.5-6) [39].

4.6. Differential Abundance Analysis

Metastats [40] was employed to identify differentially abundant taxa between CF and WT groups at various taxonomical ranks (phylum, class, order, family, genus, and species). The p-values generated at each taxonomical rank were, respectively, adjusted by a Benjamini–Hochberg false discovery rate (FDR) correction [41]. Significant differences were defined at FDR <= 0.1.

4.7. Functional Analysis

We used PICRUSt [15] to predict the functional profiles of the fecal bacteria communities in the CF and WT rabbit models based on 16S rRNA data. PICRUSt uses phylogenetic modeling to predict the metagenome of a microbiome community based on 16S rRNA data and reference microbiome genome databases, including Greengenes [36] and IMG [42]. The metagenome prediction results in an annotated table of predicted gene family abundance for each sample, where gene families can be functionally classified as orthologous groups in terms of KEGG orthology (KO) [43]. The relative abundances (in percentages) of predicted KO terms were compared between the CF and WT groups using a Wilcoxon rank sum test. The nominal p-values were adjusted by a Benjamini–Hochberg FDR correction [41]. Significant differences were defined at FDR <= 0.1.

Supplementary Materials: The following are available online at https://www.mdpi.com/2075-4426/11/2/132/s1, Figure S1: Rarefaction curves for the CF and WT rabbits, Table S1: Summary statistics of processing pair-end 16S rRNA sequencing data, Table S2: Summary statistics of merged tags from pre-processed read pairs, Table S3: Differentially abundant taxa between CF and WT groups at various taxonomic ranks.

Author Contributions: J.X. and Z.Z. conceived the idea. X.L., J.-P.J., Z.Z., and J.X. designed the experiments. X.L., M.B., X.H., J.S., and J.X. conducted experiments. X.L., K.Z., K.H., J.-P.J., Z.Z., and J.X. analyzed the data. K.Z., J.-P.J., Z.Z., and J.X. wrote the manuscript. All authors have read and agreed to the published version of the manuscript.

Funding: National Institutes of Health: HL133162.

Acknowledgments: This work was supported by National Institutes of Health (Grant# HL133162 to J.-P.J. and J.X.).

Conflicts of Interest: The authors declare that the research was conducted in the absence of any conflict of interest.

References

1. Wang, Y.; Wrennall, J.A.; Cai, Z.; Li, H.; Sheppard, D.N. Understanding how cystic fibrosis mutations disrupt CFTR function: From single molecules to animal models. *Int. J. Biochem. Cell Biol.* **2014**, *52*, 47–57. [CrossRef]
2. Stoltz, D.A.; Meyerholz, D.K.; Welsh, M.J. Origins of cystic fibrosis lung disease. *New Engl. J. Med.* **2015**, *372*, 351–362. [CrossRef] [PubMed]
3. Bear, C.E. A Therapy for Most with Cystic Fibrosis. *Cell* **2020**, *180*, 211. [CrossRef] [PubMed]
4. Cystic fibrosis. *Nat. Rev. Dis Primers* **2015**, *1*, 15049. [CrossRef] [PubMed]
5. Sathe, M.; Houwen, R. Meconium ileus in Cystic Fibrosis. *J. Cyst. Fibros.* **2017**, *16* (Suppl. 2), S32–S39. [CrossRef] [PubMed]
6. Galante, G.; Freeman, A.J. Gastrointestinal, Pancreatic, and Hepatic Manifestations of Cystic Fibrosis in the Newborn. *Neoreviews* **2019**, *20*, e12–e24. [CrossRef]
7. Van der Doef, H.P.; Kokke, F.T.; van der Ent, C.K.; Houwen, R.H. Intestinal obstruction syndromes in cystic fibrosis: Meconium ileus, distal intestinal obstruction syndrome, and constipation. *Curr. Gastroenterol. Rep.* **2011**, *13*, 265–270. [CrossRef] [PubMed]
8. Hadjiliadis, D.; Khoruts, A.; Zauber, A.G.; Hempstead, S.E.; Maisonneuve, P.; Lowenfels, A.B. Cystic Fibrosis Colorectal Cancer Screening Task Force. Cystic Fibrosis Colorectal Cancer Screening Consensus Recommendations. *Gastroenterology* **2018**, *154*, 736–745.e714. [CrossRef]
9. Miragoli, F.; Federici, S.; Ferrari, S.; Minuti, A.; Rebecchi, A.; Bruzzese, E.; Buccigrossi, V.; Guarino, A.; Callegari, M.L. Impact of cystic fibrosis disease on archaea and bacteria composition of gut microbiota. *FEMS Microbiol. Ecol.* **2017**, *93*, fiw230. [CrossRef]
10. Antosca, K.M.; Chernikova, D.A.; Price, C.E.; Ruoff, K.L.; Li, K.; Guill, M.F.; Sontag, N.R.; Morrison, H.G.; Hao, S.; Drumm, M.L.; et al. Altered Stool Microbiota of Infants with Cystic Fibrosis Shows a Reduction in Genera Associated with Immune Programming from Birth. *J. Bacteriol.* **2019**, *201*, e00274-19. [CrossRef]
11. Coffey, M.J.; Nielsen, S.; Wemheuer, B.; Kaakoush, N.O.; Garg, M.; Needham, B.; Pickford, R.; Jaffe, A.; Thomas, T.; Ooi, C.Y. Gut Microbiota in Children with Cystic Fibrosis: A Taxonomic and Functional Dysbiosis. *Sci. Rep.* **2019**, *9*, 18593. [CrossRef]
12. Xu, J.; Livraghi-Butrico, A.; Hou, X.; Rajagopalan, C.; Zhang, J.; Song, J.; Jiang, H.; Wei, H.G.; Wang, H.; Bouhamdan, M.; et al. Phenotypes of CF rabbits generated by CRISPR/Cas9-mediated disruption of the CFTR gene. *JCI Insight* **2021**, *6*, e139813.
13. Lozupone, C.A.; Hamady, M.; Kelley, S.T.; Knight, R. Quantitative and qualitative beta diversity measures lead to different insights into factors that structure microbial communities. *Appl. Environ. Microbiol.* **2007**, *73*, 1576–1585. [CrossRef]
14. Cox, T.F.; Cox, M.A.A. *Multidimensional Scaling*, 2nd ed.; Chapman & Hall/CRC: Boca Raton, FL, USA, 2001.

15. Langille, M.G.; Zaneveld, J.; Caporaso, J.G.; McDonald, D.; Knights, D.; Reyes, J.A.; Clemente, J.C.; Burkepile, D.E.; Vega Thurber, R.L.; Knight, R.; et al. Predictive functional profiling of microbial communities using 16S rRNA marker gene sequences. *Nat. Biotechnol.* **2013**, *31*, 814–821. [CrossRef] [PubMed]
16. Lynch, S.V.; Goldfarb, K.C.; Wild, Y.K.; Kong, W.; De Lisle, R.C.; Brodie, E.L. Cystic fibrosis transmembrane conductance regulator knockout mice exhibit aberrant gastrointestinal microbiota. *Gut Microbes* **2013**, *4*, 41–47. [CrossRef]
17. Bazett, M.; Honeyman, L.; Stefanov, A.N.; Pope, C.E.; Hoffman, L.R.; Haston, C.K. Cystic fibrosis mouse model-dependent intestinal structure and gut microbiome. *Mamm. Genome* **2015**, *26*, 222–234. [PubMed]
18. Meeker, S.M.; Mears, K.S.; Sangwan, N.; Brittnacher, M.J.; Weiss, E.J.; Treuting, P.M.; Tolley, N.; Pope, C.E.; Hager, K.R.; Vo, A.T.; et al. CFTR dysregulation drives active selection of the gut microbiome. *Plos Pathog* **2020**, *16*, e1008251. [CrossRef]
19. Sun, X.; Olivier, A.K.; Yi, Y.; Pope, C.E.; Hayden, H.S.; Liang, B.; Sui, H.; Zhou, W.; Hager, K.R.; Zhang, Y.; et al. Gastrointestinal pathology in juvenile and adult CFTR-knockout ferrets. *Am. J. Pathol.* **2014**, *184*, 1309–1322. [CrossRef]
20. Magne, F.; Gotteland, M.; Gauthier, L.; Zazueta, A.; Pesoa, S.; Navarrete, P.; Balamurugan, R. The Firmicutes/Bacteroidetes Ratio: A Relevant Marker of Gut Dysbiosis in Obese Patients? *Nutrients* **2020**, *12*, 1474. [CrossRef] [PubMed]
21. Alexander, C.; Rietschel, E.T. Bacterial lipopolysaccharides and innate immunity. *J. Endotoxin Res.* **2001**, *7*, 167–202. [CrossRef] [PubMed]
22. Trinh, N.T.; Bilodeau, C.; Maillé, E.; Ruffin, M.; Quintal, M.-C.; Desrosiers, M.-Y.; Rousseau, S.; Brochiero, E. Deleterious impact of Pseudomonas aeruginosa on cystic fibrosis transmembrane conductance regulator function and rescue in airway epithelial cells. *Eur. Respir. J.* **2015**, *45*, 1590–1602. [CrossRef]
23. Stanton, B.A.; Coutermarsh, B.; Barnaby, R.; Hogan, D. Pseudomonas aeruginosa Reduces VX-809 Stimulated F508del-CFTR Chloride Secretion by Airway Epithelial Cells. *PLoS ONE* **2015**, *10*, e0127742. [CrossRef]
24. Laselva, O.; Stone, T.A.; Bear, C.E.; Deber, C.M. Anti-Infectives Restore ORKAMBI((R)) Rescue of F508del-CFTR Function in Human Bronchial Epithelial Cells Infected with Clinical Strains of P. aeruginosa. *Biomolecules* **2020**, *10*, 334.
25. Verhelst, X.; Dias, A.M.; Colombel, J.F.; Vermeire, S.; Van Vlierberghe, H.; Callewaert, N.; Pinho, S.S. Protein Glycosylation as a Diagnostic and Prognostic Marker of Chronic Inflammatory Gastrointestinal and Liver Diseases. *Gastroenterology* **2020**, *158*, 95–110. [CrossRef] [PubMed]
26. Blomme, B.; van Steenkiste, C.; Callewaert, N.; van Vlierberghe, H. Alteration of protein glycosylation in liver diseases. *J. Hepatol.* **2009**, *50*, 592–603. [PubMed]
27. Mollica, M.P.; Mattace Raso, G.; Cavaliere, G.; Trinchese, G.; De Filippo, C.; Aceto, S.; Prisco, M.; Pirozzi, C.; Di Guida, F.; Lama, A.; et al. Butyrate Regulates Liver Mitochondrial Function, Efficiency, and Dynamics in Insulin-Resistant Obese Mice. *Diabetes* **2017**, *66*, 1405–1418. [CrossRef]
28. Den Besten, G.; van Eunen, K.; Groen, A.K.; Venema, K.; Reijngoud, D.-J.; Bakker, B.M. The role of short-chain fatty acids in the interplay between diet, gut microbiota, and host energy metabolism. *J. Lipid Res.* **2013**, *54*, 2325–2340. [CrossRef] [PubMed]
29. Tang, Q.; Jin, G.; Wang, G.; Liu, T.; Liu, X.; Wang, B.; Cao, H. Current Sampling Methods for Gut Microbiota: A Call for More Precise Devices. *Front. Cell Infect. Microbiol.* **2020**, *10*, 151. [CrossRef] [PubMed]
30. Fadrosh, D.W.; Ma, B.; Gajer, P.; Sengamalay, N.; Ott, S.; Brotman, R.M.; Ravel, J. An improved dual-indexing approach for multiplexed 16S rRNA gene sequencing on the Illumina MiSeq platform. *Microbiome* **2014**, *2*, 6. [CrossRef]
31. Magoc, T.; Salzberg, S.L. FLASH: Fast length adjustment of short reads to improve genome assemblies. *Bioinformatics* **2011**, *27*, 2957–2963. [PubMed]
32. Edgar, R.C. Search and clustering orders of magnitude faster than BLAST. *Bioinformatics* **2010**, *26*, 2460–2461. [CrossRef]
33. Edgar, R.C. UPARSE: Highly accurate OTU sequences from microbial amplicon reads. *Nat. Methods* **2013**, *10*, 996–998. [CrossRef]
34. Edgar, R.C.; Haas, B.J.; Clemente, J.C.; Quince, C.; Knight, R. UCHIME improves sensitivity and speed of chimera detection. *Bioinformatics* **2011**, *27*, 2194–2200. [CrossRef] [PubMed]
35. Wang, Q.; Garrity, G.M.; Tiedje, J.M.; Cole, J.R. Naive Bayesian classifier for rapid assignment of rRNA sequences into the new bacterial taxonomy. *Appl. Environ. Microbiol.* **2007**, *73*, 5261–5267. [CrossRef] [PubMed]
36. DeSantis, T.Z.; Hugenholtz, P.; Larsen, N.; Rojas, M.; Brodie, E.L.; Keller, K.; Huber, T.; Dalevi, D.; Hu, P.; Andersen, G.L. Greengenes, a chimera-checked 16S rRNA gene database and workbench compatible with ARB. *Appl. Environ. Microbiol.* **2006**, *72*, 5069–5072. [CrossRef] [PubMed]
37. Schloss, P.D.; Westcott, S.L.; Ryabin, T.; Hall, J.R.; Hartmann, M.; Hollister, E.B.; Lesniewski, R.A.; Oakley, B.B.; Parks, D.H.; Robinson, C.J.; et al. Introducing mothur: Open-source, platform-independent, community-supported software for describing and comparing microbial communities. *Appl. Environ. Microbiol.* **2009**, *75*, 7537–7541.
38. Caporaso, J.G.; Kuczynski, J.; Stombaugh, J.; Bittinger, K.; Bushman, F.D.; Costello, E.K.; Fierer, N.; Pena, A.G.; Goodrich, J.K.; Gordon, J.I.; et al. QIIME allows analysis of high-throughput community sequencing data. *Nat. Methods* **2010**, *7*, 335–336.
39. Anderson, M.J. A New Method for Non-parametric Multivariate Analysis of Variance. *Austral. Ecol.* **2001**, *26*, 32–46.
40. White, R.; Nagarajan, N.; Pop, M. Statistical methods for detecting differentially abundant features in clinical metagenomic samples. *PLoS Comput. Biol.* **2009**, *5*, e1000352. [CrossRef]
41. Benjamini, Y.; Hochberg, Y. Controlling the False Discovery Rate: A Practical and Powerful Approach to Multiple Testing. *J. R. Stat. Soc. Ser. B (Methodol.)* **1995**, *57*, 289–300. [CrossRef]

42. Markowitz, V.M.; Chen, I.A.; Palaniappan, K.; Chu, K.; Szeto, E.; Grechkin, Y.; Ratner, A.; Jacob, B.; Huang, J.; Williams, P.; et al. IMG: The Integrated Microbial Genomes database and comparative analysis system. *Nucleic Acids Res.* **2012**, *40*, D115–D122. [CrossRef] [PubMed]

43. Kanehisa, M.; Goto, S.; Sato, Y.; Furumichi, M.; Tanabe, M. KEGG for integration and interpretation of large-scale molecular data sets. *Nucleic Acids Res.* **2012**, *40*, D109–D114. [CrossRef] [PubMed]

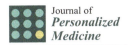

Systematic Review

Fecal Microbiota Transplantation in Allogeneic Hematopoietic Stem Cell Transplantation Recipients: A Systematic Review

Andrea Pession [1], Daniele Zama [1], Edoardo Muratore [1,*], Davide Leardini [1], Davide Gori [2], Federica Guaraldi [2,3], Arcangelo Prete [1], Silvia Turroni [4], Patrizia Brigidi [5] and Riccardo Masetti [1]

1. Pediatric Oncology and Hematology "Lalla Seràgnoli", Pediatric Unit—IRCCS Azienda Ospedaliero-Universitaria di Bologna, 40138 Bologna, Italy; andrea.pession@unibo.it (A.P.); daniele.zama@aosp.bo.it (D.Z.); davide.leardini3@gmail.com (D.L.); arcangelo.prete@aosp.bo.it (A.P.); riccardo.masetti5@unibo.it (R.M.)
2. Department of Biomedical and Neuromotor Sciences (DIBINEM), University of Bologna, 40126 Bologna, Italy; davide.gori4@unibo.it (D.G.); federica.guaraldi@yahoo.it (F.G.)
3. IRCCS Istituto delle Scienze Neurologiche di Bologna, 40126 Bologna, Italy
4. Department of Pharmacy and Biotechnology (FABIT), University of Bologna, 40126 Bologna, Italy; silvia.turroni@unibo.it
5. Department of Medical and Surgical Sciences (DIMEC), University of Bologna, 40126 Bologna, Italy; patrizia.brigidi@unibo.it
* Correspondence: edoardo.muratore@studio.unibo.it; Tel.: +39-051-214-4665

Citation: Pession, A.; Zama, D.; Muratore, E.; Leardini, D.; Gori, D.; Guaraldi, F.; Prete, A.; Turroni, S.; Brigidi, P.; Masetti, R. Fecal Microbiota Transplantation in Allogeneic Hematopoietic Stem Cell Transplantation Recipients: A Systematic Review. *J. Pers. Med.* **2021**, *11*, 100. https://doi.org/10.3390/jpm11020100

Academic Editor: Lucrezia Laterza
Received: 15 December 2020
Accepted: 2 February 2021
Published: 4 February 2021

Publisher's Note: MDPI stays neutral with regard to jurisdictional claims in published maps and institutional affiliations.

Copyright: © 2021 by the authors. Licensee MDPI, Basel, Switzerland. This article is an open access article distributed under the terms and conditions of the Creative Commons Attribution (CC BY) license (https://creativecommons.org/licenses/by/4.0/).

Abstract: The disruption of gut microbiota eubiosis has been linked to major complications in allogeneic hematopoietic stem cell transplantation (allo-HSCT) recipients. Various strategies have been developed to reduce dysbiosis and related complications. Fecal microbiota transplantation (FMT) consists of the infusion of fecal matter from a healthy donor to restore impaired intestinal homeostasis, and could be applied in the allo-HSCT setting. We conducted a systematic review of studies addressing the use of FMT in allo-HSCT patients. In the 23 papers included in the qualitative synthesis, FMT was used for the treatment of recurrent *Clostridioides difficile* infections or as a therapeutic strategy for steroid-resistant gut aGvHD. FMT was also performed with a preventive aim (e.g., to decolonize from antibiotic-resistant bacteria). Additional knowledge on the biological mechanisms underlying clinical findings is needed in order to employ FMT in clinical practice. There is also concern regarding the administration of microbial consortia in immune-compromised patients with altered gut permeability. Therefore, the safety profile and efficacy of the procedure must be determined to better assess the role of FMT in allo-HSCT recipients.

Keywords: hematopoietic stem cell transplantation; fecal microbiota transplantation; gut microbiota; aGvHD; antibiotic-resistant bacteria

1. Introduction

Allogeneic hematopoietic stem cell transplantation (allo-HSCT) is a potential curative strategy for many oncological, hematological, metabolic and immunological diseases [1–3]. Despite advances in transplantation technology and supportive care, the procedure is still associated with marked morbidity and mortality, mainly due to the recurrence of the primary disease or transplant-related complications [4]. Infections and acute Graft versus Host Disease (aGvHD) represent two of the main transplant-related complications after allo-HSCT [5].

Chemo and radiotherapy prior to transplant ablate circulating white blood cells and damage the gut epithelium, enabling the translocation of microbes through the intestinal mucosa and eventually into the bloodstream [6]. Therefore, potentially life-threatening bacterial infections can occur during the early neutropenic post-transplant phase, with the burden of antibiotic-resistant bacteria (ARB) being a critical issue in the management of these patients [7].

aGvHD is characterized by the response of alloreactive donor T cells to host organs including the skin, gut and liver. Multiple signals interact with lymphocytes and antigen-presenting cells to regulate the allo-immune response, such as the level of inflammatory cytokines and the presence of damage- and pathogen-associated molecular patterns [8]. Corticosteroids represent the first line therapy for aGvHD treatment, but their administration results in complete remission in less than half of the patients [9,10]. Over the last few years, numerous novel agents have been developed and investigated for the management of steroid-refractory or steroid-dependent disease, but no definitive consensus has been reached on the optimal second-line therapy for aGvHD [9,10].

Among the numerous factors known to be involved in the development of these complications, the recipient gut microbiome (GM) is emerging as a key determinant. The advent of large-scale genomic sequencing studies has greatly improved our ability to characterize the complex microbial communities hosted by our organism and enhanced our comprehension of the relationship between GM, immunity and intestinal epithelium [11,12]. In particular, the GM is recognized as an integral part of the host immune system, capable of fine-tuning immune responses, thus strongly contributing to homeostasis. Moreover, through the production of a plethora of bioactive molecules, the GM may also signal to various extraintestinal organs, having a system-level impact on human health. In this regard, the increasing use of the so-called omics approaches, including metagenomics, metatranscriptomics, metaproteomics, metabolomics and not least, culturomics, is starting to shed some light on the biological processes underpinning the crosstalk between the GM and the host [7,11].

HSCT and related procedures (i.e., conditioning regimen, antibiotic exposure, diet, antiacid prophylaxis) represent a combination of upsetting events that profoundly modifies the GM structure, leading to disruption of the mutualistic asset, with the establishment of the so-called dysbiosis [13,14]. Lower alpha diversity of the GM at the time of neutrophil engraftment was associated with higher transplantation-related mortality and lower overall survival [15]. Moreover, specific GM compositional layouts were associated with clinical allo-HSCT outcomes. For example, decreased amounts of beneficial bacteria belonging to the order Clostridiales (e.g., the genus *Blautia*) and a shift towards an enteropathogenic community with predominance of Gram-negative Enterobacteriales (*Escherichia coli, Klebsiella, Enterobacter* spp.) along with Gram-positive Lactobacillales (*Lactobacillus, Enterococcus* and *Streptococcus* spp.) were correlated with increased incidence of aGvHD and aGvHD-related mortality [16,17]. Intestinal dominance by individual taxa, defined as a single bacterial taxon comprising 30% or more of the GM, often precedes the development of a corresponding bloodstream infection [18]. However, the main limitation of these studies is their observational nature, and so they can only demonstrate correlations and not causative relationships.

This increasing knowledge on the GM role in the pathophysiology of the main allo-HSCT complications has led to fascinating ideas for modulating the intestinal ecosystem in order to improve clinical outcomes. Recently, numerous therapeutic strategies have been proposed in the literature to prevent the damage or restore GM integrity, including the optimization of antibiotic administration [19], the route of nutritional support [20–22] and the use of prebiotics [23]. GM can also be modulated using live microorganisms or microbial consortia, from traditional probiotics or next-generation candidates to fecal microbiota transplantation (FMT). FMT consists of the infusion of fecal matter from a healthy donor into the gastrointestinal tract of a recipient harboring a dysbiotic GM. The source of fecal material could be autologous, with stools collected before the onset of dysbiosis, or from a related or unrelated healthy donor. Because of genetic similarity and shared environment, a related FMT donor may have a closer GM composition, which may be inadvisable in certain cases. Stools can be handled and prepared as fresh fecal material, or frozen and stored in a stool bank. FMT can be delivered via the upper gastrointestinal tract using esophagogastroduodenoscopy, nasogastric or nasoduodenal tube and oral capsule, or via colonoscopy and enema [24]. This procedure directly modifies the host GM composition in an attempt to restore GM diversity and gut homeostasis [25]. FMT was first shown to be successful in the treatment of recurrent *Clostridioides difficile* infections (rCDI) and is now recommended in patients with rCDI in whom appropriate antibiotic treatments failed [26]. Thanks to its potential to re-establish an eubiotic GM layout in the recipient, FMT has been proposed for the treatment of other conditions, including inflammatory bowel disease, with promising preliminary findings [27].

In this context, there is a growing interest for FMT in allo-HSCT as a potential preventive or therapeutic strategy, mainly regarding aGvHD and infections [28]. However, many practical and safety issues arise in this setting, which have limited its application in recent years. Different FMT protocols could be applied, varying with regards to donor selection and screening, preparation of recipients and route of infusion [24]. Safety concerns have been raised regarding its use in immune-compromised patients with impaired gut permeability [29]. Indeed, a case of bacteremia caused by a multidrug-resistant *E. coli* transmitted through FMT has recently been reported, which led to the patient's death [30].

Numerous publications have reviewed this topic, either as the main focus of the paper or as a part of a more comprehensive view on the role of GM in transplantation, but this is the first systematic review on this issue. The aim of this study is to provide an up-to-date systematic review regarding the evolving evidence on the use of FMT in allo-HSCT recipients, summarizing the present literature and providing insights for future investigations.

2. Methods

A systematic review was conducted according to the Preferred Reporting Items for Systematic Reviews and Meta-Analyses (PRISMA) guidelines [31]. Electronic databases, including PubMed (https://pubmed.ncbi.nlm.nih.gov) and Trip (https://www.tripdatabase.com) were searched to identify relevant studies published up to October 2020. The following string was used to perform the literature search: (Bone Marrow transplant * OR BMT OR stem cell transplant * OR SCT OR hematopoietic transplant * OR haematopoietic transplant * OR hematopoietic stem cell transplant * OR haematopoietic stem cell transplant * OR hematopoietic cell transplant * OR haematopoietic cell transplant * OR HCT OR HSCT OR blood disorders OR leukemia OR immunocompromised) AND (fecal microbiota transplant * OR faecal microbiota transplant * OR FMT).

The search was restricted to English-language studies involving human subjects undergoing allo-HSCT receiving FMT for any indication. Two reviewers (EM, DL) independently identified potentially eligible studies by screening titles and abstracts. The same authors assessed the full-texts of potentially relevant studies for inclusion and consulted the reference lists of previously published primary and secondary papers to manually search for additional relevant papers. Any disagreement regarding eligibility and inclusion in the systematic review was resolved through discussion and consensus between the two readers. If consensus was not reached, the opinion of a third author (RM) who acted as a "blind" final arbiter was requested. Investigators and corresponding authors were contacted for studies with incomplete data in order to obtain additional information if needed.

3. Results
3.1. Literature Search

The literature search strategy yielded 673 references (301 in PubMed, 371 in Trip and one identified through manual search).

As shown in Figure 1, the number of potentially relevant papers identified by titles was 49. Among these 49 studies, 25 were excluded from the systematic review because they were reviews or did not address the role of FMT in the allo-HSCT setting. One paper was excluded because the etiology of diarrhea, reported as the reason for FMT, was not clear [32]. Of the 23 studies assessed, 15 were case reports or retrospective case series [30,33–46], seven were prospective cohorts [47–53], while only one completed randomized controlled trial was found in the literature [54].

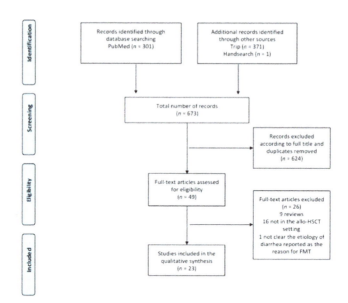

Figure 1. Preferred Reporting Items for Systematic Reviews and Meta-Analyses (PRISMA) flow diagram of the search strategy and included studies. The relevant number of papers at each point is given.

In the following sections, we will present evidence on the use of FMT in allo-HSCT recipients. In the papers included in this qualitative synthesis, FMT was performed either with a therapeutic aim, both in the context of rCDI and as a second-line agent for gut aGvHD, or as a preventive strategy, in order to reduce dysbiosis or decolonize from ARB. A brief overview of the risks of FMT reported in the literature in this peculiar population will also be provided.

3.2. rCDI

Five studies evaluated FMT for the treatment of allo-HSCT recipients with rCDI. Neeman et al. and De Castro et al. first reported two successful case reports, in which FMT was performed by injecting fecal material via a nasojejunal tube from a related donor, or with material from two different donors delivered by means of push enteroscopy [39,40].

Since then, three small series have been published. Webb et al. analyzed seven allo-HSCT recipients who underwent FMT via nasojejunal tube or colonoscopy from an unrelated donor, with five of these patients still under immunosuppressive therapy. Six patients had no relapse, while one needed another FMT to obtain remission [41]. Another series reported FMT administration in three pediatric patients from related and unrelated donors via a gastric tube or colonoscopy, with only one achieving rCDI remission [42]. Moss et al. delivered FMT to eight patients as oral encapsulated therapy from unrelated donors. Resolution from rCDI was achieved in all patients at eight weeks, and only one had a recurrence at a later time. A metagenomic analysis of the stools showed a modification of the gut resistome (i.e., the set of genes conferring antibiotic resistance in the GM), with a reduction in the burden of antibiotic resistance genes by >50% following FMT, which persisted for more than one year. Conversely, the analysis of the dynamics of microbial communities highlighted the limited durability of the specific bacterial consortium introduced with FMT, with short-term similarity and long-term dissimilarity between donor and recipient GM composition [43].

3.3. Steroid-Resistant Gut aGvHD

Nine papers explored FMT as a potential therapeutic strategy for steroid-resistant or steroid-dependent gut GvHD (Table 1), defined as progression within 3–5 days or incomplete response by 7–14 days of treatment (steroid resistance) or recurrence after initial dose reduction (steroid dependence) [5].

Table 1. Summary of included studies regarding FMT as a therapeutic strategy for steroid-refractory or dependent gut aGvHD.

First Author	Year	Number of Patients	Route of Administration	Donor	CR	PR	CR/Patients %	CR + PR/Patients %	Comments
Kakihana	2016	4	Nasoduodenal tube	Relative or Spouse	3	1	75%	100%	Response assessed within 7–14 days; in three cases a second FMT was needed.
Spindelboeck	2017	3	Colonoscopy	Unrelated or Related	2	1	67%	100%	Two patients achieved complete response with multiple FMT, one obtained a partial response after a single FMT with persistent grade I GVHD
Qi	2018	8	Nasoduodenal tube	Unrelated	5	1	63%	75%	The FMT recipients exhibited improved progression-free survival within 90 days after the diagnosis, compared with an historical control group, but no difference in overall survival.
Kaito	2018	1	Oral capsules	Related	-	1	-	100%	Digestive symptoms improved soon after initiation of FMT. aGvHD improved to stage 1 after the second cycle of FMT with the improvement of endoscopic findings.
Shouval	2018	7	Oral capsules	Unrelated	2	1	29%	43%	-
Zhong	2019	1 child	Jejunal tube under gastro-duodenoscopy guidance	Unrelated	1	-	100%	100%	-
Biernat	2020	2	Nasogastric tube	Unrelated	1	1	50%	100%	In one case complete remission was achieved, but the patient later died due to liver aGvHD and bloodstream infections. In the second case only temporary reduction and death occurred by multiorgan failure.
Mao	2020	1	Oral capsules	Unrelated	1	-	100%	100%	Complete remission after the first cycle of FMT. Recurrence 11 days later, but remission achieved with a second cycle.
Von Lier	2020	15	Nasoduodenal tube	Unrelated	10	-	67%	67%	Response assessed at 28 days after FMT. In six of the 10 complete responders, immunosuppression was successfully tapered within six months. In the other four, GvHD symptoms returned upon tapering of immunosuppressive therapy
Total	-	42	-	-	25	6	60%	74%	-

aGvHD: Graft versus Host Disease; allo-HSCT: allogeneic hematopoietic stem cells transplantation; CR: Complete Response; FMT: Fecal Microbiota Transplantation; PR: Partial Response.

Kakihana et al. reported for the first time the use of FMT in patients with steroid-resistant or dependent gut aGvHD [45]. They administered FMT from a related donor by nasoduodenal tube in four patients. All patients responded, with three complete responses and one partial response, but in three cases a second FMT was needed. Improvement of the gastrointestinal symptoms was observed within several days, combined with an increase in peripheral effector regulatory T cells [47].

In a subsequent report, three patients received FMT delivered by colonoscopy for refractory grade IV gut GvHD from related and unrelated donors. A clinical response with stool volume reduction was observed in all patients. Two achieved complete response with multiple FMT after 73 and 29 days from the first fecal infusion, while the other obtained a partial response, still presenting with grade I GvHD after one course of FMT. Based on 16S rRNA gene analysis of the pre- and post-FMT GM, restoration of microbial diversity and richness correlated with clinical improvement [44].

Another study involved eight patients with refractory grade IV gut GvHD receiving one or two courses of FMT from unrelated donors via a nasoduodenal tube. Symptoms were relieved in all patients, and five of them experienced complete response and no relapse. One week after FMT, the GM analysis of patients showed improved bacterial diversity and enrichment in health-promoting taxa, particularly *Bacteroides* and *Ruminococcaceae* [48].

Von Lier et al. reported 15 patients who received a single FMT via nasoduodenal infusion from an unrelated donor. A total of 10 patients showed complete remission within one month after FMT, without additional interventions to alleviate GvHD symptoms. In six of them, immunosuppressant drug therapy was successfully tapered within six months. In the other four individuals undergoing a complete response, GvHD symptoms returned upon the tapering of immunosuppressive therapy. The positive clinical response was accompanied by an increase in GM alpha diversity and partial engraftment of donor bacterial species. Moreover, increased relative abundance of short-chain fatty acid-producing bacteria, including Clostridiales members and particularly *Blautia*, was observed in the recipient's stool [49].

Two other cases of allo-HSCT patients receiving multiple FMT from unrelated healthy donors via a nasogastric tube were reported. One patient experienced complete remission of gastrointestinal symptoms, but died more than one month later due to liver aGvHD and bloodstream infections related to the indwelling catheter. The other had only a temporary reduction in symptoms; diarrhea recurred one week after the last FMT and the patient died from multiorgan failure [45].

Kaito et al. reported the first case in which FMT from a related donor was performed by the administration of oral capsules in a patient with refractory gut GvHD [46]. A subsequent case series enrolled seven patients who received one to three FMT from unrelated donors, administered orally by capsules. After FMT, the introduction of new bacteria and an increase in microbial diversity was found in the recipient's stool, with a strong reduction in the rate of bacterial dominance. Only two patients achieved complete remission, and one a partial response [50]. In the case report by Mao et al., after two cycles of oral FMT capsules from unrelated donor, intestinal aGvHD was gradually controlled and did not recur during the two-month follow-up. The diversity and structure of the GM after FMT were closer to those of healthy donors. Moreover, the amount of *Blautia* in the GM increased after FMT, which may explain the clinical improvement. Consistent with Kaito's report, repeated doses of FMT brought continuous improvement of the gastrointestinal aGvHD symptoms. In this case, the symptoms improved but recurred after the first course of capsule FMT, while the second dose was effective in achieving complete remission [33].

The first report of FMT for refractory aGvHD in children was provided by Zhong et al. in 2019.

FMT was performed twice via a nasojejunal tube from an unrelated donor, and resulted in symptom remission. Taxonomic analysis of GM showed gradual reduction in Proteobacteria and increase in Firmicutes after FMT, and the restoration of diversity [34].

3.4. FMT as a Preventive Strategy

FMT was used as a preventive strategy in allo-HSCT in seven studies. In five of them, the aim was to decolonize from ARB strains, while in the other two the aim was to prevent and reduce GM dysbiosis (Table 2).

J. Pers. Med. **2021**, *11*, 100

Table 2. Summary of included studies regarding FMT as a preventive strategy in allo-HSCT patients.

First Author	Year	Indication	Number of Patients	Route of Administration	Donor	Main Results
Bilinski	2017	ARB decolonization	20 with blood disorders (10 neutropenic, 4 aGvHD, 2 chronic GvHD)	Nasoduodenal tube	Unrelated	60% of patients achieved complete ARB decolonization at one month after FMT.
Innes	2017	ARB decolonization	1 before allo-HSCT	Nasogastric tube	Unrelated	By day +16 after FMT, no ARB was detected on rectal screening swabs.
Taur	2018	Dysbiosis reduction	25 (14 received FMT; 11 control group with no intervention)	Enema	Autologous	FMT patients had boosted microbial diversity and reestablishment of the intestinal microbiota composition they had before antibiotic treatment and allo-HSCT.
DeFililpp	2018	Dysbiosis reduction	13	Oral capsules	Unrelated	Improved intestinal microbiome diversity associated with expansion of stool-donor taxa.
Battipaglia	2019	ARB decolonization	10 (6 before and 4 after allo-HSCT)	Enema or nasogastric tube	Unrelated or Relative	Decolonization was achieved in 7 out of 10 patients.
Merli	2020	ARB decolonization	5 children before allo-HSCT	Esophagogastroduodenoscopy	Unrelated	Long-term decolonization was not achieved in four out of five patients.
Ghani	2020	ARB decolonization	11 with blood disorders (8 before allo-HSCT)	Nasogastric tube	Unrelated	Decolonization in 41% of patients. Reduction in bloodstream infections.

ARB: antibiotic-resistant bacteria; allo-HSCT: allogeneic hematopoietic stem cells transplantation; FMT: Fecal Microbiota Transplantation.

Bilinski at al. examined patients with blood disorders (40% neutropenic patients, 16% patients with aGvHD and 8% with chronic GvHD) colonized with ARB who underwent FMT via a nasoduodenal tube from unrelated donors; 60% of patients achieved complete decolonization one month after FMT [51]. Innes et al. described a case in which FMT was performed before HSCT to extensively eradicate drug-resistant organisms [35]. After these two encouraging reports, ten adult patients colonized by multidrug-resistant strains received FMT after ($n = 6$) or before ($n = 4$) HSCT from related or unrelated donors, delivered via enema or nasogastric tube. Three patients needed a second transplant from the same donor due to the initial failure of the procedure. Decolonization was achieved in seven out of ten patients. Interestingly, one case of grade III gut aGvHD still occurred after FMT performed before HSCT [36]. Ghani et al. delivered FMT from unrelated donors using a nasogastric tube in eleven patients with an underlying hematologic disorder, colonized by multidrug-resistant bacteria, of which eight underwent allo-HSCT after FMT. Although only 41% of patients were no longer colonized on rectal screening following FMT, there was a significant reduction in bloodstream infections by resistant and nonresistant strains compared to the control group. Moreover, shorter inpatient stays and fewer days of carbapenems administration were observed. Interestingly one patient developed bacteremia caused by a multidrug-resistant strain, but different from the previous colonizing microorganisms, and was treated effectively with a shorter antibiotic course [52].

Merli et al. carried out the only study with this aim in the pediatric population. They performed one course of FMT via esophagogastroduodenoscopy in five pediatric patients before allo-HSCT using samples from the same donor, to induce ARB decolonization. Eighty percent of patients tested negative for ARB strains within one week from FMT, but long-term decolonization was not achieved in four out of five patients [37].

Two other studies addressed FMT use to prevent and reduce dysbiosis. Autologous FMT after allo-HSCT was performed in a randomized controlled clinical trial. Compared with the control group, 16S rRNA gene sequencing of 14 patients after FMT revealed boosted microbial diversity and reestablishment of the GM composition they had before antibiotic treatment and allo-HSCT. In particular, important commensal groups, typically dominant in a healthy-like adult GM, such as *Lachnospiraceae*, *Ruminococcaceae* and Bacteroidetes members, were successfully re-established. According to a metagenomic analysis, auto-FMT also appeared to have reversed alterations in the functional content of the GM, mainly regarding genes involved in microbial virulence and metabolism [54]. In a subsequent analysis, they observed, during the first 100 days after engraftment, higher counts of neutrophils, lymphocytes and monocytes in the peripheral blood of auto-FMT recipients [12].

A similar result was obtained using FMT from unrelated donors, administered orally in 13 patients in the period immediately after neutrophil engraftment. FMT resulted in improved GM diversity associated with expansion of stool-donor taxa, including Clostridiales, and increased urinary levels of the tryptophan metabolite 3-indoxyl sulfate, recently proposed as a marker of GM eubiosis, associated with favorable outcome after allo-HSCT [55]. Notably, the subset of patients who received broad-spectrum antibiotics appeared to have attained the largest gains in terms of GM diversity. Two patients subsequently developed grade III–IV gut aGvHD, with one of them presenting concurrent bacteremia and subsequent multiorgan failure. There were no additional cases of bloodstream infections after FMT, but one case of CDI was observed [53].

3.5. Safety Issues in Allo-HSCT Recipients

The majority of the included studies report FMT as a generally well tolerated procedure, with no serious adverse events [32–37,39–52,54]. Interestingly, in the case series of Shouval et al. two patients developed bacteremia after the infusion, but targeted metagenomic sequencing demonstrated that the bacterial strains did not originate from the FMT inoculum [50]. DeFilipp et al. observed only one serious treatment-related adverse event (grade three abdominal pain) that resolved within 24 h of capsule administration [53]. Two studies specifically addressed the risks of FMT in allo-HSCT recipients. One patient enrolled in a trial to preemptively administer FMT oral capsules before allo-HSCT developed febrile neutropenia eight days after the last FMT dose, and died from severe sepsis two days later. The final results of blood cultures showed an extended-spectrum beta-lactamase-producing *E. coli* strain. The same strain was found in the lots of capsules from the donor, with a similar, but not identical, resistance pattern. Fecal samples of the recipient before FMT were negative for extended-spectrum beta-lactamase-producing microorganisms. Genomic relatedness between samples taken from the donor and blood cultures was calculated by means of whole-genome sequencing and single-nucleotide polymorphism-based analysis, and revealed that the bacterium was transmitted through FMT [30]. In another report, FMT was performed to decolonize from ARB before allo-HSCT. After ten days from allo-HSCT, Norovirus gastroenteritis was diagnosed, and it was later complicated by aGvHD. The symptoms resolved after a course of steroids and a second FMT from another donor with Norovirus-free stools. Fecal samples from the first FMT were analyzed and found to contain genotype II Norovirus, the same type identified in the patient's stool. The authors speculated that Norovirus-induced colitis damaged the intestinal mucosa and "exposed" host antigens. Combined with increased gut permeability to molecules of a dysbiotic GM and an inflammatory milieu, this led to sensitization of allo-reactive lymphocytes and triggered aGvHD [38].

4. Discussion

In this systematic review we summarized the present literature on the use of FMT in the allo-HSCT setting. The role of FMT in the treatment of rCDI is established [24], and can be considered effective also in patients undergoing allo-HSCT [56]. Numerous studies evaluated FMT as a treatment for steroid-resistant gut aGvHD, providing encouraging preliminary data regarding feasibility and efficacy that need to be confirmed in larger prospective studies. However, diagnosis of aGvHD was not documented by biopsies in all cases in five studies [34,45,47,48,50], and this may have led to the inclusion of patients with other causes of diarrhea. The necessity of histological confirmation should be carefully taken into account in designing future studies, considering the invasiveness of the procedure especially in pediatric patients.

Moreover, steroid-resistant aGvHD carries a dismal prognosis, and the role of FMT in holding down the allo-immune response and improving survival could be less effective in patients with an already deteriorated clinical status and deeply altered GM and gut mucosa [28]. For this reason, FMT has been proposed to prevent the unavoidable dysbiosis occurring after HSCT and potentially reduce the incidence of GM-related complications, such as aGvHD and infections [57,58]. However, designing a study with the aim of improving gut eubiosis is challenging because it is difficult to evaluate efficacy while there are still no clear clinical and GM-related endpoints to assess [14].

The results of FMT in decolonizing patients from ARB are also promising, but the rates of decolonization vary from 20% to 70%.

Proposed mechanisms by which FMT can mediate clinical benefits include direct competition of the commensal microbiota delivered by FMT with pathogens, restoration of secondary bile acid and short-chain fatty acid metabolism, repair of the gut barrier and modulation of the mucosal and systemic immune system. However, further studies are needed to fill the gap in the comprehension of the exact mechanisms underlying FMT action [25,59].

Another primary issue that should be addressed while discussing the results of FMT is the heterogeneity of key practical aspects that could influence clinical effectiveness, namely donor type, timing of infusion, delivery mode, stool screening, number of infusions and antibiotic policy (Figure 2). For example, to date no study exists in the literature comparing the results of related vs. unrelated donors of fecal material [60]. The use of frozen capsules from unrelated donors instead of siblings could reduce costs and waiting times, and consent a broader screening of fecal material, but they may be difficult to administer due to mucositis in the early phase after allo-HSCT [29,46]. Autologous FMT may also have the advantage of simple preparation and control during donor procedures, as well as reducing the risk of potentially transmitting pathogens from a third-party donor GM. However, a baseline healthy sample may not always be available. [11,54]. Repeated FMTs could increase the chance of durable modification of the gut ecosystem, thus improving the long-term achievement of clinical outcomes [37]. Antibiotics practice also influences the outcome of the procedure. Some studies discontinued them prior to the FMT procedure for a variable amount of time and routinely administered no specific pre-FMT antibiotic regimen, while others used oral colistin or vancomycin and neomycin before FMT to improve decolonization efficacy [35,37]. The use of antibiotics after FMT could also have a major impact. In the study by Val Lier et al., all the patients with secondary failure after a complete remission of gut aGvHD received antibiotics shortly after donor FMT, and the authors speculated that this may have interfered with a lasting response [49]. Bilinski et al. observed that patients who did not receive antibiotics within seven days after FMT achieved complete decolonization in a significantly higher proportion compared with those who did receive antibiotics [51].

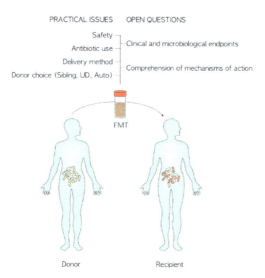

Figure 2. Practical issues and open questions to address in the design of future FMT intervention. UD: Unrelated Donor.

Considering the risk of life-threatening infections in immunocompromised patients, antimicrobial treatment is pivotal, and the decision to withhold antibiotic therapy for any period of time to allow successful engraftment of the transplanted GM should be approached with caution. The relationship between timing of antibiotic course and FMT outcomes must therefore be a focus of research in the near future.

Despite the strong scientific rationale and the emerging potential clinical utility of FMT in allo-HSCT patients, the risk of infections resulting from the delivery of living microbial consortia to an immunocompromised host with impaired gut permeability must be of utmost concern [29]. While most studies deem FMT as a safe procedure in allo-HSCT recipients, some reports raised the concern of potentially transmitting pathogens from the fecal donor to recipients. This must prompt better efforts in extending donor stool screenings to rule out all potentially transmittable pathogens. Furthermore, correlating adverse events to FMT in these patients affected by multiple comorbidities is sometimes a difficult task, and advanced microbial analysis may be necessary [30,50]. The few data on the use of FMT in pediatric populations could raise specific concerns regarding the possible transmission of disease-related GM configurations and the long-term effects of GM manipulation [61,62], such as the occurrence of weight gain [63], irritable bowel syndrome [64] or long-lasting colonization by ARB [30].

5. Conclusions and Future Directions

FMT is a promising and potentially useful strategy with different purposes in allo-HSCT recipients. The microbiome could therefore be considered as a target of new individualized therapies, potentially guiding therapeutical decisions in the near future based on the patient's GM signature. This fits into the medical model of personalized medicine, which stratifies people into different groups—with medical decisions, practices, and interventions being tailored to the individual patient based on the predicted response or risk of disease.

There is still much work to be done to understand if FMT can be implemented in clinical practice, both in terms of effectiveness and safety. Biological studies should provide novel insights into the comprehension of the mechanisms underlying the clinical findings. In particular, metagenomic and metabolomic analysis could help us to understand the effect of the administration of complex microbial consortia on the damaged gut ecosystem.

From a practical point of view, FMT should be performed in a selected center equipped with the required facilities to store, analyze and deliver the fecal material. A committed multidisciplinary team comprising hematologist, gastroenterologist, microbiologist, infectious disease physician and trained nurse is required to address the clinical complexity of the procedure.

Larger clinical trials are needed to definitively address the safety and effectiveness of this procedure for different purposes, and to define the main determinants of clinical response to FMT, such as the recipient's basal GM layout and donor GM composition, antibiotic practice and the immune status of the host [65,66].

Author Contributions: R.M., D.Z., E.M., D.L. and A.P. (Andrea Pession) conceptualized the study design. D.G. contributed to developing the review protocol. E.M. and D.L. performed the literature search and data collection. S.T., P.B., F.G., A.P. (Arcangelo Prete) and A.P. (Andrea Pession) contributed in data interpretation. E.M., D.Z., R.M. and D.L. wrote the first draft of the manuscript and produced the tables and figures. All authors contributed to reviewing and editing the final version. E.M. had responsibility for final submission of the article. All authors have read and agreed to the published version of the manuscript.

Funding: This study was supported by research funding from the Italian Ministero della Salute (Bando Ricerca Finalizzata 2013, Giovani Ricercatori section, code GR-2013-02357136) to R.M.

Institutional Review Board Statement: Not applicable.

Informed Consent Statement: Not applicable.

Conflicts of Interest: The authors declare no conflict of interest.

References

1. Jenq, R.R.; van den Brink, M.R.M. Allogeneic haematopoietic stem cell transplantation: Individualized stem cell and immune therapy of cancer. *Nat. Rev. Cancer* **2010**, *10*, 213–221. [CrossRef] [PubMed]
2. Copelan, E.A. Hematopoietic Stem-Cell Transplantation. *N. Engl. J. Med.* **2006**, *354*, 1813–1826. [CrossRef]
3. Dini, G.; Zecca, M.; Balduzzi, A.; Messina, C.; Masetti, R.; Fagioli, F.; Favre, C.; Rabusin, M.; Porta, F.; Biral, E.; et al. Associazione Italiana Ematologia ed Oncologia Pediatrica–Hematopoietic Stem Cell Transplantation (AIEOP-HSCT) Group. No difference in outcome between children and adolescents transplanted for acute lymphoblastic leukemia in second remission. *Blood* **2011**, *118*, 6683–6690. [CrossRef]
4. Henig, I.; Zuckerman, T. Hematopoietic Stem Cell Transplantation—50 Years of Evolution and Future Perspectives. *Rambam Maimonides Med. J.* **2014**, *5*, e0028. [CrossRef]
5. Carreras, E.; Dufour, C.; Mohty, M.; Kröger, N. *The EBMT Handbook: Hematopoietic Stem Cell Transplantation and Cellular Therapies*; Springer International Publishing AG: Cham, Switzerland, 2019.
6. Balletto, E.; Mikulska, M. Bacterial Infections in Hematopoietic Stem Cell Transplant Recipients. *Mediterr. J. Hematol. Infect. Dis.* **2015**, *7*, e2015045. [CrossRef]
7. D'Amico, F.; Soverini, M.; Zama, D.; Consolandi, C.; Severgnini, M.; Prete, A.; Pession, A.; Barone, M.; Turroni, S.; Biagi, E.; et al. Gut resistome plasticity in pediatric patients undergoing hematopoietic stem cell transplantation. *Sci. Rep.* **2019**, *9*, 1–7. [CrossRef] [PubMed]
8. Zeiser, R.; Blazar, B.R. Acute Graft-versus-Host Disease-Biologic Process, Prevention, and Therapy. *N. Engl. J. Med.* **2017**, *377*, 2167–2179. [CrossRef] [PubMed]
9. Ferrara, J.L.M.; Levine, J.E.; Reddy, P.; Holler, E. Graft-versus-host disease. *Lancet* **2009**, *373*, 1550–1561. [CrossRef]
10. Dignan, F.L.; Clark, A.; Amrolia, P.; Cornish, J.; Jackson, G.S.; Mahendra, P.; Scarisbrick, J.J.; Taylor, P.C.; Hadzic, N.; Shaw, B.E.; et al. Diagnosis and management of acute graft-versus-host disease. *Br. J. Haematol.* **2012**, *158*, 30–45. [CrossRef]
11. Andermann, T.M.; Peled, J.U.; Ho, C.; Reddy, P.; Riches, M.; Storb, R.; Teshima, T.; van den Brink, M.R.M.; Alousi, A.; Balderman, S.; et al. The Microbiome and Hematopoietic Cell Transplantation: Past, Present, and Future. *Biol. Blood Marrow Transpl.* **2018**, *24*, 1322–1340. [CrossRef] [PubMed]
12. Schluter, J.; Peled, J.; Taylor, B.P.; Markey, K.A.; Smith, J.A.; Taur, Y.; Niehus, R.; Staffas, A.; Dai, A.; Fontana, E.; et al. The gut microbiota is associated with immune cell dynamics in humans. *Nature* **2020**, *588*, 303–307. [CrossRef]
13. Masetti, R.; Zama, D.; Leardini, D.; Muratore, E.; Turroni, S.; Prete, A.; Brigidi, P.; Pession, A. The gut microbiome in pediatric patients undergoing allogeneic hematopoietic stem cell transplantation. *Pediatr. Blood Cancer* **2020**, *67*, e28711. [CrossRef] [PubMed]
14. Zama, D.; Bossù, G.; Leardini, D.; Muratore, E.; Biagi, E.; Prete, A.; Pession, A.; Masetti, R. Insights into the role of intestinal microbiota in hematopoietic stem-cell transplantation. *Ther. Adv. Hematol.* **2020**, *11*, 204062071989696. [CrossRef]

15. Peled, J.U.; Gomes, A.L.; Devlin, S.M.; Littmann, E.R.; Taur, Y.; Sung, A.D.; Weber, D.; Hashimoto, D.; Slingerland, A.E.; Slingerland, J.B.; et al. Microbiota as predictor of mortality in allogeneic hematopoietic-cell transplantation. *N. Engl. J. Med.* **2020**, *382*, 822–834. [CrossRef] [PubMed]
16. Jenq, R.R.; Taur, Y.; Devlin, S.M.; Ponce, D.M.; Goldberg, J.D.; Ahr, K.F.; Littmann, E.R.; Ling, L.; Gobourne, A.C.; Miller, L.C.; et al. Intestinal Blautia Is Associated with Reduced Death from Graft-versus-Host Disease. *Biol. Blood Marrow Transpl.* **2015**, *21*, 1373–1383. [CrossRef]
17. Zama, D.; Biagi, E.; Masetti, R.; Gasperini, P.; Prete, A.; Candela, M.; Brigidi, P.; Pession, A. Gut microbiota and hematopoietic stem cell transplantation: Where do we stand? *Bone Marrow Transpl.* **2017**, *52*, 7–14. [CrossRef]
18. Taur, Y.; Xavier, J.B.; Lipuma, L.; Ubeda, C.; Goldberg, J.; Gobourne, A.; Lee, Y.J.; Dubin, K.A.; Socci, N.D.; Viale, A.; et al. Intestinal domination and the risk of bacteremia in patients undergoing allogeneic hematopoietic stem cell transplantation. *Clin. Infect. Dis.* **2012**, *55*, 905–914. [CrossRef]
19. Bekker, V.; Zwittink, R.D.; Knetsch, C.W.; Sanders, I.M.; Berghuis, D.; Heidt, P.J.; Vossen, J.M.; De Vos, W.M.; Belzer, C.; Bredius, R.G.; et al. Dynamics of the Gut Microbiota in Children Receiving Selective or Total Gut Decontamination Treatment during Hematopoietic Stem Cell Transplantation. *Biol. Blood Marrow Transpl.* **2019**. [CrossRef]
20. D'Amico, F.; Biagi, E.; Rampelli, S.; Fiori, J.; Zama, D.; Soverini, M.; Barone, M.; Leardini, D.; Muratore, E.; Prete, A.; et al. Enteral Nutrition in Pediatric Patients Undergoing Hematopoietic SCT Promotes the Recovery of Gut Microbiome Homeostasis. *Nutrients* **2019**, *11*, 2958. [CrossRef]
21. Andersen, S.; Staudacher, H.; Weber, N.; Kennedy, G.; Varelias, A.; Banks, M.; Bauer, J. Pilot study investigating the effect of enteral and parenteral nutrition on the gastrointestinal microbiome post-allogeneic transplantation. *Br. J. Haematol.* **2019**, 2. [CrossRef] [PubMed]
22. Zama, D.; Muratore, E.; Biagi, E.; Forchielli, M.L.; Rondelli, R.; Candela, M.; Prete, A.; Pession, A.; Masetti, R. Enteral nutrition protects children undergoing allogeneic hematopoietic stem cell transplantation from blood stream infections. *Nutr. J.* **2020**, *19*, 29. [CrossRef]
23. Andermann, T.M.; Rezvani, A.; Bhatt, A.S. Microbiota Manipulation with Prebiotics and Probiotics in Patients Undergoing Stem Cell Transplantation. *Curr. Hematol. Malig. Rep.* **2016**, *11*, 19–28. [CrossRef] [PubMed]
24. Cammarota, G.; Ianiro, G.; Tilg, H.; Rajilić-Stojanović, M.; Kump, P.; Satokari, R.; Sokol, H.; Arkkila, P.; Pintus, C.; Hart, A.; et al. European consensus conference on faecal microbiota transplantation in clinical practice. *Gut* **2017**, *66*, 569–580. [CrossRef] [PubMed]
25. DeFilipp, Z.; Hohmann, E.; Jenq, R.R.; Chen, Y.-B. Fecal Microbiota Transplantation: Restoring the Injured Microbiome after Allogeneic Hematopoietic Cell Transplantation. *Biol. Blood Marrow Transpl.* **2019**, *25*, e17–e22. [CrossRef] [PubMed]
26. McDonald, L.C.; Gerding, D.N.; Johnson, S.; Bakken, J.S.; Carroll, K.C.; Coffin, S.E.; Dubberke, E.R.; Garey, K.W.; Gould, C.V.; Kelly, C.; et al. Clinical Practice Guidelines for Clostridium difficile Infection in Adults and Children: 2017 Update by the Infectious Diseases Society of America (IDSA) and Society for Healthcare Epidemiology of America (SHEA). *Clin. Infect. Dis.* **2018**, *66*, 987–994. [CrossRef] [PubMed]
27. Ianiro, G.; Bibbò, S.; Scaldaferri, F.; Gasbarrini, A.; Cammarota, G. Fecal microbiota transplantation in inflammatory bowel disease: Beyond the excitement. *Medicine* **2014**, *93*, 1–11. [CrossRef]
28. Shouval, R.; Geva, M.; Nagler, A.; Youngster, I. Fecal Microbiota Transplantation for Treatment of Acute Graft-versus-Host Disease. *Clin. Hematol. Int.* **2019**, *1*, 28. [CrossRef]
29. Wardill, H.R.; Secombe, K.R.; Bryant, R.V.; Hazenberg, M.D.; Costello, S.P. Adjunctive fecal microbiota transplantation in supportive oncology: Emerging indications and considerations in immunocompromised patients. *EBioMedicine* **2019**. [CrossRef]
30. DeFilipp, Z.; Bloom, P.P.; Soto, M.T.; Mansour, M.K.; Sater, M.R.; Huntley, M.H.; Turbett, S.; Chung, R.T.; Chen, Y.-B.; Hohmann, E.L. Drug-Resistant *E. coli* Bacteremia Transmitted by Fecal Microbiota Transplant. *N. Engl. J. Med.* **2019**, *381*, 2043–2050.
31. Moher, D.; Liberati, A.; Tetzlaff, J.; Altman, D.G.; PRISMA Group. Preferred reporting items for systematic reviews and meta-analyses: The PRISMA statement. *PLoS Med.* **2009**, *6*, e1000097. [CrossRef]
32. Zhang, J.; Ren, G.; Li, M.; Lu, P.; Yi, S. The Effects of Fecal Donors with Different Feeding Patterns on Diarrhea in a Patient Undergoing Hematopoietic Stem Cell Transplantation. *Case Rep. Hematol.* **2019**, *2019*, 1–11. [CrossRef]
33. Mao, D.; Jiang, Q.; Sun, Y.; Mao, Y.; Guo, L.; Zhang, Y.; Man, M.; Ouyang, G.; Sheng, L. Treatment of intestinal graft-versus-host disease with unrelated donor fecal microbiota transplantation capsules: A case report. *Medicine* **2020**, *99*, e22129. [CrossRef]
34. Zhong, S.; Zeng, J.; Deng, Z.; Jiang, L.; Zhang, B.; Yang, K.; Wang, W.; Zhang, T. Fecal microbiota transplantation for refractory diarrhea in immunocompromised diseases: A pediatric case report. *Ital. J. Pediatr.* **2019**, *45*, 116. [CrossRef]
35. Innes, A.J.; Mullish, B.H.; Fernando, F.; Adams, G.; Marchesi, J.R.; Apperley, J.F.; Brannigan, E.; Davies, F.; Pavlů, J. Faecal microbiota transplant: A novel biological approach to extensively drug-resistant organism-related non-relapse mortality. *Bone Marrow Transpl.* **2017**, *52*, 1452–1454. [CrossRef]
36. Battipaglia, G.; Malard, F.; Rubio, M.T.; Ruggeri, A.; Mamez, A.C.; Brissot, E.; Giannotti, F.; Dulery, R.; Joly, A.C.; Baylatry, M.T.; et al. Fecal microbiota transplantation before or after allogeneic hematopoietic transplantation in patients with hematological malignancies carrying multidrug-resistance bacteria. *Haematologica* **2019**, *104*, 1682–1688. [CrossRef] [PubMed]
37. Merli, P.; Putignani, L.; Ruggeri, A.; Del Chierico, F.; Gargiullo, L.; Galaverna, F.; Gaspari, S.; Pagliara, D.; Russo, A.; Pane, S.; et al. Decolonization of multi-drug resistant bacteria by fecal microbiota transplantation in five pediatric patients before allogeneic hematopoietic stem cell transplantation: Gut microbiota profiling, infectious and clinical outcomes. *Haematologica* **2020**. [CrossRef]

38. Bilinski, J.; Lis, K.; Tomaszewska, A.; Pechcinska, A.; Grzesiowski, P.; Dzieciatkowski, T.; Walesiak, A.; Gierej, B.; Ziarkiewicz-Wróblewska, B.; Tyszka, M.; et al. Eosinophilic gastroenteritis and graft-versus-host disease induced by transmission of Norovirus with fecal microbiota transplant. *Transpl. Infect. Dis.* **2020**. [CrossRef] [PubMed]

39. Neemann, K.; Eichele, D.D.D.; Smith, P.P.W.; Bociek, R.; Akhtari, M.; Freifeld, A. Fecal microbiota transplantation for fulminant Clostridium difficile infection in an allogeneic stem cell transplant patient. *Transpl. Infect. Dis.* **2012**, *14*, 161–165. [CrossRef] [PubMed]

40. De Castro, C.G.; Ganc, A.J.; Ganc, R.L.; Petrolli, M.S.; Hamerschlack, N. Fecal microbiota transplant after hematopoietic SCT: Report of a successful case. *Bone Marrow Transpl.* **2015**, *50*, 145. [CrossRef]

41. Webb, B.J.; Brunner, A.; Ford, C.D.; Gazdik, M.A.; Petersen, F.B.; Hoda, D. Fecal microbiota transplantation for recurrent Clostridium difficile infection in hematopoietic stem cell transplant recipients. *Transpl. Infect. Dis.* **2016**, *18*, 628–633. [CrossRef]

42. Bluestone, H.; Kronman, M.P.; Suskind, D.L. Fecal Microbiota Transplantation for Recurrent Clostridium difficile Infections in Pediatric Hematopoietic Stem Cell Transplant Recipients. *J. Pediatric. Infect. Dis. Soc.* **2018**, *7*, e6–e8. [CrossRef]

43. Moss, E.L.; Falconer, S.B.; Tkachenko, E.; Wang, M.; Systrom, H.; Mahabamunuge, J.; Relman, D.A.; Hohmann, E.L.; Bhatt, A.S. Long-term taxonomic and functional divergence from donor bacterial strains following fecal microbiota transplantation in immunocompromised patients. *PLoS ONE* **2017**, *12*, e0182585. [CrossRef]

44. Spindelboeck, W.; Schulz, E.; Uhl, B.; Kashofer, K.; Aigelsreiter, A.; Zinke-Cerwenka, W.; Mulabecirovic, A.; Kump, P.K.; Halwachs, B.; Gorkiewicz, G.; et al. Repeated fecal microbiota transplantations attenuate diarrhea and lead to sustained changes in the fecal microbiota in acute, refractory gastrointestinal graft- *versus* -host-disease. *Haematologica* **2017**, *102*, e210–e213. [CrossRef]

45. Biernat, M.M.; Urbaniak-Kujda, D.; Dybko, J.; Kapelko-Słowik, K.; Prajs, I.; Wróbel, T. Fecal microbiota transplantation in the treatment of intestinal steroid-resistant graft-versus-host disease: Two case reports and a review of the literature. *J. Int. Med. Res.* **2020**, *48*, 300060520925693. [CrossRef]

46. Kaito, S.; Toya, T.; Yoshifuji, K.; Kurosawa, S.; Inamoto, K.; Takeshita, K.; Suda, W.; Kakihana, K.; Honda, K.; Hattori, M.; et al. Fecal microbiota transplantation with frozen capsules for a patient with refractory acute gut graft-versus-host disease. *Blood Adv.* **2018**, *2*, 3097–3101. [CrossRef] [PubMed]

47. Kakihana, K.; Fujioka, Y.; Suda, W.; Najima, Y.; Kuwata, G.; Sasajima, S.; Mimura, I.; Morita, H.; Sugiyama, D.; Nishikawa, H.; et al. Fecal microbiota transplantation for patients with steroid-resistant acute graft-versus-host disease of the gut. *Blood* **2016**, *128*, 2083–2088. [CrossRef]

48. Qi, X.; Li, X.; Zhao, Y.; Wu, X.; Chen, F.; Ma, X.; Zhang, F.; Wu, D. Treating Steroid Refractory Intestinal Acute Graft-vs.-Host Disease with Fecal Microbiota Transplantation: A Pilot Study. *Front. Immunol.* **2018**, *9*, 2195. [CrossRef] [PubMed]

49. Van Lier, Y.F.; Davids, M.; Haverkate, N.J.E.; De Groot, P.F.; Donker, M.L.; Meijer, E.; Heubel-Moenen, F.C.J.I.; Nur, E.; Zeerleder, S.; Nieuwdorp, M.; et al. Donor fecal microbiota transplantation ameliorates intestinal graft-versus-host disease in allogeneic hematopoietic cell transplant recipients. *Sci. Transl. Med.* **2020**, *12*. [CrossRef] [PubMed]

50. Shouval, R.; Youngster, I.; Geva, M.; Eshel, A.; Danylesko, I.; Shimoni, A.; Beider, K.; Fein, J.A.; Sharon, I.; Koren, O.; et al. Repeated Courses of Orally Administered Fecal Microbiota Transplantation for the Treatment of Steroid Resistant and Steroid Dependent Intestinal Acute Graft Vs. Host Disease: A Pilot Study (NCT 03214289). *Blood* **2018**, *132*, 2121. [CrossRef]

51. Bilinski, J.; Grzesiowski, P.; Sorensen, N.; Mądry, K.; Muszynski, J.; Robak, K.; Wróblewska, M.; Dzieciątkowski, T.; Dulny, G.; Dwilewicz-Trojaczek, J.; et al. Fecal Microbiota Transplantation in Patients with Blood Disorders Inhibits Gut Colonization with Antibiotic-Resistant Bacteria: Results of a Prospective, Single-Center Study. *Clin. Infect. Dis.* **2017**, *65*, 364–370. [CrossRef] [PubMed]

52. Ghani, R.; Mullish, B.H.; McDonald, J.A.K.; Ghazy, A.; Williams, H.R.T.; Brannigan, E.T.; Mookerjee, S.; Satta, G.; Gilchrist, M.; Duncan, N.; et al. Disease Prevention Not Decolonization: A Model for Fecal Microbiota Transplantation in Patients Colonized With Multidrug-resistant Organisms. *Clin. Infect. Dis.* **2020**. [CrossRef] [PubMed]

53. DeFilipp, Z.; Peled, J.U.; Li, S.; Mahabamunuge, J.; Dagher, Z.; Slingerland, A.E.; Del Rio, C.; Valles, B.; Kempner, M.E.; Smith, M.; et al. Third-party fecal microbiota transplantation following allo-HCT reconstitutes microbiome diversity. *Blood Adv.* **2018**, *2*, 745–753. [CrossRef]

54. Taur, Y.; Coyte, K.; Schluter, J.; Robilotti, E.; Figueroa, C.; Gjonbalaj, M.; Littmann, E.R.; Ling, L.; Miller, L.; Gyaltshen, Y.; et al. Reconstitution of the gut microbiota of antibiotic-treated patients by autologous fecal microbiota transplant. *Sci. Transl. Med.* **2018**, *10*. [CrossRef]

55. Weber, D.; Oefner, P.J.; Hiergeist, A.; Koestler, J.; Gessner, A.; Weber, M.; Hahn, J.; Wolff, D.; Stämmler, F.; Spang, R.; et al. Low urinary indoxyl sulfate levels early after transplantation reflect a disrupted microbiome and are associated with poor outcome. *Blood* **2015**, *126*, 1723–1728. [CrossRef] [PubMed]

56. Diorio, C.; Robinson, P.D.; Ammann, R.A.; Castagnola, E.; Erickson, K.; Esbenshade, A.; Fisher, B.T.; Haeusler, G.M.; Kuczynski, S.; Lehrnbecher, T.; et al. Guideline for the management of clostridium difficile infection in children and adolescents with cancer and pediatric hematopoietic stem-cell transplantation recipients. *J. Clin. Oncol.* **2018**, *36*, 3162–3171. [CrossRef] [PubMed]

57. Khoruts, A.; Sadowsky, M.J. Understanding the mechanisms of faecal microbiota transplantation. *Nat. Rev. Gastroenterol. Hepatol.* **2016**, *13*, 508–516. [CrossRef]

58. Biagi, E.; Zama, D.; Nastasi, C.; Consolandi, C.; Fiori, J.; Rampelli, S.; Turroni, S.; Centanni, M.; Severgnini, M.; Peano, C.; et al. Gut microbiota trajectory in pediatric patients undergoing hematopoietic SCT. *Bone Marrow Transpl.* **2015**, *50*, 992–998. [CrossRef]

59. Biagi, E.; Zama, D.; Rampelli, S.; Turroni, S.; Brigidi, P.; Consolandi, C.; Severgnini, M.; Picotti, E.; Gasperini, P.; Merli, P.; et al. Early gut microbiota signature of aGvHD in children given allogeneic hematopoietic cell transplantation for hematological disorders. *BMC Med. Genom.* **2019**, *12*, 49. [CrossRef]
60. Ramai, D.; Zakhia, K.; Ofosu, A.; Ofori, E.; Reddy, M. Fecal microbiota transplantation: Donor relation, fresh or frozen, delivery methods, cost-effectiveness. *Ann. Gastroenterol.* **2019**, *32*, 30–38. [CrossRef]
61. Vindigni, S.M.; Surawicz, C.M. Fecal Microbiota Transplantation. *Gastroenterol. Clin. N. Am.* **2017**, *46*, 171–185. [CrossRef]
62. Cohen, N.A.; Maharshak, N. Novel Indications for Fecal Microbial Transplantation: Update and Review of the Literature. *Dig. Dis. Sci.* **2017**, *62*, 1131–1145. [CrossRef] [PubMed]
63. Alang, N.; Kelly, C.R. Weight gain after fecal microbiota transplantation. *Open Forum Infect. Dis.* **2015**, *2*. [CrossRef]
64. Chang, B.W.; Rezaie, A. Irritable Bowel Syndrome-Like Symptoms Following Fecal Microbiota Transplantation: A Possible Donor-Dependent Complication. *Am. J. Gastroenterol.* **2017**, *112*, 186–187. [CrossRef] [PubMed]
65. Woloszynek, S.; Pastor, S.; Mell, J.C.; Nandi, N.; Sokhansanj, B.; Rosen, G.L. Engineering Human Microbiota: Influencing Cellular and Community Dynamics for Therapeutic Applications. In *International Review of Cell and Molecular Biology*; Elsevier: Amsterdam, The Netherlands, 2016; pp. 67–124.
66. Kazemian, N.; Ramezankhani, M.; Sehgal, A.; Khalid, F.M.; Kalkhoran, A.H.Z.; Narayan, A.; Wong, G.K.-S.; Kao, D.; Pakpour, S. The trans-kingdom battle between donor and recipient gut microbiome influences fecal microbiota transplantation outcome. *Sci. Rep.* **2020**, *10*, 18349. [CrossRef] [PubMed]

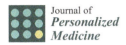

Article

Altered Gut Microbiota in Irritable Bowel Syndrome and Its Association with Food Components

Zahra A. Barandouzi [1,2], Joochul Lee [3], Kendra Maas [4], Angela R. Starkweather [2] and Xiaomei S. Cong [2,5,*]

[1] School of Nursing, Emory University, Atlanta, GA 30322, USA; zahra.barandouzi@emory.edu
[2] School of Nursing, University of Connecticut, Storrs, CT 06269, USA; angela.starkweather@uconn.edu
[3] Department of Statistics, University of Connecticut, Storrs, CT 06269, USA; joochul.lee@uconn.edu
[4] Microbial Analysis, Resources, and Services (MARS), University of Connecticut, Storrs, CT 06269, USA; kendra.maas@uconn.edu
[5] Department of Pediatrics, School of Medicine, University of Connecticut, Farmington, CT 06106, USA
* Correspondence: xiaomei.cong@uconn.edu; Tel.: +1-860-486-2694

Abstract: The interplay between diet and gut microbiota has gained interest as a potential contributor in pathophysiology of irritable bowel syndrome (IBS). The purpose of this study was to compare food components and gut microbiota patterns between IBS patients and healthy controls (HC) as well as to explore the associations of food components and microbiota profiles. A cross-sectional study was conducted with 80 young adults with IBS and 21 HC recruited. The food frequency questionnaire was used to measure food components. Fecal samples were collected and profiled by 16S rRNA Illumina sequencing. Food components were similar in both IBS and HC groups, except in caffeine consumption. Higher alpha diversity indices and altered gut microbiota were observed in IBS compared to the HC. A negative correlation existed between total observed species and caffeine intake in the HC, and a positive correlation between alpha diversity indices and dietary fiber in the IBS group. Higher alpha diversity and gut microbiota alteration were found in IBS people who consumed caffeine more than 400 mg/d. Moreover, high microbial diversity and alteration of gut microbiota composition in IBS people with high caffeine consumption may be a clue toward the effects of caffeine on the gut microbiome pattern, which warrants further study.

Keywords: irritable bowel syndrome; microbiota; microbiome; food components; nutrients

Citation: Barandouzi, Z.A.; Lee, J.; Maas, K.; Starkweather, A.R.; Cong, X.S. Altered Gut Microbiota in Irritable Bowel Syndrome and Its Association with Food Components. *J. Pers. Med.* **2021**, *11*, 35. https://doi.org/10.3390/jpm11010035

Received: 5 November 2020
Accepted: 4 January 2021
Published: 8 January 2021

Publisher's Note: MDPI stays neutral with regard to jurisdictional claims in published maps and institutional affiliations.

Copyright: © 2021 by the authors. Licensee MDPI, Basel, Switzerland. This article is an open access article distributed under the terms and conditions of the Creative Commons Attribution (CC BY) license (https://creativecommons.org/licenses/by/4.0/).

1. Introduction

Irritable bowel syndrome (IBS) is a chronic functional gastrointestinal disorder with an estimated prevalence of 10% around the globe [1]. This common functional disorder has significant impacts on patients' quality of life as well as increases enormous economic burdens of on healthcare systems [1,2]. IBS patients suffer from various ranges of symptoms, including abdominal pain/discomfort, abdominal bloating, and alteration in the bowel habits [3]. While the pathophysiology of IBS is not well understood, the interplay between diet and the gut microbiota has gained interest in recent years [4].

Diet is one of the known triggers and/or exacerbators of IBS symptoms [5]. Up to 70% of IBS patients associate their symptoms to specific foods such as dairy products, caffeine, raw vegetables, beans, peas, hot spices, fried foods, alcohol, fatty foods, as well as wheat products [3,6,7]. Although individuals may have selective food choices, dietary patterns, intake of calories, proteins, carbohydrates, and fats by patients with IBS is comparable to community controls [6].

The microbial composition in patients with IBS has been reported to be different from healthy individuals, despite the fact that their dietary patterns were found similar [6]. Studies show lower microbial diversity as well as a decrease in abundance of *Ruminococcaceae*, *Bifidobacterium*, *Faecalibacterium*, and *Erysipelotrichaceae* in IBS patients compared to healthy individuals. In addition, a higher abundance of *Lactobacillus* and *Ruminococcus* was reported in IBS patients [8,9]. Although evidence supports that IBS patients have altered gut microbiota profiles, it is still largely unknown about the microbial signature that can characterize these patients and their symptoms [6].

Diet as an important environmental factor has a strong impact on the gut microbiota enterotypes [5,6]. Diet enriched in protein and animal fat is associated with the *Bacteroides* enterotype, whereas a diet enriched in carbohydrate is related to the *Prevotella* enterotype [10]. Research also shows that the gut microbiota that belongs to the Firmicutes and Bacteriodetes phyla have an imperative role in the metabolism of carbohydrates and proteins by producing health-beneficial short-chain fatty acid (SCFAs) [11,12]. SCFAs are essential to fuel the intestinal epithelial cells and strengthen the gut barrier function [12]. In recent years, the interplay between diet and microbiota has emerged as an important pathological basis for IBS, which requires further investigation [4,13,14]. Moreover, the role of caffeine consumption on microbiome composition has been evaluated in different diseases, but limited studies have assessed the impact of caffeine in the IBS population [15,16]. Thus, in the present study, we aimed to assess the differences in nutrient intake and gut microbiota patterns between IBS and healthy control (HC) groups; meanwhile, we explored the associations between gut microbial community and food components in both IBS and HC groups.

2. Materials and Methods

2.1. Setting and Subjects

The present study was an extension of a randomized clinical trial titled "Precision Pain Self-Management in Young Adults with IBS" (P20 NR016605-01) [17]. In this trial, 80 people with IBS diagnosed by a gastroenterologist were enrolled in a longitudinal study. We used the data from the baseline session of this clinical trial and also recruited 21 healthy participants in the study. A convenience sampling method was used in the parent randomized controlled trial (RCT) and recruitment of healthy controls. A retrospective post hoc power analysis was conducted using the G-power program to examine if the sample size reached enough power to detect the effect IBS group on the alpha diversity compared to HC group. The powers of 0.86 for the total observed species (sobs) and 0.91 for Shannon index were obtained when assuming Laplace distribution of the parent response variables.

The inclusion criteria for the enrollment of IBS people were: (1) Men and women 18–29 years of age, (2) with a diagnosis of IBS from a healthcare provider using the Rome III or IV criteria, and (3) able to read and speak in English. The exclusion criteria were: (1) Having other chronic painful conditions including but not limited to fibromyalgia, chronic pelvic pain or chronic intestinal cystitis, infectious diseases (hepatitis, HIV, MRSA), celiac disease or inflammatory bowel disease, and diabetes mellitus, (2) serious mental health conditions (e.g., bipolar disorder, schizophrenia, mania), (3) women who were pregnant or post-partum 3 months, or (4) regular use of opioids, iron supplements, prebiotics/probiotics or antibiotics, and/or substance abuse. The criteria for recruitment of HC were the same as those for the IBS group, except that HC group did not have a history of IBS. The study was approved by the Institutional Review Board of the University of Connecticut. The information of the research study was explained to the participants, and all the participants provided written informed consent.

2.2. Data Collection

Both IBS and HC groups completed demographic and food frequency questionnaires via a Research Electronic Data Capture (REDCap) software/system. After receiving explicit instructions from a research team member, the participants were requested to collect their fecal samples using the OMNIgene GUT tubes (DNA Genotek Inc., Ottawa, ON, Canada) and delivered the sample to the lab via a drop-box. The fecal samples were aliquoted into bead tubes and were stored in a $-80\ ^{\circ}\text{C}$ freezer until further analysis.

2.3. Outcome Meaures

2.3.1. Assessment of Daily Food Components

The food frequency questionnaire (FFQ) [18] was used to assess the participants' dietary patterns. The questionnaire contained questions indicating the frequency of various types of foods, e.g., bread and savory biscuits, cereals, potatoes, rice and pasta, meat and fish, dairy products and fats, sweets and snacks, drinks, soups, sauces and spreads, fruits, and vegetables. The FFQ data was processed using Diet*Calc software developed by the National Institutes of Health National Cancer Institute [19] to obtain data of nutrient and food group intake. The estimation of daily food components based on 24-h dietary recall were calculated according to the portion size for participants' food energy (kcal), protein (g), total fat (g), cholesterol (mg), carbohydrate (g), dietary fiber (g), alcohol (g), and caffeine (mg).

2.3.2. Fecal Sample DNA Extraction and Microbiome Sequencing

The fecal sample processing, sequencing, and analysis were conducted at the University Center of Microbial Analysis, Resources, and Services using the protocols developed and tested by our team [20,21]. The bacterial DNA were extracted from 0.25 g of the fecal sample using the MoBio Power Soil or PowerMag Soil DNA isolation kit (MoBio Laboratories, Inc, Carlsbad, CA, USA) in accordance with the manufacturer's instruction for the Eppendorf epMotion 5076 Vac liquid handling robot or manually. Then, the V4 region of the 16S rRNA gene of the microbial community was sequenced using the Illumina platform. For the microbiome analysis, we used the Mothur software. Alpha diversity, including sobs, Simpson, and Shannon indices were used to evaluate the complexity of the whole microbial community. Beta diversity represented by Bray–Curtis dissimilarity was used to indicate the inter-subjects' variation in the bacterial composition. Multidimensional scaling (MDS) based on Bray–Curtis dissimilarity was used to identify the microbial clustering patterns and assess the relationships with food component intakes.

2.4. Statistical Analysis

The demographic characteristics of the participants were presented with frequency and percentage for categorical variables, and mean, standard deviation, and range for continuous variables. A chi-square test and Fisher's exact test were conducted to check the association between the demographic characteristics and the groups, and the Wilcoxon rank-sum test was conducted to investigate differences of age, number of household members, and daily food component intakes between the IBS and HC groups using R 3.6.0. For analysis of microbiota composition, we dropped operational taxonomic unit (OTUs) in which a ratio of zero counts was identified in more than 90% of the samples, and performed the linear discriminant analysis effect size (LEfSe) method provided at https://huttenhower.sph.harvard.edu/galaxy. An alpha level for the Kruskal–Wallis test and a threshold for the effect size were 0.05 and 2, respectively. To compare the alpha diversity between the IBS and HC groups, a Wilcoxon rank-sum test was used and the propensity score weighting method was further used to control confounding variables in weighed regression models. The Kruskal–Wallis test was utilized to identify differences in alpha diversity among groups and Spearman's rho correlation to examine the association between the alpha diversity and daily caffeine and dietary fiber intake. Lastly, based on Bray–Curtis dissimilarity, non-metric multidimensional scaling (NMDS) ordination for beta diversity was performed, and we fitted environmental variables related to food components onto the ordination to investigate the association between the beta diversity and food components using the 'vegan' package in R.

3. Results

3.1. Demographic Characteristics of the IBS and HC Groups

In total, 80 individuals with IBS and 21 HC were included in the study. There were no significant differences of age, gender, race, ethnicity, education, caregiver type, employment status, marital status, and number of household members between the IBS and healthy control groups (Table 1).

Table 1. Demographic characteristics of the participants.

Demographics	N	HC (*n* = 21)	IBS (*n* = 80)	*p*-Value
Gender				
Female	72	11 (52.38%)	61 (76.25%)	0.060
Male	29	10 (47.619%)	19 (23.75%)	
Race				
White	71	9 (42.86%)	62 (77.50%)	0.070
Asian	16	6 (28.57%)	10 (12.50%)	
African–American	12	4 (19.05%)	8 (10.00%)	
Not reported	2	2 (9.52%)	0 (0.00%)	
Ethnicity				
Non-Hispanic	84	16 (76.19%)	68 (85.00%)	0.360
Hispanic	11	4 (19.05%)	7 (8.75%)	
Not reported	6	1 (4.76%)	5 (6.25%)	
Education				
High school or lower	8	2 (9.52%)	6 (7.50%)	0.151
Some college	63	16 (76.19%)	47 (58.75%)	
Associate degree	3	1 (4.76%)	1 (1.25%)	
Bachelor degree	16	2 (9.52%)	14 (17.50%)	
Master degree	12	0 (0.00%)	12 (15.00%)	
Primary caregiver				
Parent/legal guardian	53	14 (66.67%)	39 (48.75%)	0.117
Self	46	6 (28.57%)	40 (50.00%)	
Other	2	1 (4.76%)	1 (1.25%)	
Employment status				0.269
Student	75	18 (85.71%)	57 (71.25%)	
Working now	22	2 (9.52%)	20 (25.00%)	
Unemployed	4	1 (4.76%)	3 (3.75%)	
Marital status				
Never married	98	21 (100.00%)	77 (96.25%)	1
Married	3	0 (0.00%)	3 (3.75%)	
IBS subtype				
IBS-C	9	N/A	9 (11.00%)	
IBS-D	5	N/A	5 (7.00%)	
IBS-M	66	N/A	66 (82.00%)	
Medical care setting type				
Primary	15	N/A	15 (19.00%)	
Secondary	6	N/A	6 (7.00%)	
Primary + secondary	22	N/A	22 (28.00%)	
None	37	N/A	37 (46.00%)	

	Mean (SD)		Range		
	HC	IBS	IBS	HC	*p*-value
Age (years)	20.14 (1.39)	20.39 (2.57)	18–23	18–28	0.071
Household members	4.19 (1.81)	3.29 (1.48)	1–9	1–7	0.034
Duration of IBS (years)	N/A	4.01 (2.67)	1–13	N/A	N/A

IBS-C, IBS constipation, IBS-D, IBS diarrhea, IBS-M, IBS-mixed (constipation + diarrhea), N/A, Not applicable.

3.2. Food Componnets in the IBS and HC Groups

Daily food component intakes were calculated for food energy, protein, fat, cholesterol, carbohydrate, dietary fiber, alcohol, and caffeine. There was no significant difference in daily intakes of various food components between the IBS and HC groups except in caffeine consumption (*p* = 0.024) (Figure 1). The IBS group had higher daily caffeine intake with an average of 246.42 mg/d. The details of daily food components intakes in both groups is shown in Table 2.

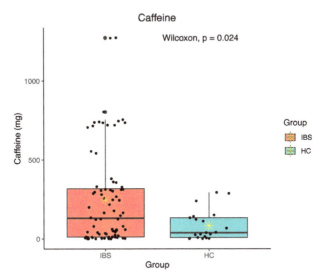

Figure 1. Difference in daily caffeine intake between irritable bowel syndrome (IBS) and healthy control (HC) groups; ✶ indicates mean.

Table 2. Daily food component intakes.

	Mean (SD)		Median (Range)	
	HC	IBS	HC	IBS
Food energy (kcal)	1965.82 (791.06)	1793.41 (761.95)	1837.46 (705.94–3768.59)	1692.51 (320.12–4223.59)
Protein (g)	83.31 (37.13)	73.29 (39.40)	83.05 (21.84–147.22)	60.48 (10.61–216.97)
Fat (g)	87.80 (41.55)	77.46 (36.56)	96.45 (21.81–182.24)	73.40 (9.90–176.68)
Cholesterol (mg)	278.76 (84.29)	228.06 (123.41)	291.71 (52.14–507.28)	205.45 (9.02–543.25)
Carbohydrate (g)	211.73 (84.29)	201.33 (84.90)	194.76 (86.60–398.42)	186.39 (27.94–453.60)
Dietary fiber (g)	19.79 (9.06)	18.44 (10.03)	16.97 (5.55–39.52)	17.31 (3.54–66.61)
Alcohol (g)	4.99 (4.56)	5.56 (5.19)	4.06 (0.01–15.60)	4.30 (0.00–19.16)
Caffeine (mg) *	82.93 (94.67)	246.42 (297.42)	38.24 (0.55–293.77)	129.92 (0.06–1273.84)

* Significant difference in median of caffeine intake ($p < 0.05$).

3.3. Fecal Microbiota Pattern in the IBS and HC Groups

3.3.1. Total Number of OTUs

A total of 483,740 OTUs were identified and analyzed in the study. Respectively, 381,900 OTUs belonged to the IBS group and 101,840 OTUs belonged to the HC group.

3.3.2. Fecal Microbiota Composition in the IBS Compared to the HC

The linear discriminant analysis effect size (LEfSe) was utilized to identify the key phylotype responsible for the differences between the IBS and HC groups (Figures 2 and 3). At the phylum level, the IBS group exhibited significantly higher abundance of *Verrucomicrobia* phylum compared to the HC group. At the class level, *Verrucomicrobia, Coriobacteriia, Bacilli,* and *Erysipelotrichia* were more abundant in the IBS group than the HC group. At the order level, we observed higher abundance of *Verrucomicrobiales, Coriobacteriales, Lactobacillales,* and *Erysipelotrichales* in the IBS group compared to the HC group. At the family level, there was higher abundance of *Coriobacteriaceae, Porphyromonadaceae, Verrucomicrobiaceae, Lachnospiraceae,* and *Erysipelotrichaceae* in the IBS group, while a higher abundance of *Prevotellaceae* was observed in the HC group. Among various genera, *Parabacteroides, Blautia, Lachnospiraceae*-unclassified 1, *Lachnospiraceae*-unclassified 2, *Veillonella, Oscillibacter, Flavonifractor, Ruminococcaceae*-unclassified, *Odoribacter, Erysipelotrichaceae*-unclassified, and *Akkermansia* were relatively more abundant in the IBS group compared to the HC. However, the abundance of *Prevotella* was more abundant in the HC group compared to the IBS group (Figures 2 and 3).

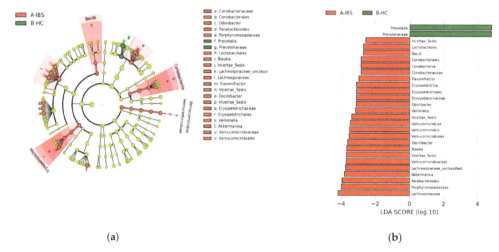

(a)　　　　　　　　　　　　　　　　(b)

Figure 2. Taxonomic differences of fecal microbiota between IBS and HC groups. (**a**) Taxonomic cladogram based on the linear discriminant analysis effect size (LEfSe) analysis. (**b**) IBS-enriched taxa are indicated with a negative linear discriminant analysis (LDA) score (red) and taxa enriched in HC have a positive score (green).

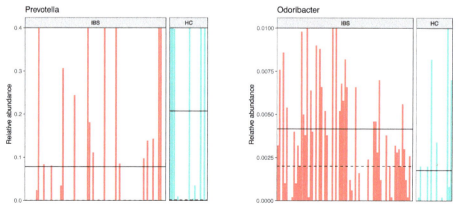

Figure 3. *Cont.*

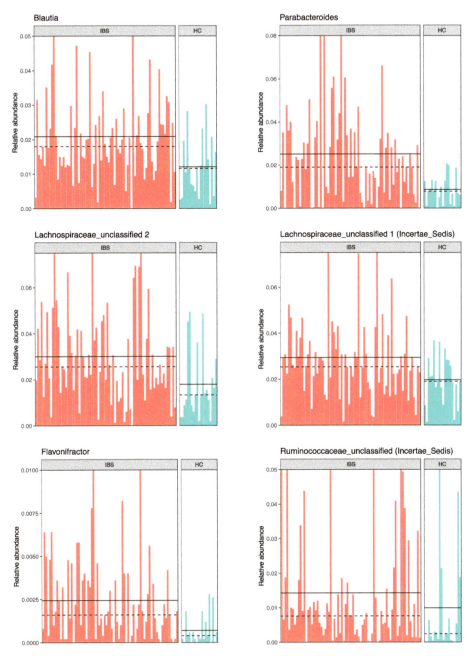

Figure 3. *Cont.*

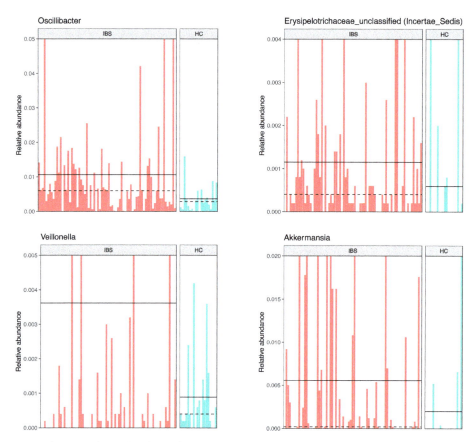

Figure 3. Relative abundance of bacterial genera in each subject of the IBS and HC groups.

3.3.3. Fecal Microbiota Diversity in the IBS Compared to the HC Group

Among various alpha diversity indices, total observed species (sobs) and the Shannon index were significantly higher in the IBS group compared to the HC group (Figures 4 and 5). However, beta-diversity using the Bray–Curtis index was not structurally different between the two groups. In order to reduce the confounding effects of demographics and food intakes on gut microbiome between the IBS and HC groups, we further applied propensity score weighting methods to give weights to all subjects and run a weighted regression model. The results consistently showed significant difference in alpha diversity indices (sobs: β = 0.188, t = 2.374, p = 0.020; Shannon: β = 1.918, t = 2.539, p = 0.013).

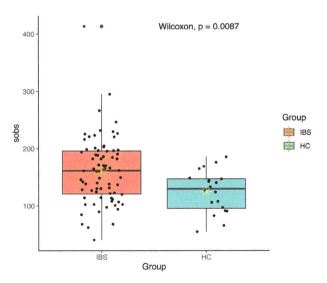

Figure 4. Total observed species (sobs) diversity between IBS and HC groups; ✱ indicates mean.

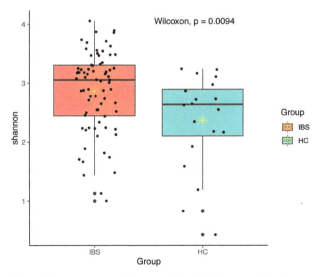

Figure 5. Shannon diversity between IBS and HC groups; ✱ indicates mean.

3.4. Associations between Fecal Microbiota Diversity and Food Component Intakes

Among different nutrient intakes, we observed a significant correlation between caffeine intake and sobs in the HC group (Figure 6). Moreover, the dietary fiber intake was significantly associated with alpha diversity indices including sobs and the Shannon index in the IBS group (Figure 7).

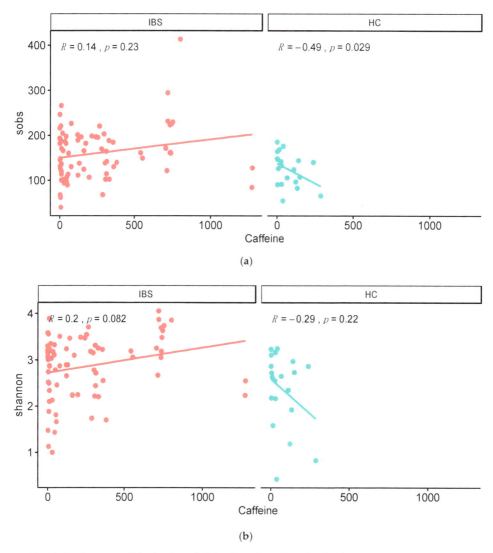

Figure 6. Correlation between caffeine intake and alpha diversity in the IBS and HC groups. (**a**) Correlation between total observed species (sobs) and caffeine intake. (**b**) Correlation between Shannon index and caffeine intake.

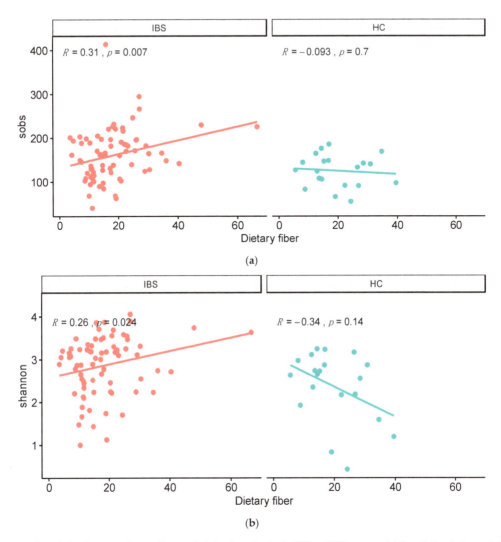

Figure 7. Correlation between dietary fiber and alpha diversity in the IBS and HC groups. (**a**) Correlation between total observed species (sobs) and dietary fiber intake. (**b**) Correlation between Shannon index and dietary fiber intake.

3.5. Fecal Microbiota Patterns Associated with the Daily Caffeine Intake

Due to the high daily consumption of caffeine in the IBS group, we further explored the impact of caffeine intake on the fecal microbiota composition and diversity. Thus, we divided the IBS group into two subgroups including High-IBS and Low-IBS. High-IBS refers to IBS people who consumed caffeine more than 400 mg/day and Low-IBS indicating IBS subjects with less than 400 mg/day caffeine consumption. This caffeine consumption cut-off was based on the US Food and Drug Administration (FDA) recommendation [22,23].

Various genera were more abundant in the High-IBS group compared to the Low-IBS and also the HC groups. Among different genera, *Parabacteroides*, *Lachnospiraceae*-unclassified, *Ruminococcaceae*-unclassified, and *Oscillibacter* had high relative abundance in IBS people with high consumption of caffeine (Figures 8 and 9).

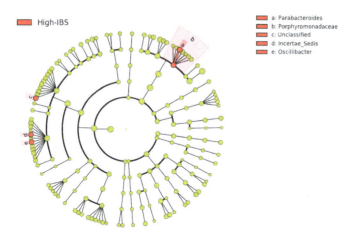

Figure 8. Taxonomic cladogram based on the LEfSe analysis. Red: Taxa enriched in High-IBS; High-IBS: Caffeine consumption more than 400 mg/day.

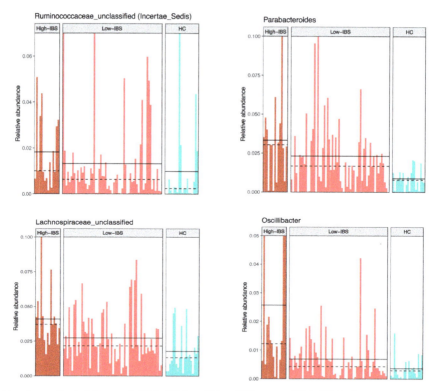

Figure 9. Abundance of bacterial genera in High-IBS, Low-IBS, and HC groups. High-IBS: Caffeine consumption more than 400 mg/day; Low-IBS: Caffeine consumption less than 400 mg/day.

The High-IBS group also had a higher alpha diversity profile compared to the Low-IBS and HC groups using the sobs and Shannon indices. Interestingly, the bacterial diversity was higher in the Low-IBS group compared to the HC (Figures 10 and 11).

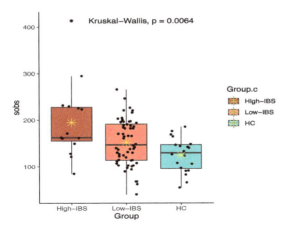

Figure 10. Total observed species (sobs) diversity among High-IBS, Low-IBS and HC groups. High-IBS: Caffeine consumption more than 400 mg/day; Low-IBS: Caffeine consumption less than 400 mg/day; ✳ indicates mean.

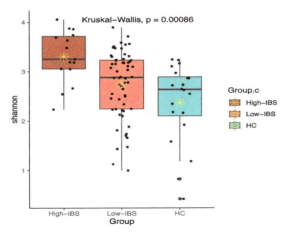

Figure 11. Shannon diversity among High-IBS, Low-IBS and HC groups. High-IBS: Caffeine consumption more than 400 mg/day; Low-IBS: Caffeine consumption less than 400 mg/day; ✳ indicates mean.

3.6. Associations between Fecal Microbiota Diversity and Food Component Intakes in the High-IBS, Low-IBS, and HC Groups

In terms of the association between bacterial diversity and food component intakes, we observed a negative correlation between sobs and caffeine intake within the HC group. However, there was no significant correlation between alpha diversity (sobs and Shannon index) and caffeine intake in both High-IBS and Low-IBS groups (Supplementary Materials Figure S1). Similarly, we did not identify any correlation between alpha diversity and dietary fiber intake in all three groups (Figure S2). No significant associations were identified among beta diversity and various food components including caffeine and dietary fiber intakes among High-IBS, Low-IBS, and HC groups (Figure S3).

4. Discussion

The results of the present study revealed that among various food components, caffeine intake was significantly different between IBS participants and the healthy controls in young adults. Moreover, the microbiome diversity and composition of IBS people were distinct from healthy controls. Correlation analysis of diet and microbiome showed a significant association between caffeine intakes with alpha diversity. Moreover, microbiome diversity was higher in the IBS group who consumed caffeine more than 400 mg/day compared to the IBS low caffeine consumption and HC groups.

4.1. Differences in Food Components between IBS and HC

The pathophysiology of IBS from the nutritional aspect is multifaceted and unsettled. IBS is a term to describe various presentations of a dysfunction and no single process can be determined as its pathophysiology [24]. There is no evidence to propose that people who developed IBS in the past had a significantly distinctive diet from healthy people [24]. This study supports evidence from previous research which shows that the intake of main food components such as carbohydrate, calories, proteins, and fats in people who currently suffer from IBS is similar to healthy adults [25,26]. While people with IBS traits may report certain food items associated with their symptoms, the overall food intake pattern is comparable to a healthy community [6].

The results of the present study showed higher daily consumption of caffeine in IBS people compared to healthy controls. In contrast to our findings, one study reported similar caffeine intake with a mean of 1.7 servings/day in people with IBS and healthy controls [27]. Caffeine's role as a trigger of IBS symptoms is unknown, but reducing its intake is recommended to improve reflux symptoms in people with IBS [6]. In addition, research shows that caffeine influences gut motility in healthy people. However, its role in people with IBS is not clear, which requires further investigations [27,28].

Current IBS dietary guidelines mainly focus on increasing dietary fiber and reduction of fat, caffeine, and alcohol intakes [29,30]. The theory behind the dietary restriction is that caffeine, high-fat food content, and alcohol may play roles in triggering IBS symptoms, and dietary fiber can help to reduce symptoms [13]. While the association between dietary restriction and IBS symptoms has been reported in studies, data regarding the manipulation of a dietary plan in IBS people are still inconsistent [30,31].

4.2. Differences in the Gut Microbiota between IBS and HC

The microbiota is an extremely diverse and metabolically active community that can play an imperative role in health and disease [32]. The host–microbiota interactions as a mutualistic ecosystem is beneficial for both host and microbiota [32,33]. A growing body of evidence is proposing gut microbiota dysbiosis as potential pathogenesis of IBS [1].

Two major phyla, *Firmicutes* and *Bacteroidetes*, constitute around 90% of the known bacteria in the gastrointestinal (GI) tract [34]. While we did not see any difference in the abundance of these phyla between IBS people and healthy controls, other studies reported contradictory results. One study found a higher abundance of *Bacteroidetes* and a lower abundance of *Firmicutes* in IBS people [35]. However, other studies reported lower abundance of *Bacteroidetes* in people with IBS [11,36]. Among other phyla, we observed a high abundance of *Verrucomicrobia*. Other studies also reported an elevated abundance of *Proteobacteria* and *Actinobacteria* in IBS people [36,37]. The variation in abundance of different phyla in IBS may be a clue toward alteration of gut microbiota that influences IBS symptoms.

Research suggests that healthy people harbor three types of enterotypes, including *Bacteroides*, *Prevotella*, and *Ruminococcus* [38]. Consistently, our results showed a higher abundance of *Prevotella* in healthy people. However, one study reported high abundance of *Ruminococcus* in people with IBS [11]. Among other genera, we observed higher abundance of *Blautia* in IBS people. Similarly, another study found a higher abundance of this genus in people with IBS [11]. Previous studies revealed *Blautia* and its belonged family, *Lachnospiraceae*, as a potential marker of imbalance in the gut, are associated with numerous diseases [39–42]. Reports of various genera in different studies suggest a large inter-individual variability in microbiota composition, which requires further studies [34].

Multiple reports have linked IBS pathogenesis with either decreased or unchanged of microbial diversity and richness [9]. Most of the studies reported lower sobs, Chao 1, and Shannon diversities in people with IBS [35,36,43]. In addition, some studies showed no distinction in terms of microbiome diversity between IBS patients and healthy people [44,45]. In contrast to the earlier findings, we observed higher sobs and Shannon diversities in IBS people compared to healthy controls. Supporting this, a study found higher microbiome diversity in IBS patients compared to healthy controls [46]. A possible explanation for these contradictory findings might be related to various techniques of DNA sequencing in different regions for specifying the diversity of the gut microbiota in studies as well as difference in the IBS population [47]. Thus, further studies using similar methodologies are required to help to distinguish IBS people from healthy ones via gut microbiota diversity.

4.3. Correlations between Food Components and the Gut Microbiota in IBS

Diet and it's macro/micronutrient components may influence the gut microbiome either directly or indirectly [48]. The majority of the recent studies have focused on the effects of low fermentable oligo-, di-, and monosaccharides and polyols (FODMAPs) diet in IBS. A low-FODMAP diet has been linked to a reduced abundance of Bifidobacteria, with potential health benefits still under debate [49]. Other studies have reported lower bacterial abundance following the introduction of a low-FODMAP diet compared with a habitual diet [50,51].

While in the low-FODMAP diet, consumption of fermentable and short-chain carbohydrate is restricted, adequate intakes of fiber is encouraged [52]. Dietary fiber has soluble and insoluble components. Though the insoluble fiber is utilized less by the gut microbiota, the soluble components of dietary fiber such as inulin and fructans are mostly used by the gut microbiota as an energy source and help to develop some beneficial bacteria, such as *Lactobacillus* and *Bifidobacteria* [53]. Research also shows the enrichment of the genus *Prevotella* in individuals with higher fiber diets [31]. *Prevotella* is a genus with a high abundance in healthy people. Thus, dietary fiber may help to develop beneficial microbiota in the human gut.

In the current study, we observed a positive correlation between dietary fiber intake and microbial diversity in people with IBS. Higher diversity and richness of the microbiota has also been shown in Agrarian vs. Western diet style communities [31,53]. Fermentation of dietary fiber by microbial fulfills some beneficial influence by production of metabolites. One of the metabolites is short-chain fatty acids (SCFA), which can reduce colonic pH and inhibits the growth of pathogens [54]. Butyrate, as another metabolite provides energy substrate to enterocytes and some bacterial species and enhances the expression of some epithelial tight junction proteins [11,54]. More research is required to determine the role of specific gut microbiota in the fermentation of fiber and the specific metabolites produced.

Our results revealed higher bacterial diversity as well as a higher abundance of some genus, including *Parabacteroides, Oscillibacter, Lachnospiraceae*-unclassified, and *Ruminococcaceae*-unclassified in the IBS group who consumed caffeine more than 400 mg/d compared to the HC. Studies on the role of caffeine consumption on microbial diversity and composition are limited. In one study, regular consumption of coffee more than 45 mL/day was associated with a higher level of *Prevotella, Bacteroides,* and *Porphyromonas* in healthy individuals [55]. In another study using a spontaneous mouse model of metabolic syndrome, daily intake of coffee or its components for 16 weeks changed the abundance of various genera such as *Coprococcus, Blautia,* and *Prevotella* in mice [56]. Caffeine, as the major water-soluble component of coffee, influences gut microbiota diversity and patterns. However, its role in the alteration of the gut microbiota remains unclear and requires further investigation [56,57].

Our study may have several limitations that need to be considered when interpreting the results. The study population was narrowed to young adults with IBS and HC. The majority of the young adults recruited in the study were students and their lifestyle may affect their diet and eventually, their gut microbiota patterns. Moreover, using Rome III or IV criteria for recruitment of IBS people might make our study population heterogonous.

The small sample size may affect the generalization of the results. Further studies with a larger sample size and more homogenous population by considering the history of diet and medication use are recommended to determine the interplay between diet and microbiota in IBS symptoms.

5. Conclusions

In summary, our result revealed similar nutrient intake patterns between IBS people and HC groups except in the daily consumption of caffeine. The gut microbiome communities were significantly different between the IBS and HC groups in terms of microbial diversity and compositions. Higher caffeine consumption in the IBS group was also associated with higher bacterial diversity as well as an alteration in microbial composition. Taken together, these results suggest the influence of caffeine on gut microbiota patterns. Further studies are necessary to investigate the interplay between caffeine intake and gut microbiota.

Supplementary Materials: The following are available online at https://www.mdpi.com/2075-442 6/11/1/35/s1, Figure S1: Correlation between caffeine intake and alpha diversity. (1) Correlation between total observed species (sobs) and caffeine intake. (2) Correlation between Shannon index and caffeine intake. High-IBS: Caffeine consumption more than 400 mg/day; Low-IBS: Caffeine consumption less than 400 mg/day. Figure S2: Correlation between dietary fiber intake and alpha diversity. (A) Correlation between total observed species (sobs) and dietary fiber intake. (B) Correlation between total Shannon index and dietary fiber intake. High-IBS: Caffeine consumption more than 400 mg/day; Low-IBS: Caffeine consumption less than 400 mg/day. Figure S3: Correlation between beta diversity and nutrient intakes in High-IBS, Low-IBS, and HC groups. High-IBS: Caffeine consumption more than 400 mg/day; Low-IBS: Caffeine consumption less than 400 mg/day; Caff: Caffeine; Fiber: Fiber; and HC groups: High-IBS: Caffeine consumption more than 400 mg/day; Low-IBS: Caffeine consumption less than 400 mg/day; Caff: caffeine; Fiber: Fiber.

Author Contributions: Conceptualization, Z.A.B., A.R.S., and X.S.C.; formal analysis, J.L. and K.M.; funding acquisition, Z.A.B., A.R.S., and X.S.C.; methodology, Z.A.B., J.L., and X.S.C.; project administration, A.R.S., X.S.C.; software, J.L. and K.M.; supervision, A.R.S. and X.S.C.; writing—original draft, Z.A.B.; writing—review and editing, A.R.S. and X.S.C. All authors have read and agreed to the published version of the manuscript.

Funding: The present study was funded by P20 NR016605-01 (PI: A.R.S; pilot PI: X.S.C) and the American Nurses Foundation (PI: Z.A.B).

Institutional Review Board Statement: The study was conducted according to the guidelines of the Declaration of Helsinki, and approved by the Institutional Review Board of the University of Connecticut (Protocol #H16-152; July, 2016).

Informed Consent Statement: Informed consent was obtained from all subjects involved in the study.

Data Availability Statement: The data presented in this study are available on request from the corresponding author. The data are not publicly available due to ongoing data analysis.

Acknowledgments: The authors acknowledge the support from the University of Connecticut School of Nursing, P20 Center for Accelerating Precision Pain Self-Management. The authors also acknowledge people who participated in the study.

Conflicts of Interest: The authors declare no conflict of interest.

References

1. Herndon, C.C.; Wang, Y.; Lu, C.-L. Targeting the gut microbiota for the treatment of irritable bowel syndrome. *Kaohsiung J. Med. Sci.* **2020**, *36*, 160–170. [CrossRef]
2. Dimidi, E.; Rossi, M.; Whelan, K. Irritable bowel syndrome and diet: Where are we in 2018? *Curr. Opin. Clin. Nutr. Metab. Care* **2017**, *20*, 456–463. [CrossRef]
3. Mazzawi, T.; El-Salhy, M. Effect of diet and individual dietary guidance on gastrointestinal endocrine cells in patients with irritable bowel syndrome. *Int. J. Mol. Med.* **2017**, *40*, 943–952. [CrossRef]

4. Valeur, J.; Småstuen, M.C.; Knudsen, T.; Lied, G.A.; Røseth, A.G. Exploring Gut Microbiota Composition as an Indicator of Clinical Response to Dietary FODMAP Restriction in Patients with Irritable Bowel Syndrome. *Dig. Dis. Sci.* **2018**, *63*, 429–436. [CrossRef]
5. Rajilić-Stojanović, M.; Jonkers, D.M.; Salonen, A.H.; Hanevik, K.; Raes, J.; Jalanka, J.; De Vos, W.M.; Manichanh, C.; Golic, N.; Enck, P.; et al. Intestinal Microbiota And Diet in IBS: Causes, Consequences, or Epiphenomena? *Am. J. Gastroenterol.* **2015**, *110*, 278–287. [CrossRef]
6. El-Salhy, M.; Hatlebakk, J.G.; Hausken, T. Diet in Irritable Bowel Syndrome (IBS): Interaction with Gut Microbiota and Gut Hormones. *Nutrients* **2019**, *11*, 1824. [CrossRef]
7. Altobelli, E.; Del Negro, V.; Angeletti, P.M.; Latella, G. Low-FODMAP Diet Improves Irritable Bowel Syndrome Symptoms: A Meta-Analysis. *Nutrients* **2017**, *9*, 940. [CrossRef]
8. Pozuelo, M.; Panda, S.; Santiago, A.; Mendez, S.; Accarino, A.; Santos, J.; Guarner, F.; Azpiroz, F.; Manichanh, C. Reduction of butyrate- and methane-producing microorganisms in patients with Irritable Bowel Syndrome. *Sci. Rep.* **2015**, *5*, 12693. [CrossRef]
9. Chong, P.P.; Chin, V.K.; Looi, C.Y.; Wong, W.F.; Madhavan, P.; Yong, V.C. The Microbiome and Irritable Bowel Syndrome—A Review on the Pathophysiology, Current Research and Future Therapy. *Front. Microbiol.* **2019**, *10*, 1136. [CrossRef]
10. Wu, G.D.; Chen, J.; Hoffmann, C.; Bittinger, K.; Chen, Y.Y.; Keilbaugh, S.A.; Bewtra, M.; Knights, D.; Walters, W.A.; Knight, R.; et al. Linking Long-Term Dietary Patterns with Gut Microbial Enterotypes. *Science* **2011**, *334*, 105–108. [CrossRef]
11. Rajilić-Stojanović, M. Function of the microbiota. *Best Pract. Res. Clin. Gastroenterol.* **2013**, *27*, 5–16. [CrossRef]
12. Parada Venegas, D.; De la Fuente, M.K.; Landskron, G.; González, M.J.; Quera, R.; Dijkstra, G.; Harmsen, H.J.M.; Faber, K.N.; Hermoso, M.A. Short chain fatty acids (SCFAs)-mediated gut epithelial and immune regulation and its relevance for inflammatory bowel diseases. *Front. Immunol.* **2019**, *10*, 277. [CrossRef]
13. Ooi, S.L.; Correa, D.; Park, S.C. Probiotics, prebiotics, and low FODMAP diet for irritable bowel syndrome—What is the current evidence? *Complement. Ther. Med.* **2019**, *43*, 73–80. [CrossRef]
14. Harris, L.A.; Baffy, N. Modulation of the gut microbiota: A focus on treatments for irritable bowel syndrome. *Postgrad. Med.* **2017**, *129*, 872–888. [CrossRef]
15. Mansour, A.; Mohajeri-Tehrani, M.R.; Karimi, S.; Sanginabadi, M.; Poustchi, H.; Enayati, S.; Asgarbeik, S.; Nasrollahzadeh, J.; Hekmatdoost, A. Short term effects of coffee components consumption on gut microbiota in patients with non-alcoholic fatty liver and diabetes: A pilot randomized placebo-controlled, clinical trial. *EXCLI J.* **2020**, *19*, 241–250. [PubMed]
16. Gurwara, S.; Dai, A.; Ajami, N.; El-Serag, H.B.; Graham, D.Y.; Jiao, L. 196 Caffeine Consumption and the Colonic Mucosa-Associated Gut Microbiota. *Am. J. Gastroenterol.* **2019**, *114*, S119–S120. [CrossRef]
17. Cong, X.; Ramesh, D.; Perry, M.; Xu, W.; Bernier, K.M.; Young, E.E.; Walsh, S.; Starkweather, A. Pain self-management plus nurse-led support in young adults with irritable bowel syndrome: Study protocol for a pilot randomized control trial. *Res. Nurs. Health* **2018**, *41*, 121–130. [CrossRef]
18. Kristal, A.R.; Feng, Z.; Coates, R.J.; Oberman, A.; George, V. Associations of race/ethnicity, education, and dietary intervention with the validity and reliability of a food frequency questionnaire: The Women's Health Trial Feasibility Study in Minority Populations. *Am. J. Epidemiol.* **1997**, *146*, 856–869. [CrossRef]
19. (NIH), National Institutes of Health. Diet History Questionnaire II (DHQ II): Diet*Calc Software. 2020. Available online: https://epi.grants.cancer.gov/dhq2/dietcalc/ (accessed on June 2020).
20. Cong, X.; Judge, M.; Xu, W.; Diallo, A.; Janton, S.; Brownell, E.A.; Maas, K.; Graf, J. Influence of Feeding Type on Gut Microbiome Development in Hospitalized Preterm Infants. *Nurs. Res.* **2017**, *66*, 123–133. [CrossRef]
21. Cong, X.; Xu, W.; Janton, S.; Henderson, W.A.; Matson, A.; McGrath, J.M.; Maas, K.; Graf, J. Gut Microbiome Developmental Patterns in Early Life of Preterm Infants: Impacts of Feeding and Gender. *PLoS ONE* **2016**, *11*, e0152751. [CrossRef]
22. (FDA), U.S.; Food and Drug Administration. Spilling the Beans: How Much Caffeine Is Too Much. 30 October 2020. Available online: https://www.fda.gov/consumers/consumer-updates/spilling-beans-how-much-caffeine-too-much (accessed on June 2020).
23. Cho, H.-W. How Much Caffeine is Too Much for Young Adolescents? *Osong Public Health Res. Perspect.* **2018**, *9*, 287–288. [CrossRef] [PubMed]
24. Harper, A.; Naghibi, M.M.; Garcha, D. The Role of Bacteria, Probiotics and Diet in Irritable Bowel Syndrome. *Foods* **2018**, *7*, 13. [CrossRef] [PubMed]
25. El-Salhy, M.; Østgaard, H.; Hausken, T.; Gundersen, D. Diet and effects of diet management on quality of life and symptoms in patients with irritable bowel syndrome. *Mol. Med. Rep.* **2012**, *5*, 1382–1390. [CrossRef]
26. Saito, Y.A.; Locke, G.R.; Weaver, A.L.; Zinsmeister, A.R.; Talley, N.J. Diet and Functional Gastrointestinal Disorders: A Population-Based Case-Control Study. *Am. J. Gastroenterol.* **2005**, *100*, 2743–2748. [CrossRef]
27. Reding, K.W.; Cain, K.C.; Jarrett, M.E.; Eugenio, M.D.; Heitkemper, M.M. Relationship Between Patterns of Alcohol Consumption and Gastrointestinal Symptoms Among Patients with Irritable Bowel Syndrome. *Am. J. Gastroenterol.* **2013**, *108*, 270–276. [CrossRef]
28. Heizer, W.D.; Southern, S.; McGovern, S. The Role of Diet in Symptoms of Irritable Bowel Syndrome in Adults: A Narrative Review. *J. Am. Diet. Assoc.* **2009**, *109*, 1204–1214. [CrossRef]
29. Böhn, L.; Störsrud, S.; Liljebo, T.M.; Collin, L.; Lindfors, P.; Törnblom, H.; Simrén, M. Diet Low in FODMAPs Reduces Symptoms of Irritable Bowel Syndrome as Well as Traditional Dietary Advice: A Randomized Controlled Trial. *Gastroenterology* **2015**, *149*, 1399–1407.e2. [CrossRef]

30. Eswaran, S.; Muir, J.; Chey, W.D. Fiber and Functional Gastrointestinal Disorders. *Am. J. Gastroenterol.* **2013**, *108*, 718–727. [CrossRef]
31. Staudacher, H.M.; Whelan, K. Altered gastrointestinal microbiota in irritable bowel syndrome and its modification by diet: Probiotics, prebiotics and the low FODMAP diet. *Proc. Nutr. Soc.* **2016**, *75*, 306–318. [CrossRef]
32. Backhed, F. Host-Bacterial Mutualism in the Human Intestine. *Science* **2005**, *307*, 1915–1920. [CrossRef]
33. Cong, X.; Xu, W.; Romisher, R.; Poveda, S.; Forte, S.; Starkweather, A.; Henderson, W.A. Gut microbiome and infant health: Brain-gut-microbiota axis and host genetic factors. *Yale J. Biol. Med.* **2016**, *89*, 299. [PubMed]
34. Qin, J.; Li, R.; Raes, J.; Arumugam, M.; Burgdorf, K.S.; Manichanh, C.; Nielsen, T.; Pons, N.; Levenez, F.; Yamada, T.; et al. A human gut microbial gene catalogue established by metagenomic sequencing. *Nature* **2010**, *464*, 59–65. [CrossRef] [PubMed]
35. Zhuang, X.; Tian, Z.; Li, L.; Zeng, Z.; Chen, M.; Xiong, L. Fecal Microbiota Alterations Associated With Diarrhea-Predominant Irritable Bowel Syndrome. *Front. Microbiol.* **2018**, *9*, 1600. [CrossRef]
36. Rangel, I.; Sundin, J.; Fuentes, S.; Repsilber, D.; De Vos, W.M.; Brummer, R.J. The relationship between faecal-associated and mucosal-associated microbiota in irritable bowel syndrome patients and healthy subjects. *Aliment. Pharmacol. Ther.* **2015**, *42*, 1211–1221. [CrossRef] [PubMed]
37. Ringel-Kulka, T.; Benson, A.K.; Carroll, I.M.; Kim, J.; Legge, R.M.; Ringel, Y. Molecular characterization of the intestinal microbiota in patients with and without abdominal bloating. *Am. J. Physiol. Liver Physiol.* **2016**, *310*, G417–G426. [CrossRef]
38. Arumugam, M.; Raes, J.; Pelletier, E.; Le Paslier, D.; Yamada, T.; Mende, D.R.; Fernandes, G.R.; Tap, J.; Bruls, T.; Batto, J.M.; et al. Enterotypes of the human gut microbiome. *Nature* **2011**, *473*, 174–180. [CrossRef]
39. Tap, J.; Furet, J.; Bensaada, M.; Philippe, C.; Roth, H.; Rabot, S.; Lakhdari, O.; Lombard, V.; Henrissat, B.; Corthier, G.; et al. Gut microbiota richness promotes its stability upon increased dietary fibre intake in healthy adults. *Environ. Microbiol.* **2015**, *17*, 4954–4964. [CrossRef]
40. Nishino, K.; Nishida, A.; Inoue, R.; Kawada, Y.; Ohno, M.; Sakai, S.; Inatomi, O.; Bamba, S.; Sugimoto, M.; Kawahara, M.; et al. Analysis of endoscopic brush samples identified mucosa-associated dysbiosis in inflammatory bowel disease. *J. Gastroenterol.* **2018**, *53*, 95–106. [CrossRef]
41. Jackson, M.A.; Verdi, S.; Maxan, M.-E.; Shin, C.M.; Zierer, J.; Bowyer, R.C.E.; Martin, T.; Williams, F.M.K.; Menni, C.; Bell, J.T.; et al. Gut microbiota associations with common diseases and prescription medications in a population-based cohort. *Nat. Commun.* **2018**, *9*, 2655. [CrossRef]
42. Brunkwall, L.; Ericson, U.; Nilsson, P.M.; Orho-Melander, M.; Ohlsson, B. Self-reported bowel symptoms are associated with differences in overall gut microbiota composition and enrichment of Blautia in a population-based cohort. *J. Gastroenterol. Hepatol.* **2020**. [CrossRef]
43. Jeffery, I.B.; Das, A.; O'Herlihy, E.; Coughlan, S.; Cisek, K.; Moore, M.; Bradley, F.; Carty, T.; Pradhan, M.; Dwibedi, C.; et al. Differences in Fecal Microbiomes and Metabolomes of People With vs Without Irritable Bowel Syndrome and Bile Acid Malabsorption. *Gastroenterology* **2020**, *158*, 1016–1028.e8. [CrossRef] [PubMed]
44. Hugerth, L.W.; Andreasson, A.; Talley, N.J.; Forsberg, A.M.; Kjellström, L.; Schmidt, P.T.; Agreus, L.; Engstrand, L. No distinct microbiome signature of irritable bowel syndrome found in a Swedish random population. *Gut* **2019**, *69*, 1076–1084. [CrossRef] [PubMed]
45. Pittayanon, R.; Lau, J.T.; Yuan, Y.; Leontiadis, G.I.; Tse, F.; Surette, M.; Moayyedi, P. Gut Microbiota in Patients With Irritable Bowel Syndrome—A Systematic Review. *Gastroenterology* **2019**, *157*, 97–108. [CrossRef] [PubMed]
46. Labus, J.S.; Hollister, E.B.; Jacobs, J.P.; Kirbach, K.; Oezguen, N.; Gupta, A.; Acosta, J.; Luna, R.A.; Aagaard, K.M.; Versalovic, J.; et al. Differences in gut microbial composition correlate with regional brain volumes in irritable bowel syndrome. *Microbiome* **2017**, *5*, 49. [CrossRef]
47. Lee, B.J.; Bak, Y.T. Irritable Bowel Syndrome, Gut Microbiota and Probiotics. *J. Neurogastroenterol. Motil.* **2011**, *17*, 252–266. [CrossRef]
48. Singh, R.K.; Chang, H.-W.; Yan, D.; Lee, K.M.; Ucmak, D.; Wong, K.; Abrouk, M.; Farahnik, B.; Nakamura, M.; Zhu, T.H.; et al. Influence of diet on the gut microbiome and implications for human health. *J. Transl. Med.* **2017**, *15*, 73. [CrossRef]
49. Staudacher, H.M.; Lomer, M.C.E.; Anderson, J.L.; Barrett, J.S.; Muir, J.G.; Irving, P.M.; Whelan, K. Fermentable Carbohydrate Restriction Reduces Luminal Bifidobacteria and Gastrointestinal Symptoms in Patients with Irritable Bowel Syndrome. *J. Nutr.* **2012**, *142*, 1510–1518. [CrossRef]
50. Shepherd, S.J.; Parker, F.C.; Muir, J.G.; Gibson, P.R. Dietary Triggers of Abdominal Symptoms in Patients With Irritable Bowel Syndrome: Randomized Placebo-Controlled Evidence. *Clin. Gastroenterol. Hepatol.* **2008**, *6*, 765–771. [CrossRef]
51. Halmos, E.P.; Christophersen, C.T.; Bird, A.R.; Shepherd, S.J.; Gibson, P.R.; Muir, J.G. Diets that differ in their FODMAP content alter the colonic luminal microenvironment. *Gut* **2015**, *64*, 93–100. [CrossRef]
52. Barrett, J.S. How to institute the low-FODMAP diet. *J. Gastroenterol. Hepatol.* **2017**, *32*, 8–10. [CrossRef]
53. James, S.C.; Fraser, K.; Young, W.; McNabb, W.C.; Roy, N.C. Gut Microbial Metabolites and Biochemical Pathways Involved in Irritable Bowel Syndrome: Effects of Diet and Nutrition on the Microbiome. *J. Nutr.* **2020**, *150*, 1012–1021. [CrossRef] [PubMed]
54. Kannampalli, P.; Shaker, R.; Sengupta, J.N. Colonic butyrate-algesic or analgesic? *Neurogastroenterol. Motil.* **2011**, *23*, 975–979. [CrossRef] [PubMed]
55. González, S.; Salazar, N.; Ruiz-Saavedra, S.; Gómez-Martín, M.; Reyes-Gavilán, C.G.D.L.; Gueimonde, M. Long-Term Coffee Consumption is Associated with Fecal Microbial Composition in Humans. *Nutrients* **2020**, *12*, 1287. [CrossRef] [PubMed]

56. Nishitsuji, K.; Watanabe, S.; Xiao, J.; Nagatomo, R.; Ogawa, H.; Tsunematsu, T.; Umemoto, H.; Morimoto, Y.; Akatsu, H.; Inoue, K.; et al. Effect of coffee or coffee components on gut microbiome and short-chain fatty acids in a mouse model of metabolic syndrome. *Sci. Rep.* **2018**, *8*, 16173. [CrossRef]
57. Sato, Y.; Itagaki, S.; Kurokawa, T.; Ogura, J.; Kobayashi, M.; Hirano, T.; Sugawara, M.; Iseki, K. In vitro and in vivo antioxidant properties of chlorogenic acid and caffeic acid. *Int. J. Pharm.* **2011**, *403*, 136–138. [CrossRef]

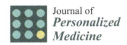

Article

Differential Microbial Pattern Description in Subjects with Autoimmune-Based Thyroid Diseases: A Pilot Study

Isabel Cornejo-Pareja [1,2,†], Patricia Ruiz-Limón [1,2,†], Ana M. Gómez-Pérez [1], María Molina-Vega [1], Isabel Moreno-Indias [1,2,*] and Francisco J. Tinahones [1,2,3]

[1] Unidad de Gestión Clínica de Endocrinología y Nutrición, Instituto de Investigación Biomédica de Málaga (IBIMA), Hospital Clínico Virgen de la Victoria, 29010 Málaga, Spain; isabelmaria_cornejo@hotmail.com (I.C.-P.); patriciaruizlimon@ibima.eu (P.R.-L.); anamgp86@gmail.com (A.M.G.-P.); molinavegamaria@gmail.com (M.M.-V.); fjtinahones@uma.es (F.J.T.)
[2] CIBER Fisiopatología de la Obesidad y Nutrición (CIBEROBN), Instituto de Salud Carlos III, 28029 Madrid, Spain
[3] Department of Medicine and Dermatology, University of Málaga, 29010 Málaga, Spain
* Correspondence: isabel.moreno@ibima.eu; Tel.: +34-95-103-2647
† These authors share first authorship.

Received: 15 September 2020; Accepted: 20 October 2020; Published: 26 October 2020

Abstract: The interaction between genetic susceptibility, epigenetic, endogenous, and environmental factors play a key role in the initiation and progression of autoimmune thyroid diseases (AITDs). Studies have shown that gut microbiota alterations take part in the development of autoimmune diseases. We have investigated the possible relationship between gut microbiota composition and the most frequent AITDs. A total of nine Hashimoto's thyroiditis (HT), nine Graves–Basedow's disease (GD), and 11 otherwise healthy donors (HDs) were evaluated. 16S rRNA pyrosequencing and bioinformatics analysis by Quantitative Insights into Microbial Ecology and Phylogenetic Investigation of Communities by Reconstruction of Unobserved States (PICRUSt) were used to analyze the gut microbiota. Beta diversity analysis showed that gut microbiota from our groups was different. We observed an increase in bacterial richness in HT and a lower evenness in GD in comparison to the HDs. GD showed a significant increase of *Fusobacteriaceae*, *Fusobacterium* and *Sutterella* compared to HDs and the core microbiome features showed that *Prevotellaceae* and *Prevotella* characterized this group. *Victivallaceae* was increased in HT and was part of their core microbiome. *Streptococcaceae*, *Streptococcus* and *Rikenellaceae* were greater in HT compared to GD. Core microbiome features of HT were represented by *Streptococcus*, *Alistipes*, *Anaerostipes*, *Dorea* and *Haemophilus*. *Faecalibacterium* decreased in both AITDs compared to HDs. PICRUSt analysis demonstrated enrichment in the xenobiotics degradation, metabolism, and the metabolism of cofactors and vitamins in GD patients compared to HDs. Moreover, correlation studies showed that some bacteria were widely correlated with autoimmunity parameters. A prediction model evaluated a possible relationship between predominant concrete bacteria such as an unclassified genus of *Ruminococcaceae*, *Sutterella* and *Faecalibacterium* in AITDs. AITD patients present altered gut microbiota compared to HDs. These alterations could be related to the immune system development in AITD patients and the loss of tolerance to self-antigens.

Keywords: Graves–Basedow's diseases; Hashimoto's thyroiditis; autoimmunity; gut microbiota

1. Introduction

Autoimmune thyroid diseases (AITDs) are the most common organ-specific autoimmune disorders. Within AITDs, Hashimoto's thyroiditis and Graves–Basedow's disease are the most frequent conditions.

Hashimoto's thyroiditis (HT) is identified by lymphocytes infiltration in the thyroid gland which leads to the destruction of thyroid follicles, and the production of autoantibodies against thyroid peroxidase (TPO, 90–95%) and thyroglobulin (TG, 20–50%) [1,2].

On the other hand, Graves' disease (GD) is identified by the production of autoantibodies of the immunoglobulin G1 subclass that are directed against the thyrotropin receptor which induces thyroid hormone overproduction and also causing hypertrophy and hyperplasia of thyroid cells [3].

The etiology of AITDs is thought to be multifactorial, arising from an interaction between genetic susceptibility, epigenetic, and various endogenous and environmental factors [4].

Several studies have provided evidence for genetic factors, however, the concordance rate for AITDs among monozygotic twins is in the range of 35–55% compared with 3% in dizygotic twins, emphasizing that other important factors, such as the environment, are implicated in the pathogenesis of AITD [5–7].

Gut microbiota takes part in the homeostasis of the host, and especially in the regulation of the immune system. Gut microbiota is a promising agent for the development of personalized medicine as it collects information about its host, like diet or environmental factors [8]. Recent evidence suggest that the alteration of gut microbiota may have connection with autoimmune diseases [9–12].

Notwithstanding, the pathogenic link between gut microbiota and AITDs has not been fully elucidated, with only a few studies in humans [13–15]. Zhao et al., demonstrated that HT patients had an altered gut microbiota profile compared with the healthy population and this profile correlated with clinical parameters [16].

In the present study, we aimed to investigate the gut microbiota profile in patients affected by AITD, both HT and GD; and its relationship with autoimmunity markers.

2. Materials and Methods

2.1. Participants

A total of 18 AITD patients (nine GD patients and nine HT patients) were recruited at the Department of Endocrinology and Nutrition of Virgen de la Victoria University Hospital (Málaga, Spain). Moreover, we included 11 otherwise healthy donors (HDs) with similar anthropometric features as study groups, without thyroid disease and without family history of thyroid disease. These HDs were euthyroid and goiter was not evident on physical examination. Individuals were included from those who were attended at the hospital during the first half of 2018.

All participants with GD were receiving synthetic antithyroid (Neo-tomizol, 5–20 mg of dose) and HT patients were receiving levothyroxine treatment (Eutirox, 50–175 µg of dose) and presented an acceptable control of the disease which allowed us to focus on the pathophysiology of autoimmunity and not on thyroid dysfunction. The exclusion criteria were: pregnancy; type 1 or type 2 diabetes mellitus; other autoimmune disease; and chronic and/or severe gastrointestinal disorders. We also excluded patients and HDs with extreme diets, those exposed to antibiotic therapy (current or previous 3 months), chronic drugs different to AITDs medication that alter microbiota profile, those taking probiotic agents, and the non-acceptance of informed consent.

The study protocol was approved by the Medical Ethics Committee of Virgen de la Victoria University Hospital and conducted according to principals of the Declaration of Helsinki. All participants enrolled provided their written informed consent and were also verbally informed of the characteristics of the study.

2.2. Anthropometric and Laboratory Measurements

Anthropometric measurements, including body weight, height, and waist and hip circumferences, were collected. Peripheral venous blood samples were obtained after 8 hours of fasting. The serum was centrifuged at 4000 rpm for 15 min at 4 °C and frozen at −80 °C until analysis. Levels of cholesterol, triglycerides, HDL-cholesterol, and glucose were analyzed by enzymatic methods (Randox Laboratories Ltd., Crumlin, UK) and glycosylated hemoglobin (HbA1c) was determined by Dimension Vista autoanalyzer (Siemens Healthcare Diagnostics, Munich, Germany).

Laboratory markers of autoimmunity [thyroid stimulating immunoglobulin (TSI), anti- thyroperoxidase (Anti-TPO)] and thyroid profile [thyroid-stimulating hormone (TSH), free thyroxine (FT4), free triiodothyronine (FT3)] were quantified as part of the routine patient management in the case of AITD patients, with exception of HDs. Reference ranges were for TSH 0.4–5 µIU/mL; FT4 11–22 pmol/L; and FT3 2–5 pmol/L. TSI was measured by Elecsys Anti-TSHR test following the manufacturer's protocols (Roche, Basel, Switzerland) in a Roche electrochemiluminometric analyzer (Cobas e 801, Roche, Basel, Switzerland). Anti-TPO was detected by Atellica IM Anti-Thyroid Peroxidase assay (SIEMENS Healthineers, Erlangen, Germany) using the Atellica IM Analyzer (SIEMENS Healthineers, Erlangen, Germany). Reference ranges were for TPO-Ab > 60 IU/mL and TSI-Ab > 2 IU/mL.

2.3. DNA Extraction from Faecal Samples

Faecal samples were obtained by the volunteers, immediately refrigerated, and carried to the laboratory, where they were stored at −80 °C for subsequent analysis.

DNA was extracted from 200 mg of stool using the QIAamp DNA stool Mini kit (Qiagen, Hilden, Germany) according to the manufacturer's protocols. DNA concentration was measured by absorbance at 260 nm, and the purity was verified by determining the A260/A280 ratio with a Nanodrop spectrophotometer (Nanodrop Technologies, Wilmington, DE, USA).

2.4. Sequencing of 16S rRNA and Bioinformatic Analysis

The Ion 16S Metagenomics Kit (Thermo-Fisher Scientific Inc., Waltham, MA, USA) was used to amplified the ribosomal 16S rRNA gene region from stool DNA, with two primer sets (V2–4–8 and V3–6, 7–9) covering the most of the hypervariable regions of the 16S rRNA region in bacteria. The libraries were created using the Ion Plus Fragment Library Kit (Thermo Fisher Scientific, Waltham, MA, USA). Barcodes were added to each sample using the Ion Xpress Barcode Adapters kit (Thermo Fisher Scientific, Waltham, MA, USA). Emulsion PCR and sequencing of the amplicon libraries were carried out on an Ion 520 chip (Ion 520TM Chip Kit) using the Ion Chef System and Torrent S5TM system, respectively, using the Ion 520TM/530TM Kit-Chef (Thermo Fisher Scientific, Waltham, MA, USA) according to the manufacturer's instructions. Torrent Suite™ Server software (Thermo Fisher Scientific, Waltham, MA, USA), version 5.4.0, with default parameters for the 16S Target Sequencing (bead loading ≤30, key signal ≤30, and usable sequences ≤30) was used to base calling and run demultiplexing. Raw data is stored at the public repository SRA database (NCBI) with the BioProject PRJNA666641.

The open-source Quantitative Insights into Microbial Ecology (QIIME2, version 2019.7) software was used to analyze the quality sequences [17,18] and also was used for diversity analysis and subsequent taxonomic analysis through clustering with search [19] and the reference base Greengenes version 13_8 at 97% of identity.

Metagenome function was predicted by Phylogenetic Investigation of Communities by Reconstruction of Unobserved States (PICRUSt) analysis through picking operational taxonomic units (OTUs) from the Greengenes database, as described elsewhere [20]. The resulting OTU table was employed to predict the metagenome at three different Kyoto Encyclopedia of Genes and Genomes (KEGG) Orthology (KO) levels (level (L) 1 to L3).

2.5. Statistical Analysis

The open-source Statistical Analysis of Metagenomic Profiles [STAMP (v 2.1.3)] [21] was used to compare the differential abundances of taxa, KEGG categories, and subcategories, with the White's non-parametric test. α- and β-diversities were analyzed within QIIME2, through the diversity plugin: β-diversity metrics employed a permutational multivariate analysis of variance (PERMANOVA) with 999 permutations, while α-diversity metrics involved a Kruskal–Wallis test.

Anthropometric and clinical characteristics were analyzed with the IBM SPSS Statistics 25 (IBM, Armonk, NY, USA). The relationship between gut microbiota and thyroid variables was analyzed using Spearman's correlations models. Binary logistic regression models were fitted to assess the relationship between thyroid profile and autoimmunity markers with particular features as independent predictors. To control for potential confounding factors, their results were adjusted by age (years), sex (male or female) and body mass index (BMI, kg/m^2). The results were described as mean and dispersion (standard deviation, SD) for quantitative variables and as a proportion for qualitative variables. Statistical significance was established at $p < 0.05$. p values were corrected for multiple comparisons using the Benjamini–Hochberg method at 0.1, and reported as q-value, when appropriate.

3. Results

3.1. Clinical Data Study

All subjects ($n = 29$) were of Spanish nationality and born and grown in the Andalusian community. The study groups showed similar clinical characteristics about age, sex, anthropometric parameters, or metabolic profile, without finding statistically significant differences ($p > 0.05$). Our AITD patients had normalized thyroid function by medical treatment, substitution with levothyroxine in HT patients, or antithyroid drugs in patients with GD. However, we found significant differences in autoimmunity between the three study groups. TPO-Ab was significantly increased in HT and TSI-Ab was significantly increased in GD. HDs values of TPO-Ab resulted in slightly increased levels than expected for healthy individuals. In addition, according to serum TSH range our HDs were euthyroid. These demographic and clinical data of the subjects are summarized in Table 1.

Table 1. Clinical and demographic characteristics of patients and healthy donors.

Parameters	HT Patients ($n = 9$)	GD Patients ($n = 9$)	HDs ($n = 11$)	p-Value
Sex (M/F, % F)	(0/10, 100)	(2/7, 77.8)	(4/7, 63.5)	0.113
Age (years, mean ± SD)	40.3 ± 9.6	46.2 ± 8.6	48.8 ± 6.2	0.062
Smokers (%)	30	44.4	——	0.515
Family history of Thyroid disease (%)	50	33.3	——	0.484
Time of evolution of thyroid disease (months, mean ± SD)	134.4 ± 101.3	16.4 ± 22.6	——	0.001 *
Anthropometry				
Weight (kg, mean ± SD)	63.4 ± 11.7	66.6 ± 13.0	69.5 ± 8.1	0.354
BMI (kg/m^2, mean ± SD)	24.9 ± 5.8	25.2 ± 4.7	25.0 ± 2.0	0.831
Waist c. (cm, mean ± SD)	81.4 ± 13.8	86.1 ± 10.9	87.9 ± 8.4	0.321
Hip c. (cm, mean ± SD)	98.3 ± 10.7	101.6 ± 11.3	97.0 ± 4.1	0.391
Blood pressure				
Systolic (mmHg, mean ± SD)	121.6 ± 11.3	119.6 ± 16.2	128.8 ± 17.3	0.636
Diastolic (mmHg, mean ± SD)	75.3 ± 5.1	75.0 ± 15.4	78.6 ± 8.7	0.449
Analytical metabolic				
Glucose (mg/dL, mean ± SD)	86.6 ± 6.5	93.4 ± 4.1	91.0 ± 8.3	0.078
HbA1c (%, mean ± SD)	5.1 ± 0.3	5.3 ± 0.4	5.3 ± 0.3	0.29
Total-C (mg/dL, mean ± SD)	178.5 ± 44.7	192.2 ± 29.6	192.4 ± 47.8	0.568
LDL-c (mg/dL, mean ± SD)	107.7 ± 39.1	109.4 ± 10.2	110.1 ± 38.1	0.758
HDL-c (mg/dL, mean ± SD)	56.8 ± 11.7	65.6 ± 22.2	60.5 ± 12.9	0.666
TGs (mg/dL, mean ± SD)	70.1 ± 16.6	85.2 ± 31.9	108.8 ± 59.0	0.132
CRP (mg/dL, mean ± SD)	3.1 ± 0.0	3.2 ± 0.4	4.1 ± 1.4	0.116
Thyroid profile				

Table 1. *Cont.*

Parameters	HT Patients (n = 9)	GD Patients (n = 9)	HDs (n = 11)	p-Value
TSH (μIU/mL, mean ± SD)	2.6 ± 2.8	3.3 ± 8.5	2.2 ± 1.0	0.030 *
FT4 (pmol/L, mean ± SD)	15.4 ± 2.2	15.2 ± 3.1	15.2 ± 1.3	0.76
FT3 (pmol/L, mean ± SD)	3.8 ± 0.2	5.5 ± 2.3	4.8 ± 0.4	0.002 *
TPO-Ab (IU/mL, mean ± SD)	1186.7 ± 358.4	792.0 ± 621.7	160.3 ± 381.3	0.001 *
TPO-Ab > 60 IU/mL (P/N, % P)	(10/0, 100)	(6/3, 66.7)	(2/9, 18.2)	0.000 *
TSI-Ab (IU/mL, mean ± SD)	3.5 ± 7.2	16.8 ± 34.1	0.8 ± 0.1	0.000 *
TSI-Ab > 2 IU/mL (P/N, % P)	(1/9, 10)	(9/0, 100)	(0/11, 0)	0.000 *

BMI, body mass index; CRP, C-reactive protein; FT3, free triiodothyronine; FT4, free thyroxine; GD, Graves–Basedow's disease; HDs, healthy donors; HDL-c, high-density lipoprotein; Hip c. hip circumference; HT, Hashimoto's thyroiditis; LDL-c, low-density lipoprotein cholesterol; M/F, male/female; P/N, positive/negative ratio; TGs, triglycerides; Total-C, total cholesterol; TPO-Ab, thyroperoxidase antibody; TSI-Ab thyroid stimulating immunoglobulin antibody; Waist c. waist circumference. * Significant differences $p < 0.05$.

3.2. Gut Microbiota Diversity in AITD Patients

After the quality assessment, a total of 2,785,614 quality 16S rRNA gene sequences with an average of 26,056 ± 29,024 sequences per sample passed the filters. In order to compare the populations of the different groups, dimensional Principal Coordinates Analysis plots of UniFrac distances were used. Qualitative (Unweighted UniFrac distance) and quantitative (Weighted Unifrac distance) relationships showed differences among the groups ($p = 0.003$ and $p = 0.002$, respectively) (Figure 1A,B). Further analysis showed that our AITD patients did not show significant differences ($p > 0.05$), but they showed statistically significant differences with respect to HDs ($p < 0.05$ in groups, AITD patients related to HDs) (Figure S1).

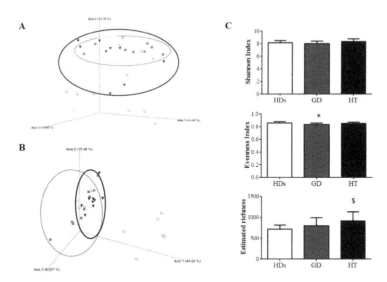

Figure 1. Estimation of diversity in healthy donors (HDs), Graves–Basedow's disease (GD) patients, and Hashimoto's thyroiditis (HT) patients. Clustering of fecal bacterial communities according to the different study groups by PCoA using unweighted and weighted UniFrac distances. Statistical differences were observed between groups. (**A**) Unweighted UniFrac distances, $p = 0.003$; and (**B**) Weighted UniFrac distances, $p = 0.002$. Dots belong to the HDs group; square to GD patients and cone to HT patients. (**C**) Shannon Diversity and Evenness indexes and estimated richness among different groups were compared. All values are mean ± SD. * $p < 0.05$ GD patients vs. HDs; $ $p < 0.05$ HT patients vs. HDs. Circles belong to the HDs; squares to GD patients and triangles to HT patients.

Alpha diversity was assessed using rarefaction curves. Richness, estimated by the observed features index, demonstrated a significant increase in HT patients versus HDs ($p = 0.022$), while no differences were found between the other groups. Evenness, calculated by the Pielou index, showed a significant decreased in GD patients compared with HDs ($p = 0.03$) and no significant differences among the other groups. Finally, biodiversity, estimated by the Shannon index, suggested no significant differences among the study groups (Figure 1C).

3.3. Gut Microbiota Profile in AITD Patients

Dominant bacterial phyla were Bacteroidetes and Firmicutes, while Proteobacteria, Actinobacteria, and Tenericutes shared smaller proportions, between 1–10%, in the different study groups. No differences were observed between our study groups at this taxa level (Figure 2A).

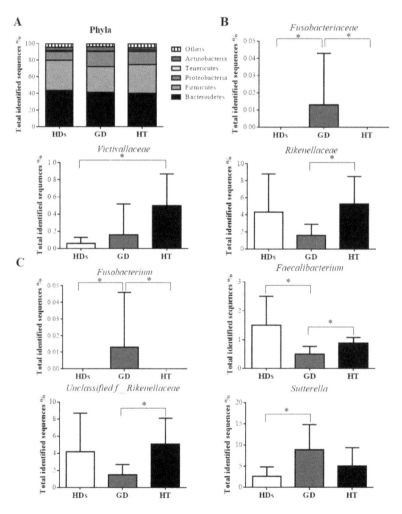

Figure 2. (**A**) Microbiota profile of faecal samples from the study groups at the phylum level. (**B**) Families statistically significant between the study groups. (**C**) Genera statistically significant between the study groups. * Indicates significant differences between groups, q < 0.1 (q = *p*-FDR-corrected).

At the family level, *Fusobacteriaceae* was significantly increased in GD patients when compared with HT patients and HDs (q = 0.01). Furthermore, a significantly higher abundance was found in HT patients when compared with HDs for *Victivallaceae* (q = 0.03). In addition, *Rikenellaceae* was significantly decreased in GD patients compared with HT patients (q = 0.04) (Figure 2B).

Finally, at the genus level, *Fusobacterium* was significantly higher in GD patients compared with HDs and also compared with HT patients (q = 0.02 and q = 0.009, respectively). *Faecalibacterium* was significantly lower in GD patients compared to HDs and also compared with HT patients (q = 0.02 and q = 0.07, respectively). An unclassified genus of the family *Rikenellaceae* was significantly lower in GD patients compared to HT patients (q = 0.03). The genus *Sutterella* was significantly higher in GD patients compared to HDs (q = 0.10) (Figure 2C).

3.4. Core Microbiome in AITD Patients and HDs

After studying the differences between groups, we wondered if each group was characterized by a concrete core gut microbiome. We investigated the core microbiome of each group, meaning those features that were shared among the 85% of the samples of each study group. At the family level, we observed that a total of 15 identified families were shared by all the volunteers of the study (See the complete list in Table S1). Interestingly, *Pasteurellaceae* was only shared between AITD patients. *Victivallaceae* and *Streptococcaceae* were characteristic of the HT group and *Prevotellaceae* of GD group; while *Christensenellaceae* seemed to be characteristic of the HDs group (Figure 3A). On the other hand, 12 identified genera were shared between the three groups (See the complete list in Table S1). *Collinsella* and *Roseburia* belonged to the core microbiome of both AITDs, while *Butyricimonas* was shared by GD patients and HDs. HT patients were the group with a greater number of characteristic features: *Streptococcus*, *Alistipes*, *Anaerostipes*, *Dorea* and *Haemophilus*; while *Prevotella* was characteristic of the GD group. No characteristic genus was found in the HDs group (Figure 3B).

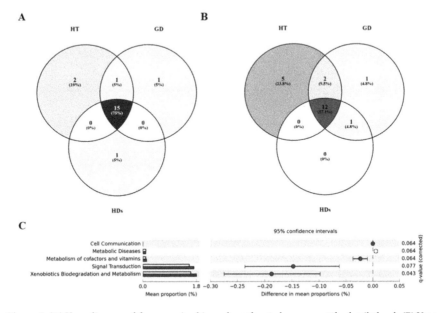

Figure 3. (**A**) Venn diagram of the core microbiome from the study groups at the family level. (**B**) Venn diagram of the core microbiome from the study groups at the genus level. (**C**) Significant differences in predicted functional composition at level 2 of Kyoto Encyclopedia of Genes and Genomes (KEGG) Pathways of the gut microbiota among HDs (white) and GD patients (dark grey). Only functional capacities with $p < 0.1$ are shown; q = *p*-value FDR-corrected.

3.5. Differences in the Metabolic Profiles of Gut Microbiota between AITD Patients and HDs

PICRUSt metagenome predictions were used to identify those microbial functions that were enriched or degraded in AITD patients and HDs. In tier 2 of the KO categories, we observed no significant differences between HT patients and HDs or between both pathologies. However, we found pathways significantly different between GD patients and HDs at this level (Figure 3C).

Moreover, in tier 3 of the KO categories, we have not observed changes between HT patients and HDs. Nevertheless, we have detected a high number of pathways significantly different between GD patients and HDs at this level. The 27 pathways can be observed in detail in Figure S2.

3.6. AITDs Could Be Related to Bacterial Profile

Correlation studies were performed to establish a relationship between the thyroid autoimmunity of the study groups and their gut microbiota. Significant univariate correlations were found between the number of specific bacteria with thyroid autoimmunity markers like thyroperoxidase antibody (TPO-ab) (positive correlation with *Alistipes*; *Ruminococcaceae* unclassified and *Enterobacteriaceae*, so negative correlation with *Faecalibacterium*) and thyroid stimulating immunoglobulin antibody (TSI-ab) (positive correlation with *Lactobacillus* and *Pasteurellaceae* and negative correlation with *Faecalibacterium*) (Table 2).

Table 2. Simple linear correlation relationship of autoimmunity and thyroid profile with gut microbiota (taxa abundances: samples at phylum, family, and genus levels).

Plylum Level	Family or Genus Level	TPO-Ab	TSI-Ab
Bacteroidetes		—	—
	Alistipes	$r = 0.432; p = 0.019$	—
Firmicutes		—	—
	Lactobacillaceae	—	$r = 0.517; p = 0.006$
	Lactobacillus	—	$r = 0.517; p = 0.006$
	Faecalibacterium	$r = -0.453; p = 0.014$	$r = -0.406; p = 0.036$
	Ruminococcaceae unclasificated	$r = 0.408; p = 0.028$	—
Proteobacteria		—	—
	Enterobacteriaceae	$r = 0.416; p = 0.025$	—
	Pasteurellaceae	—	$r = 0.441; p = 0.021$

TPO-Ab, thyroperoxidase antibody; TSI-Ab, thyroid stimulating immunoglobulin antibody.

When we evaluated the possible implication of the gut microbial community in global AITDs, we found that an unclassified genus of *Ruminococcaceae* was associated with a 49.4% rise in the odds of the TPO-ab presence in the crude model. This trend was also maintained in the adjusted model by BMI, age, and sex (Table 3). Likewise, we found that *Sutterella* could influence in TSI-ab presence, with a 35.1% increase in either the crude model or the adjusted model. However, *Faecalibacterium* was associated with a decrease of 94.1% in the odds of presenting positive TSI autoimmunity in the crude model, so this relationship is maintained in the adjusted model (Table 4).

Table 3. Adjusted model for autoimmunity thyroid profile (Positive TPO-Ab >60 IU/mL)—Gut microbiota community.

Positive TPO Autoimmunity (TPO-Ab >60 IU/mL)		
	Ruminococcaeae unclassified	
	OR (CI)	*p*
Crude model	1.494 (1.041–2.145)	0.029
Model 1	1.474 (1.026–2.413)	0.038

Binary logistic regression analysis: Odds ratio (OR) and 95% confidence interval (CI) for the association between positive thyroid autoimmunity and gut microbiota. Positive levels of TPO antibody were defined as a level >60 IU/mL. Dependent variable: positive TPO autoimmunity—TPO-Ab levels <60 IU/mL (0) vs. TPO-Ab levels >60 IU/mL (1). Model 1: adjusted for sex, age, and BMI.

Table 4. Adjusted model for autoimmunity thyroid profile (Positive TSI-Ab >2 IU/mL)—Gut microbiota community.

	Positive TSI Autoimmunity (TSI-Ab >2 IU/mL)			
	Sutterella		*Faecalibacterium*	
	OR (CI)	*p*	OR (CI)	*p*
Crude model	1.351 (1.053–1.734)	0.018	0.059 (0.004–0.958)	0.047
Model 1	1.499 (1.041–2.158)	0.030	0.025 (0.001–0.900)	0.044

Binary logistic regression analysis: ddds ratio (OR) and 95% confidence interval (CI) for the association between positive thyroid autoimmunity and gut microbiota. Positive levels of TSI antibody were defined as a level >2 IU/mL. Dependent variable: positive TSI autoimmunity—TSI-Ab levels <2 IU/mL (0) vs. TSI-Ab levels >2 IU/mL (1). Model 1: adjusted for sex, age, and BMI.

4. Discussion

Our study has pointed out that the AITDs share common as well as particular gut microbiome profile features that differ from the stool profile of HDs and those dysbiotic amounts of particular taxa could be related with the development of the disease.

Autoimmune disease initiation has been linked to gut microbiota dysbiosis by different mechanisms such as molecular mimicry, the by-stander activation, and the epitope spreading. In recent years, patients bearing with an already established AITDs have also been reported to show alterations of the gut microbial composition [22–24].

Gut microbiome profiles from our study groups are different according to beta diversity analysis. However, further comparisons showed that the main differences belonged to the microbiota populations of HDs and each one of the AITDs studied. Thus, AITDs could share some patterns of their microbiota profiles. AITDs microbial changes have been classically attributed to morphological changes. Interestingly, patients with HT presented ultrastructural morphological changes of distal duodenum enterocytes, a variation in microvillus thickness, and a leaky gut condition [22]. On the other hand, GD frequently impacts the hollow organs with lower levels of gastric acid production, increased the intestinal motility which along with autoimmune gastritis contributing to diarrhea. Thus, GD might reshape the intestinal microbial composition through intestinal physiological modifications [7].

The increased bacterial richness that we have observed in our HT patients might be related to the bacterial overgrowth in the intestinal tract of these hypothyroid patients [25,26]. On the other hand, our GD patients showed a lower evenness in their microbiota populations in comparison to the HDs, which could indicate that in this population, could be dominant features. However, biodiversity did not show any significant differences among our study groups, which was aligned with reported works [15,27,28].

Our core microbiome results have demonstrated that the identified features at family and genus levels were mainly shared by our three study groups. However, despite this apparent normality, we have found some specific bacteria characteristic of each particular condition.

Taking together the differences in the feature abundances of each group and their respective core microbiomes, we have found important trends associated with each study group. About GD patients, we found a significant increase in the *Fusobacteriaceae* family and its *Fusobacterium* genus in GD. *Fusobacterium* is a well-recognized pro-inflammatory bacterium [29] and *Fusobacterium nucleatum* has been already reported in GD patients [30]. *Sutterella* was found higher in abundance in GD patients than in HDs. *Sutterella* has been positively related to prediabetes and inflammatory bowel disease [31,32] and it has an immunomodulatory role and pro-inflammatory capacity in the human gastrointestinal tract [33]. Moreover, we have also found a remarkable relationship between *Prevotellaceae* family and *Prevotella* genus with GD group through the core microbiome analysis. *Prevotella* has been linked with GD patients [27] and other autoimmune diseases like rheumatoid arthritis [34]. Thus, *Fusobacterium*, *Sutterella* and *Prevotella*, features relative to GD disease, have been linked to processes related to inflammation and autoimmunity.

In the case of HT patients, the family *Victivallaceae* is increased and is part of their core microbiome. Nevertheless, the role of these bacteria is little known, only some reports linking *Victivallaceae* with diet and obesity [35]. Another member of the core microbiome is the family *Streptococcaceae* and its genus *Streptococcus* that in combination with *Rikenellaceae*, which has been found increased in the HT patients concerning GD, have been reported to take part in the decrease in alpha-diversity in type 1 diabetes, with the capacity to behave as pathogens [36]. This is also the case of *Haemophilus*, which most of its species are considered pathobionts. *H. influenzae* has been reported to induce autoimmune disease by molecular mimicry of an epitope [37]. Furthermore, other core microbiome features of HT like *Alistipes*, *Anaerostipes* or *Dorea* could also be treated as pathobionts that within the disease environment could develop the capacity to damage the host. Together these results suggest that it could be possible that with a larger study these pathobionts from the core microbiome of the tested groups could reach a statistical significance between them.

About HDs related to AITDs, the core microbiome launched that *Christensenellaceae* was characteristic of this group. This result is compatible with studies that identify *Christensenellaceae* family as an important player in human health, associated with human longevity [38] and with lower levels of BMI [39]. As in the other groups, maybe a longer study could trigger differences in the abundance of *Christensenellaceae* with respect to the AITDs. Moreover, our study showed that *Faecalibacterium* genus decreases in autoimmune thyroid conditions compared to HDs, which is aligned with previous works [16,27]. It is important to remark that, although HDs were appropriate for the comparison with the other groups attending to their anthropometric and biochemical variables (no differences were observed with respect to the tested groups), the election of volunteers with a lower BMI could be beneficial for greater differences with respect to the tested groups. This fact could be also considered about the election of volunteers without TPO-Ab, although it is known that low levels are not relevant for the clinical practice if they are not accompanied by other variables [40]. These issues will be considered in future studies.

According to the PICRUSt analysis, GD disease is characterized by enrichment in xenobiotics degradation and metabolism as well as the metabolism of cofactors and vitamins in comparison to HDs. This could be related to the fact that GD patients are characterized by hypermetabolism [41] and could be translated into their microbiota profiles. Moreover, the enrichment in xenobiotics degradation could be related to the fact of these patients are medicated. This result could be indicative of some kind of intervention of the gut microbiota in the medication action, as it has been reported with other drugs [42].

Further analysis was performed to establish a possible relationship between autoimmunity parameters and specific features. Our analyses showed a positive correlation of TSI-ab with *Pasteurellaceae* family shared by AITDs patients. *Pasteurellaceae* family has been previously correlated with GD patients [27]. Thus, our correlation studies showed that some members of the gut microbiota were widely correlated with autoimmunity parameters, indicating that the gut microbiota might be closely related to the AITDs. Our findings may support future research on the interaction of the gut microbiota to the development of the AITDs. Likewise, a prediction model evaluated a possible relationship between predominant concrete bacteria in the AITDs. An unclassified genus of the *Ruminococcaeae* family and *Sutterella* were related to HT patients and GD patients, increasing the risk of presenting positive TPO-ab and TSI-ab, respectively. On one hand, *Ruminococcaceae* has been found as a part of the shared core microbiome of our volunteers [43]. On the other hand, we have already shown the implication of *Sutterella* in inflammatory conditions.

The most promising feature seems to be *Faecalibacterium*. *Faecalibacterium* has been related to a decrease of 94.1% in TSI immunity. In addition, inflammatory processes like inflammatory bowel diseases and colorectal cancer are favored when *Faecalibacterium* is decreased [44,45]. Moreover, in our study, *Faecalibacterium* has been shown as a protective factor, reducing the probability of presenting TSI-ab related to GD patients. The decrease of *Faecalibacterium* could indicate a real dysbiosis in these patients.

Although this study has several strengths, as the complete characterization of the microbiota, several limitations to this research must be acknowledged, like the low number of subjects because of the pilot study nature of our investigation. In this manner, this fact has been advertized throughout the document. Although further longitudinal investigations are necessary to evaluate the progression of the AITDs, these results contribute to the increase in scarce knowledge about the relationship between the gut microbiota and AITDs.

5. Conclusions

In this pilot study, our observations demonstrated a gut dysbiosis in AITD patients, may be able to contribute to thyroid disease development. Thus, gut dysbiosis might be related to the immune system development in AITD patients and the loss of tolerance to self-antigens including thyroglobulin and the autoimmunity that triggers AITD. Even though the studies of microbiome and their association to predict disease states are useful for personalized medicine, a deeper understanding of the microbiome might be necessary for the development of evidence-based microbial therapeutics in AITDs. Furthermore, studies with a greater number of subjects and longitudinal studies investigations might be required to evaluate the progression of the AITDs. Nevertheless, our results contribute to the increase in scarce knowledge about the relationship between the gut microbiota and AITDs.

Supplementary Materials: The following are available online at http://www.mdpi.com/2075-4426/10/4/192/s1, Table S1: Shared families and genera from each core microbiomes of the study group. Figure S1: Clustering of fecal bacterial communities according to the different study groups by PCoA using unweighted and weighted UniFrac distances. Figure S2: Significant differences in predicted functional composition at the level 3 of KEGG Pathways of the gut microbiota among HDs and GD patients.

Author Contributions: Conceptualization, I.C.-P., P.R.-L., I.M.-I. and F.J.T.; methodology, I.C.-P., P.R.-L., I.M.-I. and F.J.T.; validation, I.C.-P., P.R.-L., A.M.G.-P., M.M.-V., I.M.-I. and F.J.T.; formal analysis, I.C.-P., P.R.-L., A.M.G.-P., M.M.-V., I.M.-I. and F.J.T.; investigation, I.C.-P., P.R.-L., A.M.G.-P., M.M.-V., I.M.-I. and F.J.T.; resources, I.C.-P., P.R.-L., A.M.G.-P., M.M.-V., I.M.-I. and F.J.T.; data curation, I.C.-P., P.R.-L., I.M.-I. and F.J.T.; writing—original draft preparation, I.C.-P., P.R.-L., I.M.-I. and F.J.T.; writing—review and editing, I.C.-P., P.R.-L., A.M.G.-P., M.M.-V., I.M.-I. and F.J.T.; visualization, I.C.-P., P.R.-L., I.M.-I. and F.J.T.; supervision, I.M.-I. and F.J.T.; project administration, I.C.-P., P.R.-L., I.M.-I. and F.J.T.; funding acquisition, I.M.-I. and F.J.T. All authors have read and agreed to the published version of the manuscript.

Funding: This work was supported by Instituto de Salud Carlos III co-founded by Fondo Europeo de Desarrollo Regional—FEDER (CP16/00163, PI18/01160), Madrid, Spain. ICP was supported by Rio Hortega and now for Juan Rodes from the Spanish Ministry of Economy and Competitiveness (ISCIII) and cofounded by Fondo Europeo de Desarrollo Regional-FEDER (CM 17/00169, JR 19/00054). PRL was supported by the "Sara Borrell" program from ISCIII; Madrid, Spain and cofounded by Fondo Europeo de Desarrollo Regional—FEDER (CD19/00216). AMGP was supported by a research contract from Servicio Andaluz de Salud (B-0033-2014). MMV was supported by Rio Hortega from the Spanish Ministry of Economy and Competitiveness (ISCIII) and cofounded by Fondo Europeo de Desarrollo Regional-FEDER (CM18/00120). IMI was supported by the "MS type I" program from ISCIII; Madrid, Spain, cofounded by Fondo Europeo de Desarrollo Regional—FEDER (CP16/00163).

Acknowledgments: The authors thank the Metagenomic Platform of the CIBER Physiopathology of Obesity and Nutrition (CIBERobn), ISCIII, Madrid, Spain, especially to Pablo Rodríguez.

Conflicts of Interest: The authors declare no conflict of interest.

References

1. Pearce, E.N.; Farwell, A.P.; Braverman, L.E. Thyroiditis. *N. Engl. J. Med.* **2003**, *348*, 2646–2655. [CrossRef] [PubMed]
2. Devdhar, M.; Ousman, Y.H.; Burman, K.D. Hypothyroidism. Endocrinol. *Metab. Clin. North Am.* **2007**, *36*, 595–615. [CrossRef] [PubMed]
3. De Leo, S.; Lee, S.Y.; Braverman, L.E. Hyperthyroidism. *Lancet* **2016**, *388*, 906–918. [CrossRef]
4. Hasham, A.; Tomer, Y. Genetic and epigenetic mechanisms in thyroid autoimmunity. *Immunol. Res.* **2012**, *54*, 204–213. [CrossRef] [PubMed]
5. Tozzoli, R.; Barzilai, O.; Ram, M.; Villalta, D.; Bizzaro, N.; Sherer, Y.; Shoenfeld, Y. Infections and autoimmune thyroid diseases: Parallel detection of antibodies against pathogens with proteomic technology. *Autoimmun. Rev.* **2008**, *8*, 112–115. [CrossRef] [PubMed]

6. Prummel, M.F.; Strieder, T.; Wiersinga, W.M. The environment and autoimmune thyroid diseases. *Eur. J. Endocrinol.* **2004**, *150*, 605–618. [CrossRef] [PubMed]

7. Ebert, E.C. The Thyroid and the Gut. *J. Clin. Gastroenterol.* **2010**, *44*, 402–406. [CrossRef] [PubMed]

8. Behrouzi, A.; Nafari, A.H.; Siadat, S.D. The significance of microbiome in personalized medicine. *Clin. Transl. Med.* **2019**, *8*, 16. [CrossRef]

9. Leiva-Gea, I.; Sánchez-Alcoholado, L.; Martín-Tejedor, B.; Castellano-Castillo, D.; Moreno-Indias, I.; Urda-Cardona, A.; Tinahones, F.J.; Fernández-García, J.C.; Queipo-Ortuño, M.I. Gut Microbiota Differs in Composition and Functionality Between Children With Type 1 Diabetes and MODY2 and Healthy Control Subjects: A Case-Control Study. *Diabetes Care* **2018**, *41*, 2385–2395. [CrossRef]

10. Vázquez, N.M.; Ruiz-Limón, P.; Moreno-Indias, I.; Manrique-Arija, S.; Tinahones, F.J.; Fernandez-Nebro, A. Expansion of Rare and Harmful Lineages is Associated with Established Rheumatoid Arthritis. *J. Clin. Med.* **2020**, *9*, 1044. [CrossRef]

11. Edwards, C.J.; Costenbader, K. Epigenetics and the microbiome: Developing areas in the understanding of the aetiology of lupus. *Lupus* **2014**, *23*, 505–506. [CrossRef] [PubMed]

12. Sellitto, M.; Bai, G.; Serena, G.; Fricke, W.F.; Sturgeon, C.; Gajer, P.; White, J.R.; Koenig, S.S.K.; Sakamoto, J.; Boothe, D.; et al. Proof of Concept of Microbiome-Metabolome Analysis and Delayed Gluten Exposure on Celiac Disease Autoimmunity in Genetically At-Risk Infants. *PLoS ONE* **2012**, *7*, e33387. [CrossRef] [PubMed]

13. Zhou, J.S.; Gill, H.S. Immunostimulatory probiotic Lactobacillus rhamnosus HN001 and Bifidobacterium lactis HN019 do not induce pathological inflammation in mouse model of experimental autoimmune thyroiditis. *Int. J. Food Microbiol.* **2005**, *103*, 97–104. [CrossRef] [PubMed]

14. Penhale, W.J.; Young, P.R. The influence of the normal microbial flora on the susceptibility of rats to experimental autoimmune thyroiditis. *Clin. Exp. Immunol.* **1988**, *72*, 288–292.

15. Ishaq, H.M.; Mohammad, I.S.; Guo, H.; Shahzad, M.; Hou, Y.J.; Ma, C.; Naseem, Z.; Wu, X.; Shi, P.; Xu, J. Molecular estimation of alteration in intestinal microbial composition in Hashimoto's thyroiditis patients. *Biomed. Pharmacother.* **2017**, *95*, 865–874. [CrossRef]

16. Zhao, F.; Feng, J.; Li, J.; Zhao, L.; Liu, Y.; Chen, H.; Jin, Y.; Zhu, B.; Wei, Y. Alterations of the Gut Microbiota in Hashimoto's Thyroiditis Patients. *Thyroid* **2018**, *28*, 175–186. [CrossRef]

17. Bolyen, E.; Rideout, J.R.; Dillon, M.R.; Bokulich, N.A.; Abnet, C.; Al-Ghalith, G.A.; Alexander, H.; Alm, E.J.; Arumugam, M.; Asnicar, F.; et al. QIIME 2: Reproducible, interactive, scalable, and extensible microbiome data science. *Nat. Biotechnol.* **2019**, *37*, 852–857. [CrossRef]

18. Callahan, B.J.; McMurdie, P.J.; Rosen, M.J.; Han, A.W.; Johnson, A.J.A.; Holmes, S.P. DADA2: High-resolution sample inference from Illumina amplicon data. *Nat. Methods* **2016**, *13*, 581–583. [CrossRef]

19. Rognes, T.; Flouri, T.; Nichols, B.; Quince, C.; Mahé, F. VSEARCH: A versatile open source tool for metagenomics. *PeerJ* **2016**, *4*, e2584. [CrossRef]

20. Benjamini, Y.; Hochberg, Y. Benjamini-1995.pdf. *J. R. Stat. Soc. B* **1995**, *57*, 289–300.

21. Parks, D.H.; Tyson, G.W.; Hugenholtz, P.; Beiko, R.G. STAMP: Statistical analysis of taxonomic and functional profiles. *Bioinformatics* **2014**, *30*, 3123–3124. [CrossRef] [PubMed]

22. Sasso, F.C.; Carbonara, O.; Torella, R.; Mezzogiorno, A.; Esposito, V.; DeMagistris, L.; Secondulfo, M.; Carratu', R.; Iafusco, D.; Cartenì, M. Ultrastructural changes in enterocytes in subjects with Hashimoto's thyroiditis. *Gut* **2004**, *53*, 1878–1880. [CrossRef]

23. Virili, C.; Fallahi, P.; Antonelli, A.; Benvenga, S.; Centanni, M. Gut microbiota and Hashimoto's thyroiditis. *Rev. Endocr. Metab. Disord.* **2018**, *19*, 293–300. [CrossRef] [PubMed]

24. Mu, Q.; Kirby, J.; Reilly, C.M.; Luo, X.M. Leaky Gut As a Danger Signal for Autoimmune Diseases. *Front. Immunol.* **2017**, *8*, 598. [CrossRef] [PubMed]

25. Lauritano, E.C.; Bilotta, A.L.; Gabrielli, M.; Scarpellini, E.; Lupascu, A.; Laginestra, A.; Novi, M.; Sottili, S.; Serricchio, M.; Cammarota, G.; et al. Association between Hypothyroidism and Small Intestinal Bacterial Overgrowth. *J. Clin. Endocrinol. Metab.* **2007**, *92*, 4180–4184. [CrossRef]

26. Ghoshal, U.C.; Shukla, R.; Ghoshal, U.; Gwee, K.-A.; Ng, S.C.; Quigley, E.M.M. The Gut Microbiota and Irritable Bowel Syndrome: Friend or Foe? *Int. J. Inflamm.* **2012**, *2012*, 1–13. [CrossRef]

27. Ishaq, H.M.; Mohammad, I.S.; Shahzad, M.; Ma, C.; Raza, M.A.; Wu, X.; Guo, H.; Shi, P.; Xu, J. Molecular Alteration Analysis of Human Gut Microbial Composition in Graves' disease Patients. *Int. J. Biol. Sci.* **2018**, *14*, 1558–1570. [CrossRef]

28. Chen, J.; Chia, N.; Kalari, K.R.; Yao, J.Z.; Novotna, M.; Soldan, M.M.P.; Luckey, D.H.; Marietta, E.V.; Jeraldo, P.R.; Chen, X.; et al. Multiple sclerosis patients have a distinct gut microbiota compared to healthy controls. *Sci. Rep.* **2016**, *6*, 28484. [CrossRef]
29. Liu, H.; Redline, R.W.; Han, Y.W. Fusobacterium nucleatum Induces Fetal Death in Mice via Stimulation of TLR4-Mediated Placental Inflammatory Response. *J. Immunol.* **2007**, *179*, 2501–2508. [CrossRef]
30. Zhou, L.; Li, X.; Ahmed, A.; Wu, D.; Liu, L.; Qiu, J.; Yan, Y.; Jin, M.; Xin, Y. Gut Microbe Analysis Between Hyperthyroid and Healthy Individuals. *Curr. Microbiol.* **2014**, *69*, 675–680. [CrossRef]
31. Allin, K.H.; Tremaroli, V.; Caesar, R.; Jensen, B.A.H.; Damgaard, M.T.F.; Bahl, M.I.; Licht, T.R.; Hansen, T.H.; Nielsen, T.; Dantoft, T.M.; et al. Aberrant intestinal microbiota in individuals with prediabetes. *Diabetologia* **2018**, *61*, 810–820. [CrossRef]
32. Lavelle, A.; Lennon, G.; O'Sullivan, O.; Docherty, N.; Balfe, A.; Maguire, A.; Mulcahy, H.E.; Doherty, G.; O'Donoghue, D.; Hyland, J.; et al. Spatial variation of the colonic microbiota in patients with ulcerative colitis and control volunteers. *Gut* **2015**, *64*, 1553–1561. [CrossRef]
33. Hiippala, K.; Kainulainen, V.; Kalliomäki, M.; Arkkila, P.; Satokari, R. Mucosal Prevalence and Interactions with the Epithelium Indicate Commensalism of Sutterella spp. *Front. Microbiol.* **2016**, *7*, 1706. [CrossRef]
34. Scher, J.U.; Sczesnak, A.; Longman, R.S.; Segata, N.; Ubeda, C.; Bielski, C.; Rostron, T.; Cerundolo, V.; Pamer, E.G.; Abramson, S.B.; et al. Expansion of intestinal Prevotella copri correlates with enhanced susceptibility to arthritis. *eLife* **2013**, *2*, e01202. [CrossRef] [PubMed]
35. Kaplan, R.C.; Wang, Z.; Usyk, M.; Sotres-Alvarez, D.; Daviglus, M.L.; Schneiderman, N.; Talavera, G.A.; Gellman, M.D.; Thyagarajan, B.; Moon, J.-Y.; et al. Gut microbiome composition in the Hispanic Community Health Study/Study of Latinos is shaped by geographic relocation, environmental factors, and obesity. *Genome Biol.* **2019**, *20*, 219–221. [CrossRef] [PubMed]
36. Kostic, A.D.; Gevers, D.; Siljander, H.; Vatanen, T.; Hyötyläinen, T.; Hämäläinen, A.-M.; Peet, A.; Tillmann, V.; Pöhö, P.; Mattila, I.; et al. The Dynamics of the Human Infant Gut Microbiome in Development and in Progression toward Type 1 Diabetes. *Cell Host Microbe* **2015**, *17*, 260–273. [CrossRef] [PubMed]
37. Croxford, J.L.; Anger, H.A.; Miller, S.D. Viral Delivery of an Epitope fromHaemophilus influenzaeInduces Central Nervous System Autoimmune Disease by Molecular Mimicry. *J. Immunol.* **2005**, *174*, 907–917. [CrossRef] [PubMed]
38. Waters, J.L.; Ley, R.E. The human gut bacteria Christensenellaceae are widespread, heritable, and associated with health. *BMC Biol.* **2019**, *17*, 1–11. [CrossRef]
39. Goodrich, J.K.; Waters, J.L.; Poole, A.C.; Sutter, J.L.; Koren, O.; Blekhman, R.; Beaumont, M.; Van Treuren, W.; Knight, R.; Bell, J.T.; et al. Human Genetics Shape the Gut Microbiome. *Cell* **2014**, *159*, 789–799. [CrossRef]
40. Prummel, M.F.; Wiersinga, W.M. Thyroid peroxidase autoantibodies in euthyroid subjects. *Best Pr. Res. Clin. Endocrinol. Metab.* **2005**, *19*, 1–15. [CrossRef]
41. Gelfand, R.A.; Hutchinson-Williams, K.A.; Bonde, A.A.; Castellino, P.; Sherwin, R.S. Catabolic effects of thyroid hormone excess: The contribution of adrenergic activity to hypermetabolism and protein breakdown. *Metabolism* **1987**, *36*, 562–569. [CrossRef]
42. Koppel, N.; Rekdal, V.M.; Balskus, E.P. Chemical transformation of xenobiotics by the human gut microbiota. *Science* **2017**, *356*, eaag2770. [CrossRef] [PubMed]
43. Punzalan, C.; Qamar, A. Probiotics for the Treatment of Liver Disease. In *The Microbiota in Gastrointestinal Pathophysiology: Implications for Human Health, Prebiotics, Probiotics, and Dysbiosis*, 1st ed.; Elsevier Inc.: London, UK, 2017; pp. 373–381. ISBN 9780128040621.
44. Louis, P.; Flint, H.J. Diversity, metabolism and microbial ecology of butyrate-producing bacteria from the human large intestine. *FEMS Microbiol. Lett.* **2009**, *294*, 1–8. [CrossRef] [PubMed]
45. Ferreira-Halder, C.V.; Faria, A.V.D.S.; Andrade, S.S. Action and function of Faecalibacterium prausnitzii in health and disease. *Best Pract. Res. Clin. Gastroenterol.* **2017**, *31*, 643–648. [CrossRef]

Publisher's Note: MDPI stays neutral with regard to jurisdictional claims in published maps and institutional affiliations.

© 2020 by the authors. Licensee MDPI, Basel, Switzerland. This article is an open access article distributed under the terms and conditions of the Creative Commons Attribution (CC BY) license (http://creativecommons.org/licenses/by/4.0/).

MDPI
St. Alban-Anlage 66
4052 Basel
Switzerland
Tel. +41 61 683 77 34
Fax +41 61 302 89 18
www.mdpi.com

Journal of Personalized Medicine Editorial Office
E-mail: jpm@mdpi.com
www.mdpi.com/journal/jpm

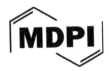